Basic Pharmacology

Basic Pharmacology

Editors
R W Foster and B Cox

With

J R Carpenter	H Schnieden
M J Dascombe	A P Silverman
M Hollingsworth	R C Small
N P Keaney	Janet Vale
G E Mawer	A H Weston
I D Morris	E T Whalley
P W Mullen	T R Wilson
J M H Rees	

The Department of Pharmacology, Materia Medica
and Therapeutics, The University of Manchester

Butterworths
London Boston Durban Singapore Sydney Toronto Wellington

First published 1980
Reprinted 1983
© University of Manchester, Department of Pharmacology,
Materia Medica and Therapeutics 1980
ISBN 0 407 00170 0

British Library Cataloguing in Publication Data

Basic pharmacology.
  1. Pharmacology
  I. Foster, R W   II. Cox, Barry, *b. 1937*
  615'.1   RM300   80-49873

  ISBN 0-407-00170-0

Typeset by Scribe Design, Gillingham, Kent
Printed and bound by Redwood Burn Limited, Trowbridge

Preface

In the thirteenth century Roger Bacon, writing in *De Erroribus Medicorum,* alleged that the typical medical man of the day was ignorant of his own simple medicine and put himself in the hands of unlearned apothecaries. There are those who would make similar allegations about the prescribers and dispensers of today's medicines. Accordingly, this book is offered in the hope that it will provide sufficient information about the drugs in current use to render such allegations groundless.

As authors of this book, the staff of the Department of Pharmacology, Materia Medica and Therapeutics at Manchester University have been able to draw on experience developed during 15 years of teaching pharmacology to students of several different disciplines. This experience gained from teaching is tempered by the fact that, as a group, the authors have variously prescribed, dispensed, scientifically investigated and even been on the receiving end of a selection of the compounds mentioned in their text.

The organization of this book is simple in concept. It is divided into sections, each section following a particular theme and being introduced by the relevant general principles — anatomical, biochemical or pharmacological. In each section the major groups of drugs relevant to the theme are discussed with detailed reference to important 'type' substances. Drugs of lesser importance are placed in proper context.

Though the format of the book is simple in concept, the realization of its content proved a formidable task. By way of example, the writing of the section concerning the actions of drugs on the central nervous system posed particular problems. This is an area where, despite a current spate of research activity, our knowledge of basic drug actions is very imprecise and to relate such actions to behavioural changes is necessarily difficult. The authors' final product for this and other sections is the result of many hours of discussion and debate.

As outlined in the introduction, this book is addressed to a wide spectrum of readers. It is to be hoped that no reader will fail to appreciate that selective toxicity (that is, the ability to chemically influence one type of biological activity without modifying any other) is the central theme of pharmacology.

Most importantly, the reader should appreciate that selective toxicity can never be absolute. Harold Kaminetsky perhaps put the dangers of chemotherapy into proper perspective yet left us with a message of hope when he suggested that there can be no really safe biologically active drugs — but there can be safe physicians.

H. Schnieden

Introduction

This book is intended for all who embark on the study of pharmacology. Most of its readers will be students of either medicine or pharmacy, whilst a few will regard pharmacology as their main or second subject. We teach all such students ourselves, think we know their needs and have attempted to satisfy the requirements of each of these groups in a single text. They have two things in common; an interest in the uses to which the drugs they study are put, and the fact that they are embarking on the study of pharmacology. Thus, we have provided a textbook which begins at the beginning, assuming only a modicum of chemistry, biology and physiology as prerequisites. It proceeds in the direction of paramedical or therapeutic rather than chemical pharmacology, assuming that the student will have access to further biology or physiology during his study. It goes far enough to cover all the introductory material; in other words, it should cover the first year of study by any of the above groups and still leave some material to launch a second year. Although newly published it has had the benefit of passing through several stages of evolution and refinement. In the form of extensive lecture notes it has been used by Manchester students for some years and we thank all our previous students who have consciously or unconsciously suggested improvements.

Perhaps the major problem encountered in the teaching of pharmacology is the large and ever-increasing number of drug names. Certainly the most frequent criticism levelled by new students is that of too many drug names. The complaint is not simply about weight of numbers but also about the apparent similarity in the names of drugs from different pharmacological groups, which for the inexperienced leads to misunderstanding and confusion. Therefore, in this book we have first defined a rigorous policy on drug names (*see below*) and, secondly, attempted an approach to the teaching of pharmacology which places a premium on understanding and reduces rote memorization to an essential minimum. This approach we call the Thematic Approach.

Rather than talk about individual chemical or therapeutic drug groups as in the traditional or systematic treatments of pharmacology, we have divided our book into sections with a common theme. We have also considered carefully the order in which these themes are presented. Thus, the book starts with a section which has as its theme the mechanisms by which drugs act at the efferent peripheral nervous system and its effectors. This is the chosen starting point because it is in this area that mechanism of drug action is probably best understood. Also, a high proportion of the drugs mentioned in this section have therapeutic potential and the system can be used as a model to predict or infer the mechanism of action of drugs in other less well understood areas (for example central nervous system, CNS). From this starting point of drug action at a discrete well defined site the theme changes to a consideration of mechanism of drug action on tissues under endocrine or local hormonal influence. Thus, the principle of drug interaction with chemical mediators is still the theme but now a greater variety of effectors and of time scales of action is considered. The next section is that of drug action on the CNS. First, the theme is again interactions with chemical mediators, which relies heavily on the principles and concepts presented in the preceding two sections, but then a second theme is introduced, that of non-specific interactions where drug effects other than those of interaction via a specific receptor site are considered. So far the themes have been drug interactions with endogenous systems, but in the next section the theme changes to a consideration of the mechanism of drug action on parasitic cells, be they microorganisms or neoplasms. The emphasis is now on mechanisms by which parasitic cell growth or survival is selectively inhibited. At this point the student has been provided with sufficient information in pharmacology so that drugs are no longer simply names. The theme changes from that of drug action to that of drug disposition and metabolism so that an appreciation of how these factors influence drug action can be gained. At the end of the book the theme changes once again so that the Applied Section considers the practical application of drugs and illustrates how an appreciation of mechanism of action can be put to a therapeutic use. This section also brings together drugs from different sections and so hopefully counteracts compartmentalization of information, a condition to which students seem to be innately predisposed.

With the plethora of textbooks of pharmacology which are currently available the question that might justifiably be asked is 'Why another one?'. Perhaps the answer lies in the fact that among those available we could find none which was suitable for our students who were at the beginning of a study of pharmacology. Though many excellent textbooks exist at the advanced level we felt the need for a comprehensive yet simple and concise book which adhered to our principle of understanding first and foremost, memorization last and least. Hence, our reliance heavily on comprehensive lecture note handouts (mentioned elsewhere) which have now been developed into this publication.

Policy on unfamiliar words

Words which are unfamiliar to the reader may be part of the technical language of medicine or pharmacology and all such we have defined or explained on their first occurrence. A second category exists in the ordinary stock of the English language — definitions are not provided in the text and the reader is advised to consult a dictionary.

Policy on which drugs to include

We have actively sought to limit the number of different drugs described because our primary objective has been to teach the principles of the pharmacological basis of therapeutics rather than familiarity with a rapidly ageing stock of drugs. We have therefore a narrower scope than, say, *MIMS* or the *Data Sheet Compendium* exactly as advised by the Committee of the British National Formulary. This policy is very similar to that adopted by the WHO Expert Committee reporting on The Selection of Essential Drugs.

Drugs have been categorized according to two criteria:
(1) Drugs listed in BNF (1976–78) and printed in bold type in one of the 'Notes on the use of drugs' sections are italicized, for example, *non-proprietary name.*
(2) From each pharmacological group of drugs we have chosen one which typifies the group. If its actions are understood the rest of the group, too, has been comprehended. We show these substances in sans serif type, for example, Non-proprietary name. Of course, many are also listed in the BNF and thus appear as *Non-proprietary name.*

Policy on drug names

We have used the non-proprietary names approved by the British Pharmacopoeial Commission and excluded trade names save in the very rare instances where no approved name has been assigned. For readers who are more familiar with North American terminology the US Pharmacopoeial name has been included in the index and in square brackets in the text after the first occurrence of the name. Only significant differences, however, have been declared; we have not bothered to draw special attention to systematic differences arising from different spelling conventions such as -ph- [-f-] and -oe- [-e-]. Neither did -trophin [-tropin] nor -barbitone [-barbital] seem likely to mystify our readers.

We were pleasantly surprised by the small number of significant differences; there was an era of fundamental differences, witness paracetamol [acetaminophen] and pethidine [meperidine], but modern drugs are deliberately being assigned the same name on both sides of the Atlantic.

Pharmacology, like most other scientific disciplines, is developing rapidly and the perennial problem of any text is that of keeping 'up to date'. We intend to make regular revisions of this book and will be helped in deciding the timing of these by the close connection, expressed in 'Aims and Objectives' below, with the BNF. Thus, stimuli for revision will be either a major advance in the understanding of the mechanism of action of any group of drugs, or significant therapeutic advances expressed as new inclusions in the BNF of drugs worthy of 'type substance' status.

We should be happy to receive suggestions for improvement from users of the book.

We thank John Carpenter for preparing the diagrams, and Professor Malcolm Rowland for help with Section 5, Sybil McCartney for typing the manuscript and all our colleagues for the time invested in evolving common policies and in proof reading.

AIMS AND OBJECTIVES

The aim of this book is to provide the sound pharmacological basis on which could be built a rational approach to therapeutics.

By the end of the book the reader should:

- Recognize most of the British Pharmacopoeial names of drugs (and their United States Pharmacopoeial equivalents, if different) appearing in bold type in the 'Notes on the use of drugs' section of the *British National Formulary* (BNF, latest edition),
- Be able to group together those drugs with common pharmacological properties and name one which typifies the group;
- Know the site and mechanism of action of each 'type substance';
- Know the pharmacological properties of each 'type substance' which are relevant to its therapeutic use, with special emphasis on those which can be deduced from a knowledge of the site and mechanism of action;
- Be aware of the nature (but not the detail) of the therapeutic application of each group of drugs;
- Know the common or serious side (or toxic) effects of each 'type substance' when used therapeutically, especially those which can be deduced from the pharmacological properties;
- Be able to place new drugs within the classificatory framework provided by the book.

Contents

		Page
Preface		*v*
Introduction		*vii*
List of abbreviations		*xv*

1 Drug action on the efferent peripheral nervous system and its effectors — 1

Introduction	1
Anatomy and physiology of the (efferent) peripheral nervous system and its effectors	2
The effector cells innervated by postganglionic autonomic neurones	8
The pharmacology of cholinergic axons and their terminals	15
The pharmacology of the cholinoceptor of skeletal muscle	18
The pharmacology of the cholinoceptor of ganglia	25
The pharmacology of the cholinoceptor of smooth muscle, cardiac muscle and exocrine glands	30
Cholinesterases and their inhibitors	35
The pharmacology of noradrenergic neuroeffector transmission	39
The adrenal medulla	55
Local anaesthetics	56
Anti-arrhythmic drugs	60
Appendix (dose response relationship; receptor theory; antagonism)	65

2 Endocrine pharmacology — 73

Hypothalamo—pituitary axis	74
Gonadotrophins	75
Oestrogens, progestogens and androgens	80
The thyroid gland and drugs used in thyroid abnormalities	89
Insulin and glucagon	93
The adrenal cortex and the corticosteroids	98
Angiotensin	101
Diuretics	102
Local hormones	106
The pharmacology of inflammation	115
Anticoagulant compounds	120

3 Drug action on the central nervous system — 125

Chemical transmission in the CNS	126

Classification of mental disorders 132
Screening of new drugs 133
Antidepressants 134
Neuroleptics 139
Narcotic analgesics and their antagonists 143
Stimulants and hallucinogens 150
Antipyretic analgesics 154
The state of consciousness and the non-specific depressants 156

4 *Antiparasitic chemotherapy* 169
Biochemical selectivity 170
Distributional selectivity 179
Drug resistance in parasites 183
Chemotherapy of metazoal infestations 184
Chemotherapy of protozoal infections 186
Chemotherapy of fungal infections 190
Chemotherapy of bacterial infections 192
Chemotherapy of viral infections 202
Chemotherapy of malignant neoplasms 203

5 *Drug disposition and metabolism* 209
Drug absorption 210
Distribution 213
Elimination 219
Model simulation of drug disposition 225
Pharmacokinetic terms and equations 225
Pharmacokinetics and dosage regimens 227
Water-soluble drugs 231
Drugs with intermediate solubility 233
Lipid-soluble drugs 236
Acidic drugs 242
Basic drugs 245
Summary 250

6 *Applied pharmacology* 251
Abuse of drugs 251
Toxicity 255
Developmental toxicity 259
Adverse drug interactions 264
Acute poisoning 267
Gastrointestinal complaints 269
Cardiac glycosides 275
Heart failure 276
Hypertension and antihypertensive drugs 279
Angina of effort 285
Asthma 287
Headache and migraine 292
Mental disorders and drugs which alleviate them 295
Nausea, retching and vomiting 299
Epilepsy 301

Family planning   306
Drugs and appetite   310
Drugs and the blood   312
Drugs in joint disease   316
Drugs and the skin   319
'Coughs and colds'   325

Suggested further reading   326

Index   327

List of abbreviations

ACh	acetylcholine
AChE	acetylcholinesterase
ACTH	adrenocorticotrophic hormone, corticotrophin
ADH	antidiuretic hormone
ATP	adenosine triphosphate
AV	atrioventricular
bd	(lit bis die) twice daily
BNF	*British National Formulary*
BP	blood pressure
C.	Corynebacterium
cAMP	cyclic adenosine monophosphate
cf	(lit confer) compare
ChE	cholinesterase
Ci	Curie
Cl.	Clostridium
CNS	central nervous system
CoA	coenzyme A
COMT	catechol O-methyl transferase
CSF	cerebrospinal fluid
CTZ	chemosensitive trigger zone
DHF	dihydrofolate
DNA	desoxyribonucleic acid
DOPA	dihydroxyphenylalanine
E.	Escherichia
EC50	concentration of drug evoking a half maximal effect
ECF	extracellular fluid
ECT	electroconvulsive therapy
EEG	electroencephalogram
epp	end plate potential
epsp	excitatory post-synaptic potential
FEV_1	forced expiratory volume in one second
FFA	free fatty acid
FSH	follicle stimulating hormone

g	gram
GABA	γ-aminobutyric acid
GFR	glomerular filtration rate
GH	growth hormone
H.	Haemophilus
h	hour
HCG	human chorionic gonadotrophin
HMG	human menopausal gonadotrophin
5-HT	5-hydroxytryptamine
HWY	hundred woman years
Hz	Hertz (1 Hertz is 1 cycle per second)
Ig-	immunoglobulin-
im	intramuscular
IUD	intrauterine device
iv	intravenous
k-	kilo- (10^3)
ℓ	litre
LH	luteinizing hormone
lit	literally
log	logarithm
LSD	lysergic acid diethylamide
M.	Mycobacterium
m	metre
m-	milli-(10^{-3})
mac	minimum anaesthetic concentration
MAO	monoamine oxidase
MFO	mixed function oxidase
mic	minimum inhibitory concentration
μ-	micro- (10^{-6})
min	minute
mol	mole (gram molecular weight)
mRNA	messenger ribonucleic acid
MW	molecular weight
N.	Neisseria
n-	nano- (10^{-9})
NA	noradrenaline
NADPH	nicotinamide adenine nucleotide phosphate (reduced)
P.	Plasmodium
P-	partial pressure
Pa-	arterial blood partial pressure
PG	prostaglandin
Ps.	Pseudomonas
qv	(lit quod vide) which see
R	registered trade name
RNA	ribonucleic acid
S.	Salmonella
SA	sino—atrial
sc	subcutaneous
SRS-A	slow-reacting substance of anaphylaxis
Staph.	Staphylococcus

Str.	Streptococcus
$t_{1/2}$	half time, half life
THC	tetrahydrocannabinol
THF	tetrahydrofolate
Tr.	Treponema
tRNA	transfer RNA
TSH	thyroid stimulating hormone, thyrotrophin
UK	United Kingdom
UV	ultraviolet
+ve	positive
—ve	negative
viz	(lit videlicet) namely
v/v	volume per unit volume
w/v	weight per unit volume

Abbreviations specific to the drug disposition section are on page 225.

1
Drug action on the efferent peripheral nervous system and its effectors

INTRODUCTION

Studies of drug effects exerted upon the peripheral nervous sytem or the cells which it innervates can provide an excellent introduction to mechanisms of drug action, the rationale behind the use of drugs as investigative tools or as therapeutic agents and the methods by which drug actions are measured. Furthermore, such studies will provide a working base from which to approach the pharmacology of other, perhaps more complex, physiological systems such as the brain.

Learning objectives

In common with other sections of this book, the drugs chosen for discussion are included in preparations listed by the BNF or constitute pharmacological tools of particular importance. For each drug mentioned you should know:

- Its mechanism of action and the changes in effector cell activity evoked both *in vitro* and *in vivo*;
- Its interactions with other pharmacological agents;
- Something of its therapeutic or scientific usage — and the rationale behind that usage;
- Something of its undesirable effects.

Consideration of these four items will not give the reader a complete understanding of the pharmacology of a given drug. By reference to other sections of this book, he should seek knowledge of the drug's handling by the body (absorption, disposition and elimination) and whether it has actions on physiological systems which are outside the scope of this section.

Clinical applications

Many of the drugs described in this section are clinically useful. They may be used:

1

(1)   To modify physiological processes and thus permit an operative or other procedure, for example, Tubocurarine (page 23);

(2)   As aids in the diagnosis of disease, for example, *Edrophonium* (page 38); and

(3)   In the symptomatic treatment of disease, for example, *Propranolol* (page 51).

It is important to realize that (with the exception of some antibiotics — *Table 1.3*) the agents mentioned in this section cannot be used to effect radical cure of disease.

Anatomy and physiology of the (efferent) peripheral nervous system and its effectors

Before we can understand how drugs produce their effects in the body we must have a thorough understanding of the anatomy and physiology of the relevant organ systems.

The nervous system can be subdivided as shown in *Figure 1.1*.

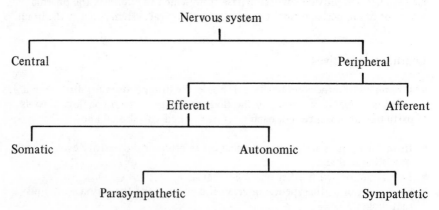

Figure 1.1   *Subdivision of the nervous system*

The central nervous system (CNS) comprises the brain and spinal cord. The peripheral nervous system lies outside the skull and vertebral column and comprises 12 pairs of nerves which emerge from the brain stem (cranial nerves) plus 31 pairs of nerves which emerge from the spinal cord (spinal nerves).

Peripheral neurones which carry impulses towards the CNS are called afferent neurones. Those which carry impulses away from the CNS are called efferent neurones.

Some cranial nerves consist of only afferent neurones, some of both afferent and efferent neurones and some of only efferent neurones. For the major part of their length, the spinal nerves consist of both afferent and efferent neurones and are thus called mixed spinal nerves. However, between its main trunk and the spinal cord, each spinal nerve breaks into a dorsal and a ventral root. Afferent neurones enter the spinal cord via the dorsal root whilst efferent fibres emerge via the ventral root (*Figure 1.5*).

The efferent peripheral nervous system can be subdivided into somatic and autonomic components.

The somatic division of the efferent peripheral nervous system comprises neurones which emerge from the spinal cord (via the ventral roots of spinal nerves) to provide excitatory innervation of skeletal muscle (*Figure 1.5*). The region where a somatic motoneurone closely approaches a skeletal muscle cell is known as the skeletal neuromuscular junction. Acetylcholine (ACh) is the chemical transmitter at this junction (*Figure 1.2*).

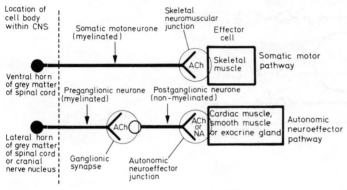

Figure 1.2   *Comparison of a somatic motor pathway with an autonomic neuroeffector pathway*

The autonomic division of the efferent peripheral nervous system provides excitatory or inhibitory innervation of cardiac muscle, smooth muscle and exocrine glands (its effector cells). The autonomic nervous pathway between the CNS and the effector cells comprises two neurones. The axon of the first neurone in the pathway emerges from the CNS (either in the course of a cranial nerve or via the ventral root of a spinal nerve) and terminates a short distance from the cell body of the second neurone in the pathway.

The gap between the two neurones is called a synapse. In many cases the synapses of autonomic pathways occur together in the course of a peripheral nerve. The collection of cell bodies in this region gives rise to a swelling of the nerve known as a ganglion. Hence the first neurone in an autonomic pathway is called the preganglionic neurone and the second cell is called the postganglionic neurone. ACh is the chemical transmitter at all autonomic ganglionic synapses (*Figure 1.2*).

The region where the axon of the postganglionic neurone closely approaches its effector cell is called an autonomic neuroeffector junction. The chemical transmitter at this junction may be ACh or Noradrenaline (NA) [norepinephrine] depending on the particular pathway under consideration (*Figure 1.2*).

The autonomic division of the efferent peripheral nervous system can be sub-divided into parasympathetic and sympathetic components according to the point of outflow of preganglionic neurones from the CNS.

THE PARASYMPATHETIC NERVOUS SYSTEM

A plan of the parasympathetic nervous system and its effectors is presented in *Figure 1.3*. Parasympathetic outflow comprises both cranial and sacral elements. Cranial parasympathetic outflow is carried in cranial nerves III (oculomotor), VII (facial), IX (glossopharyngeal) and X (vagus). Sacral parasympathetic outflow is carried in the spinal nerves of sacral segments 2, 3 and 4 of the spinal cord.

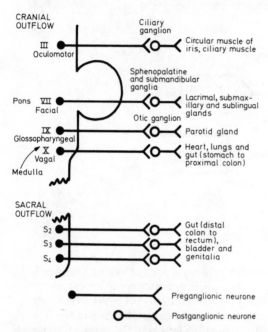

Figure 1.3   *The parasympathetic nervous system and its effectors. Parasympathetic outflow is bilaterally paired; only one side is illustrated*

Many parasympathetic ganglia are located close to, or are embedded within, the wall of the effector organ. Such ganglia are called terminal ganglia. In general, parasympathetic preganglionic neurones are long whilst the postganglionic neurones are short.

The distribution of parasympathetic innervation in the body is relatively limited — to certain effectors located within the head and to viscera within the thorax, abdomen and pelvis. The parasympathetic system does not innervate effectors located in the skin, limbs or body wall.

ACh is, in every case, the chemical transmitter between postganglionic para-sympathetic neurones and their effector cells.

4

THE SYMPATHETIC NERVOUS SYSTEM

Diagrams of the sympathetic nervous system and its effectors are presented in *Figures 1.4–1.7.*

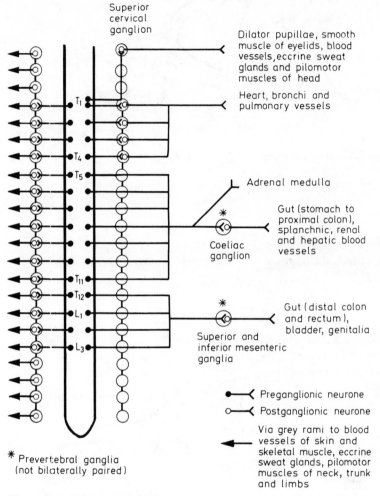

Figure 1.4 *The sympathetic nervous system and its effectors. Most pathways illustrated are bilaterally paired*

Sympathetic outflow from the CNS is described as thoracolumbar — since the preganglionic neurones emerge from the CNS in the ventral roots of the spinal nerves of the first thoracic to third lumbar segments of the spinal cord inclusive.

Sympathetic preganglionic fibres briefly join the course of the mixed spinal nerve but soon branch away to form white communicating rami (side branches of the spinal nerve) which enter the chains of paravertebral ganglia. These chains of ganglia lie on either side of the vertebrae. There are 22 ganglia in each chain. Each ganglion in a paravertebral chain is connected to the one above and the one below by nerve trunks.

5

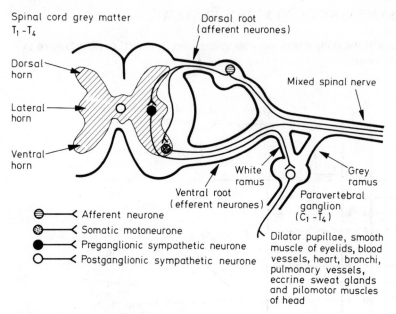

Figure 1.5 *Sympathetic outflow from the CNS. Synapse in paravertebral ganglion; distribution to sympathetically innervated structures in head and thorax*

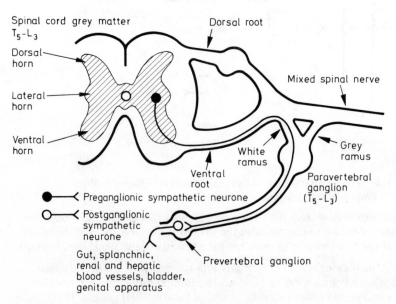

Figure 1.6 *Sympathetic outflow from the CNS. Synapse in prevertebral ganglion; distribution to sympathetically innervated structures in abdomen and pelvis*

Only 15 of the ganglia in each chain are supplied by white communicating rami. The three cervical ganglia at the top of the chain and the four sacral ganglia at the base of the chain only receive input from the CNS by neurones running upwards or downwards through the chain of ganglia by way of the interconnecting nerve trunks.

The sympathetic pathways supplying effectors located in the head and thorax are shown in *Figure 1.5*. The ganglionic synapse of these pathways occurs within the chain of paravertebral ganglia.

The sympathetic pathways supplying effectors located in the abdomen and pelvis are shown in *Figure 1.6*. In these pathways the preganglionic fibre enters the chain of paravertebral ganglia but passes straight through without synapsing. The synapse with the postganglionic neurone occurs in a prevertebral ganglion. In contrast to the paravertebral ganglia, the prevertebral ganglia are not bilaterally paired. They are ill-defined structures which form part of a neural plexus ventral to the abdominal aorta and its major branches. The coeliac and mesenteric ganglia are major components of this plexus. The adrenal medullae are embryologically and functionally equivalent to sympathetic prevertebral ganglia (page 55).

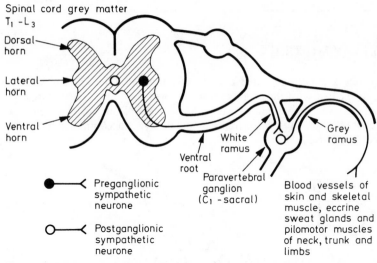

Figure 1.7   *Sympathetic outflow from the CNS. Synapse in para-vertebral ganglion; distribution through mixed spinal nerves to sympathetically innervated structures in neck, trunk and limbs*

The sympathetic pathways supplying the blood vessels of skin and skeletal muscle, and the eccrine sweat glands and pilomotor muscles of the neck, trunk and limbs are shown in *Figure 1.7*. The preganglionic neurone of these pathways forms a synapse with the postganglionic neurone with a paravertebral ganglion. The postganglionic fibre rejoins the course of the mixed spinal nerve (via the grey communicating ramus) for distribution to the effectors.

In contrast to the parasympathetic system, postganglionic sympathetic neurones are distributed almost universally throughout the body. With only a few exceptions (page 14), NA is the transmitter substance between postganglionic sympathetic neurones and their effector cells.

7

The autonomic neuroeffector junction

Postganglionic autonomic neurones branch and ramify within the effector organ to form a complex autonomic ground plexus. The number of autonomic neurones which approach an effector cell and the closeness of their approach varies greatly. Furthermore, the membranes of autonomic effector cells do not have regions which are specialized for the neuroeffector transmission process — the entire cell surface is sensitive to the action of the neurotransmitter (contrast with the motor end plate of skeletal muscle, page 18). Hence, it is often difficult to pinpoint sites of autonomic neuroeffector transmission in an electron micrograph.

The effector cells innervated by postganglionic autonomic neurones: the important effects on them of nervous activity

THE CILIARY MUSCLE

The ciliary muscle may be regarded as a ring of smooth muscle. The lens is suspended at the centre of the ring by means of ligaments. The ciliary muscle receives only parasympathetic innervation. ACh released from postganglionic neurones evokes ciliary muscle contraction and the eye is accommodated for near vision (*Figure 1.8*).

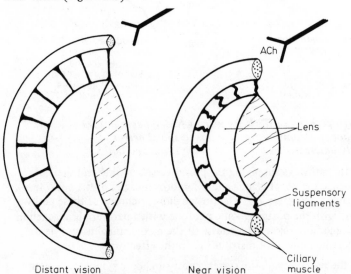

Figure 1.8 *Control of accommodation by the ciliary muscle; oblique view of sagittal section through ciliary muscle, suspensory ligament and lens*

Accommodation can be altered voluntarily, but normally the ciliary muscle is automatically regulated to keep the most distinct image of the object of fixation imposed on the retina. Activity of the ciliary muscle also aids pumping of aqueous humour from the canals of Schlemm (*Figure 1.9*) into the veins.

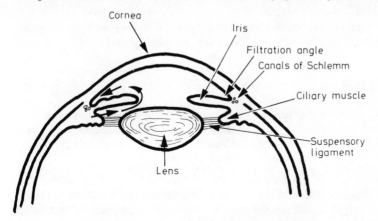

Figure 1.9   *Flow of aqueous humour from the ciliary body, through the anterior chamber of the eye; transverse section through eye*

Interference with ciliary muscle control may thus not only paralyse accommodation (cycloplegia) but may also predispose to an elevation of intraocular pressure (glaucoma).

THE IRIS

The iris contains pigment cells which give the eye its characteristic colour and render the iris opaque. The iris contains two layers of smooth muscle — the sphincter pupillae (fibres arranged concentrically around the pupil) and the dilator pupillae (fibres arranged radially).

The sphincter pupillae receives only parasympathetic innervation and ACh released from the postganglionic neurones causes contraction of the muscle fibres. The pupil thus constricts (miosis).

The dilator pupillae receives only a sympathetic innervation and NA released from the postganglionic neurones causes contraction of the muscle fibres. The pupil thus dilates (mydriasis).

Changes in the activity of the parasympathetic pathway supplying the sphincter pupillae are responsible for the pupil diameter changes associated with the light reflex. An increase in the intensity of light falling on the retina induces a reflex increase in parasympathetic discharge to the sphincter pupillae. The pupil constricts and reduces the amount of light entering the eye.

Parasympathetic discharge to the sphincter pupillae is also increased when viewing a near object. The pupillary constriction results in utilization of only the central portion of the lens. The spherical and chromatic aberration of the lens is thus minimized and its depth of focus is increased.

Paralysis of the sphincter pupillae can lead to photophobia and also a narrowing of the angle (filtration angle) between the base of the iris and the inner surface of the cornea. This may predispose to impaired drainage of aqueous humour into the canals of Schlemm and hence to a rise in intraocular pressure (glaucoma) (*Figure 1.9*).

The dilator pupillae plays little part in the light reflex. Sympathetic discharge in response to fright or other emotional states may evoke mydriasis.

THE EYELIDS

The eyelids are largely controlled by skeletal muscle but some smooth muscle which receives only sympathetic innervation contributes. The release of NA from the postganglionic neurones evokes contraction of the smooth muscle and the eyelids retract (that is, the palpebral fissure widens).

Some mammals (for example, the cat) have a third eyelid — the nictitating membrane. This membrane can be retracted by smooth muscle attached to the nasal wall of the orbit. This smooth muscle receives only sympathetic innervation and the release of NA causes contraction of the muscle and retraction of the membrane.

Paralysis of the smooth muscle of the eyelids allows the upper eyelid to droop (ptosis) — the palpebral fissure narrows.

THE HEART

The heart receives both parasympathetic and sympathetic innervation.

Parasympathetic neurones innervate the sino—atrial (SA) node (cardiac pace-maker). The release of ACh from parasympathetic nerve terminals reduces the discharge rate of the node and the heart rate falls (bradycardia; —ve chronotropic effect).

Parasympathetic neurones also innervate the atrioventricular (AV) node. This is located on the right side of the interatrial septum and gives rise to a bundle of specialized conducting cells (Purkinje fibres) which carry the cardiac excitation wave across the AV ring and distribute the excitation wave to the ventricles. The release of ACh from parasympathetic neurone terminals depresses conduction through the AV node.

The ventricular myocardium (which performs most of the cardiac pumping work) does not receive a parasympathetic innervation.

Sympathetic neurones innervate all regions of the heart. The release of NA from these neurones increases the discharge rate of the SA node (the heart rate rises — tachycardia; +ve chronotropic effect), increases conduction through the AV node and its associated Purkinje fibres, and increases the force of contraction (+ve inotropic effect) of the ventricular myocardium.

The healthy young human heart is normally dominated by vagal tone when the subject is at rest. With increasing age, vagal tone becomes less dominant. During exercise, sympathetic tone may dominate the heart no matter what the subject's age.

RESPIRATORY SMOOTH MUSCLE

The smooth muscle of the respiratory tract receives both parasympathetic and sympathetic innervation. ACh release from parasympathetic neurone terminals evokes contraction of respiratory smooth muscle (bronchoconstriction) while NA release from sympathetic neurones evokes relaxation (bronchodilatation).

In a healthy young subject the bronchial airways are almost maximally dilated even when the subject is at rest. The activation of sympathetic pathways during exercise does not therefore evoke much more bronchodilatation. The parasympathetic pathway to respiratory smooth muscle is reflexly activated in response to the inhalation of irritant substances or particles.

GASTROINTESTINAL SMOOTH MUSCLE

The propulsive smooth muscle of the gut receives both parasympathetic and sympathetic innervation. The release of ACh from parasympathetic neurones causes smooth muscle contraction (stimulates propulsive activity) whilst NA release from sympathetic neurones causes relaxation (inhibits propulsive activity).

Under normal circumstances the propulsive smooth muscle of the gut is dominated by parasympathetic tone.

THE URINARY BLADDER

The urinary bladder comprises a capsule of smooth muscle whose function is the storage and periodic evacuation of urine. The smooth muscle of the bladder comprises the detrusor (the greater part of the capsule) and the trigone (that part bounded by the ureteric orifices and the bladder neck). An external sphincter of skeletal muscle surrounds the bladder neck (*Figure 1.10*).

The detrusor receives parasympathetic innervation only. Bladder distension is the normal stimulus for micturition (passage of urine). Bladder evacuation is normally started at will. The release of ACh from parasympathetic neurone terminals causes contraction of the detrusor and closure of the ureteric orifices. The bladder neck is shortened and widened as it is pulled upwards. This causes a fall in urethral resistance and allows the passage of urine.

The activity of skeletal muscle is involved to a variable degree in voluntary micturition. The first event may be a relaxation of the external sphincter round the bladder neck, accompanied by contraction of the diaphragm and abdominal muscles. As intraabdominal pressure rises, urine may start to flow before detrusor activity reaches its peak. However, continence and voluntary micturition are possible in the absence of skeletal muscle activity.

The trigone and bladder neck receive only sympathetic innervation but the role of this sympathetic innervation in continence and micturition is negligible.

In males the release of NA from sympathetic nerve terminals during ejaculation causes contraction of the trigone and bladder neck. This prevents the reflux of seminal fluid into the bladder.

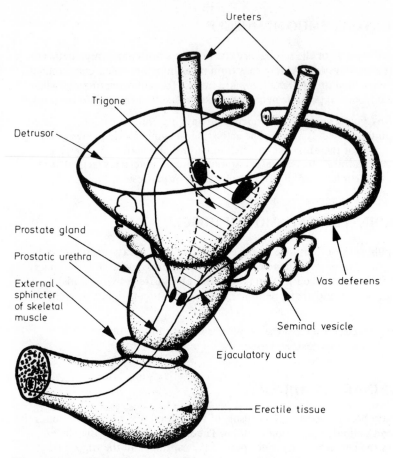

Figure 1.10 *Male genito-urinary tract*

SEMINAL VESICLE AND VAS DEFERENS

The seminal vesicle and vas deferens (*Figure 1.10*) receive only sympathetic innervation. NA release evokes contraction of the smooth muscle of these organs and hence ejaculation of spermatozoa into the prostatic urethra. Ejection of seminal fluid from the urethra (emission) is dependent on the clonic contraction of skeletal muscle.

VASCULAR SMOOTH MUSCLE

The smooth muscle of blood vessels is arranged circularly around the lumen. Most blood vessels receive sympathetic innervation only. The release of NA from the sympathetic neurone terminals causes contraction of vascular smooth muscle and hence vasoconstriction. The brain stem vasomotor centre governs the tonic discharge of the sympathetic neurones innervating blood vessels and the resultant vascular muscle tone is one of the factors responsible for the maintenance of blood pressure (BP).

Arterioles of skeletal muscle

The arterioles of skeletal muscle receive a noradrenergic, sympathetic innervation controlled by the vasomotor centre as described for other vascular muscle. In addition, they receive a second sympathetic innervation. The postganglionic neurone in this pathway, although anatomically sympathetic, releases ACh as its transmitter. The ACh causes vasodilatation of the skeletal muscle arterioles. This vasodilator pathway is activated in response to emotional shock (and so produces fainting) or in response to exercise (anticipated or current).

Arterioles of external genitalia

The arterioles of the erectile tissue of the external genitalia receive only para-sympathetic innervation. The release of ACh from the parasympathetic neurone terminals causes relaxation of the vascular muscle with resultant engorgement of the organ with blood (aided by reduced drainage due to venous compression).

PILOMOTOR MUSCLES

Pilomotor muscles are responsible for the attitude of the hair shaft. They receive only a sympathetic innervation. NA release from the sympathetic neurone terminals evokes muscle contraction and the hair shaft erects. In furry animals the pilomotor muscles play an important role in thermoregulation — in man their role is vestigial (gooseflesh).

ECCRINE SWEAT GLANDS

The eccrine sweat glands receive only a sympathetic innervation. The post-ganglionic neurones of this pathway, although anatomically sympathetic, release ACh as their transmitter. ACh release evokes sweat secretion. The eccrine sweat glands play an important role in thermoregulation; excess body heat is removed as the latent heat of vaporization of sweat.

OTHER EXOCRINE GLANDS

The lacrimal glands, salivary glands, glands of the respiratory tract and the gastric oxyntic glands receive parasympathetic innervation. The release of ACh from parasympathetic neurone terminals in each case stimulates glandular secretion.

Table 1.1 summarizes the autonomic effectors and the important effects on them of nervous activity.

13

Table 1.1 *The effector cells innervated by postganglionic autonomic nerves:*
The important effects on them of nervous activity

Sympathetic	Organ	Parasympathetic
	Eye	
No effect	Ciliary muscle	Contracted
No effect	Circular muscle of iris	Contracted
Contracted	Radial muscle of iris	No effect
Contracted	Smooth muscle of lids and nictitating membrane	No effect
No effect	*Lacrimal and salivary glands*	Secretion
	Heart	
Stimulated	SA node (rate)	Inhibited
Excited	AV node and conducting tissue	Depressed
Stimulated	Ventricular myocardium (force)	No effect
	Lung airways	
Relaxed	Smooth muscle	Contracted
No effect	Glands	Secretion
	Gut, stomach to rectum	
Inhibited	Propulsive musculature	Contracted
No effect	Gastric and pancreatic exocrine glands	Secretion
	Bladder	
No effect	Detrusor	Contracted
Contracted	Bladder neck and trigone	No effect
	Genital apparatus	
Contracted	Seminal vesicles and vas deferens (ejaculation)	No effect
No effect	Vessels of erectile tissue	Dilated
	Blood vessels	
Constricted	All	No effect
Dilated*	Those in skeletal muscle involved in fainting and exercise	No effect
	Skin	
Contracted	Pilomotor muscle	No effect
Secretion*	Eccrine sweat glands	No effect

* Cholinergic transmission occurs at this site

The pharmacology of cholinergic axons and their terminals

Revise

- Anatomy of somatic motoneurones (page 3) and anatomy of parasympathetic nerves (pages 3, 4).
- Effects of stimulating parasympathetic nerves (*Table 1.1*)
  (Acetyl) cholinergic neurones synthesize, store and release as their transmitter ACh.

They include:

- All preganglionic autonomic neurones (parasympathetic and sympathetic).
- All postganglionic parasympathetic neurones.
- A few postganglionic sympathetic neurones.
- All somatic (lower) motoneurones.
- Some neurones lying entirely within the CNS.

CHOLINERGIC TRANSMISSION

This process is basically similar at all sites in the body. It can be represented by *Figure 1.11*.

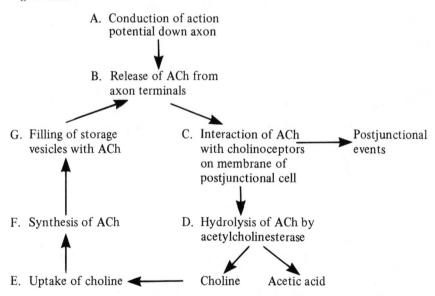

Figure 1.11 *Cholinergic neurotransmission*

Drugs which act on cholinergic axons and their terminals (i.e. drugs which interfere with stages A, B, E, F and G in *Figure 1.11*) will similarly modify cholinergic transmission at all sites. The clinical usefulness of such agents is thus limited by the diversity of their effects in the intact animal. Nevertheless, some drugs in this group (for example, the local anaesthetics) remain useful because their sphere of action in the body can be restricted by the method of administration.

Neuronal action potential conduction

Action potential conduction down the cholinergic axon may arbitrarily be regarded as the first stage in the transmission process. It can be prevented (and hence cholinergic transmission will be prevented) by local anaesthetics, for example, *Lignocaine* [lidocaine]. These agents prevent action potential conduction by membrane stabilization. They are not selective for cholinergic neurones (page 57).

Tetrodotoxin also prevents neuronal action potentials by membrane stabilization; it prevents action potential production where the upstroke of the action potential is mediated by increased membrane permeability to Na^+, for example, the action potentials of neurones and twitch skeletal muscle cells (also the early phase of the cardiac cell action potential). It does not influence the action potentials of smooth muscle since these are associated with the influx of Ca^{2+}. Hence, Tetrodotoxin can be used *in vitro* functionally to denervate smooth muscle without affecting its contractility. This is very useful in the investigation of drug action on smooth muscle to answer the question: Is the action direct or does it involve a stage where propagation of nerve action potentials is necessary?

Release of ACh from axon terminals

Two physiological mechanisms exist, as follows.

Action potential-evoked release

As an action potential invades terminal axons, membrane permeability changes occur. Na^+, Cl^- and Ca^{2+} rush into the cell and K^+ emerges. The influx of Ca^{2+} triggers mass migration of storage vesicles to the cell surface and the subsequent release of ACh by exocytosis. The empty vesicular membrane is probably retained within the cell and refilled with newly synthesized transmitter.

Since transmitter release by this mechanism requires the nerve action potential it will be prevented by local anaesthetics and Tetrodotoxin.

Transmitter release by this mechanism requires influx of Ca^{2+} and is reduced if the extracellular fluid (ECF) is deficient in this ion or contains a high concentration of Mg^{2+}.

After treatment of a tissue with Triethylcholine, action potentials release acetyltriethylcholine (a false transmitter) from cholinergic axon terminals (page 18).

Spontaneous release

This involves random migration of storage vesicles to the axon surface and release of ACh into the cleft. Although the amount of transmitter released is small, it can still influence the membrane of the postjunctional cell if the cleft width is narrow, for example, miniature end plate potentials of twitch skeletal muscle (*Figure 1.13*), spontaneous postsynaptic potentials of ganglia (*Figure 1.19*).

Since this release mechanism does not depend on the arrival of action potentials it is unaffected by Tetrodotoxin.

Triethylcholine will interfere with this release mechanism as described above.

Botulinus toxin is an exotoxin produced by *Cl. botulinum* which prevents both action potential-induced and spontaneous release of ACh from all cholinergic axons. Death in botulism results from respiratory paralysis.

Interaction of ACh with postsynaptic or postjunctional cholinoceptors

ACh in the cleft reversibly forms complexes with receptors (cholinoceptors) on the outer surface of the postsynaptic or postjunctional membrane. Some function of this interaction (page 69) determines the nature and size of the change in ionic permeability of the postsynaptic or postjunctional cell membrane.

There are three types of cholinoceptor which differ both in their affinities for drugs and in their anatomical location. Hence, this is the stage in the transmission process which offers the pharmacologist the greatest opportunity for selective interference (pages 18–35).

Hydrolysis of ACh

The enzyme acetylcholinesterase (AChE) can hydrolyse (and thus inactivate) ACh to form choline and acetic acid. The drugs which interfere with the activity of AChE are the anticholinesterases (page 36).

Uptake of choline

Choline (dietary, synthesized from ethanolamine and methionine or formed from the hydrolysis of ACh) is taken up actively by neurones.

Hemicholinium blocks the choline pump and thus produces delayed block of cholinergic transmission (preformed ACh must be used up). Hemicholinium has no clinical application. Triethylcholine competes with choline for transport into the neurone.

Synthesis of ACh (*Figure 1.12*)

Some newly synthesized ACh is immediately hydrolysed by AChE of the axonal membrane. That which is taken up into the membrane-bound storage vesicles

In mitochondria :

$$\text{Acetate} + \text{ATP} \longrightarrow \text{Adenylacetate}$$

In axonal cytoplasm :

$$\text{Adenylacetate} + \text{CoA} \xrightarrow{\text{Acetyl kinase}} \text{AcetylCoA}$$

$$\text{AcetylCoA} + \text{Choline} \xrightarrow{\text{Choline acetyltransferase}} \text{Acetylcholine} + \text{CoA}$$

Figure 1.12   *Synthesis of ACh*

is protected from hydrolysis. This ACh is stored in vesicles as a concentrated solution.

Triethylcholine competes with choline for the synthetic mechanism and acetyltriethylcholine is synthesized and stored. Since acetyltriethylcholine can be released from the nerve terminal but is much less potent than ACh on cholinoceptors it is said to function as a false transmitter. Triethylcholine thus produces delayed block of cholinergic transmission. Triethylcholine has no clinical application.

The pharmacology of the cholinoceptor of skeletal muscle

The receptor was originally designated 'nicotinic' since Nicotine could readily mimic the action of ACh at this site. Nicotinic cholinoceptors of skeletal muscle are characterized by the orders of drug potency shown in *Table 1.2*.

How do these agonists/antagonists (page 69) at the nicotinic cholinoceptor influence the development of tension by skeletal muscle? The answer depends to a certain extent on the type of muscle cell considered.

FOCALLY INNERVATED (TWITCH) SKELETAL MUSCLE

The majority of mammalian skeletal muscle cells are of this type. Each muscle cell forms only one region of close association with a somatic motoneurone terminal. Here the muscle cell membrane is specialized to form the motor end plate. Under normal circumstances this is the only part of the muscle cell membrane which has nicotinic cholinoceptors. These are located on the exterior surface.

18

Table 1.2   *Orders of drug potency at the nicotinic cholinoceptor of skeletal muscle*

(1)	*Agonists*		
	ACh		
	Carbachol	>>	Muscarine
	Nicotine		Methacholine
	Suxamethonium (succinylcholine)		
(2)	*Antagonists*		
	Tubocurarine		
	Gallamine	>>	*Atropine*
	Pancuronium		*Pentolinium*
	α-Bungarotoxin		

Note: Compounds to the left of the >> symbol are potent but not equally so, those to the right are so impotent that they may be regarded as inactive at this site.

Muscle cells of this type exhibit threshold behaviour, that is, if the cell depolarizes rapidly through a 'threshold of excitability' an action potential is triggered. The action potential normally propagates to the cell extremities without decrement, and is the electrical event which triggers the release of intracellular Ca^{2+} necessary for shortening of the myofibrils. Action potential firing (and the presence of a well developed T-tubule system and sarcoplasmic reticulum) allows the cell to develop tension quickly (twitch).

Normal sequence of events during neuromuscular transmission in twitch fibres

(1)   Arrival of action potential in the nerve terminal.
(2)   Release of ACh into the junctional cleft (width 20 nm).
(3)   Diffusion of ACh down a concentration gradient towards the motor end plate.
(4)   Association of ACh with the nicotinic cholinoceptors.
(5)   Depolarization of the motor end plate to give an end plate potential (epp).
(6)   When the epp crosses the threshold potential of excitability an action potential is triggered and this moves out from the end plate to the muscle cell extremities.
(7) Ca^{2+} release from intracellular sites causes shortening of myofibrils and the development of tension.
(8)   Dissociation of ACh/receptor complex.
(9)   Hydrolysis of ACh by AChE.
(10)   Transport of choline back into the nerve terminal.
(11)   Resynthesis of ACh.
(12)   Storage of ACh in vesicles.

Under normal circumstances a single nerve action potential releases more than sufficient ACh to depolarize the end plate to threshold; ie a safety factor exists for transmission. Normally only one muscle action potential is generated since the transmitter is hydrolysed within the refractory period of the muscle cell (*Figure 1.13*).

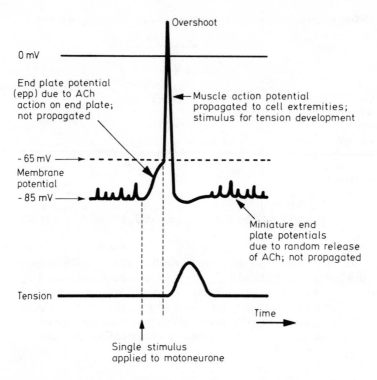

Figure 1.13 *Twitch skeletal muscle: the motor end plate electrical activity and tension development of a single fibre evoked by stimulation of its nerve supply*

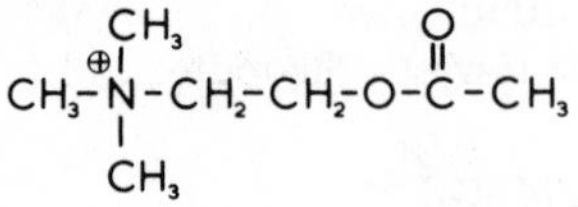

ACh

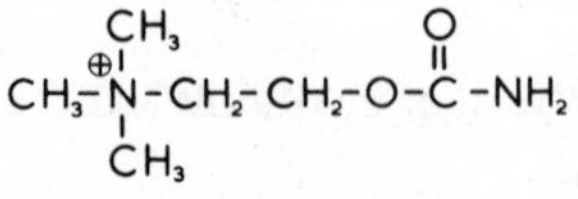

Carbachol

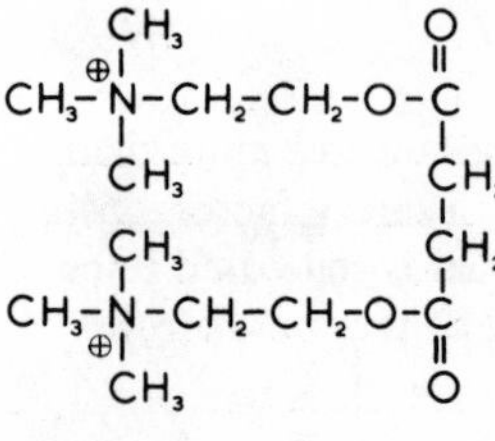

Suxamethonium

Figure 1.14 *The structures of some agonists at nicotinic cholinoceptors*

20

The effects of agonists (at nicotinic receptors) on neuromuscular transmission in twitch fibres

These agonists include ACh, *Carbachol,* Nicotine and Suxamethonium (*Figure 1.14*). They activate nicotinic receptors of the end plate and evoke a depolarization. If this depolarization is sufficiently rapid and sufficiently intense to cross the threshold of excitability, the muscle cell generates an action potential and contracts. Since these drugs are not readily hydrolysed by AChE (with the exception of ACh) the muscle cell often generates several action potentials and then enters a state where its membrane potential is less −ve than the threshold of excitability. Under such circumstances, the muscle cell becomes refractory (as regards tension development) to stimulation of its nerve supply. This is the stage of depolarizing blockade of neuromuscular transmission (*Figure 1.15*). Blockade persists until such time as the membrane of the twitch fibre has repolarized to a level more −ve than the threshold of excitability.

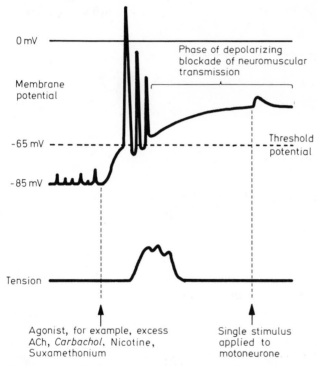

Figure 1.15   *Twitch skeletal muscle: the effects of agonists at nicotinic cholinoceptors on the motor end plate electrical activity and tension development of a single fibre*

The only agonist at nicotinic receptors used for its action on skeletal muscle is Suxamethonium. This drug is used in brief surgical or diagnostic procedures, and in electroconvulsive therapy (ECT) to produce brief (six minute) periods of paralysis. Iv injection causes asynchronous twitches of individual fibres in the body of a muscle (fasciculation) due to the early phase of action potential firing.

Then a phase of flaccid paralysis ensues due to depolarizing blockade of neuro-muscular transmission.

Suxamethonium-induced paralysis is short-lived due to rapid hydrolysis of the drug by ChE (pseudocholinesterase). Beware genetic deficiency of this enzyme (pages 35 and 257).

Effects of antagonists (at nicotinic cholinoceptors) on neuromuscular transmission in twitch fibres

Competitive antagonists (for definition of competitive antagonism, page 69) — Tubocurarine, gallamine, pancuronium. Non-competitive antagonists (for definition of non-competitive antagonism, page 70) — α-bungarotoxin.

Any of the antagonists listed above decreases the number of transmitter/receptor interactions and hence reduces the size of the epp. If the epp no longer crosses the threshold of excitability, neuromuscular transmission to that cell will fail (*Figure 1.16*).

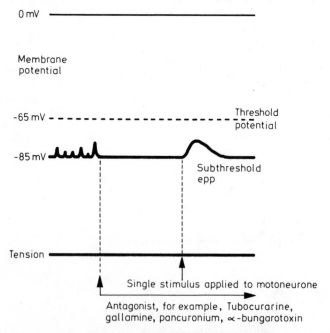

Figure 1.16   *Twitch skeletal muscle: the effects of antagonists at nicotinic cholinoceptors on the motor end plate electrical activity and tension development of a single twitch fibre*

If the effects of a neuromuscular blocking drug are observed *in vitro* or *in vivo*, a gradual depression of the twitch of the whole muscle is seen. Since transmission to a single cell is an 'all-or-none' process, this gradual effect represents the successive inactivation of individual nerve/muscle cell units.

The competitive antagonists are used to produce muscle paralysis during surgery; they allow the anaesthetist to employ a relatively light level of anaesthesia and yet have adequate muscle relaxation. They are also used in tetanus or Strychnine poisoning (page 128). In all cases where Tubocurarine-like drugs are used, there is a need to artificially ventilate the lungs. The effects of the competitive antagonists can be terminated by an anticholinesterase drug — which increases the number of transmitter/receptor interactions by increasing the concentration of transmitter.

Tubocurarine causes histamine release (*Table 2.14*) and ganglion blockade and hence lowers BP. This is not a problem with pancuronium.

α-Bungarotoxin is a component of the venom of a snake (the Taiwan banded krait — *Bungarus multicinctus*). It binds irreversibly and very specifically to the nicotinic receptors of skeletal muscle. It is not used clinically but is a very useful research tool, for example, in the localization and isolation of nicotinic cholinoceptors of muscle.

Clinically relevant interactions with neuromuscular blocking agents are shown in *Table 1.3*.

Table 1.3   *Clinically relevant interactions with neuromuscular blocking agents*

	Competitive — Tubocurarine	Depolarizing — Suxamethonium
General anaesthetics — ether, Halothane, cyclopropane	+	0
Aminosugar antibiotics — *streptomycin, neomycin, Gentamicin,* and *colistin*	+	0
Anticholinesterases — *Neostigmine*	—	+
Hypothermia	—	+

+ Increases neuromuscular blocking activity.
— Decreases neuromuscular blocking activity.
0 No pronounced effect on blocking activity.

MULTIPLY-INNERVATED (SLOW) SKELETAL MUSCLE

Each muscle cell has several neuromuscular junctions. However, the muscle cell membrane is not specialized at such sites. The nicotinic cholinoceptors, although most dense at the neuromuscular junctions, are widely distributed over the cell surface. A single nerve action potential evokes a local non-propagated depolarization of the muscle membrane and this is associated with the ionic changes which trigger a corresponding local slow contraction.

This type of muscle cell is relatively common in the muscles of birds, and certain muscles of amphibia (for example, the rectus abdominis of the frog). In mammals this type of cell is rare — intrafusal fibres of muscle spindles are one example.

The effects of agonists (at nicotinic cholinoceptors) on neuromuscular transmission in slow fibres

ACh, *Carbachol,* Suxamethonium and Nicotine all activate nicotinic cholinoceptors and thereby evoke slow, graded depolarization and slow, graded contraction of slow muscle cells. Stimulation of the nerve supply during such a response has an additive effect on both the depolarization and the tension

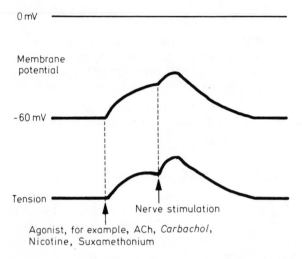

Figure 1.17   *Slow skeletal muscle: the effects of agonists at nicotinic cholinoceptors on the electrical activity and tension development of a single fibre*

development (*Figure 1.17*). Note that the phenomenon of depolarizing blockade of transmission cannot occur in slow cells since they do not exhibit threshold behaviour.

Iv injection of nicotinic agonists into birds and amphibia evokes spastic paralysis (muscle in contracted state) of any muscle containing a high proportion of slow cells.

Effects of antagonists (at nicotinic cholinoceptors) on neuromuscular transmission in slow cells

Competitive — Tubocurarine, gallamine, pancuronium.
Non-competitive — α-bungarotoxin.

By reducing the number of transmitter or agonist interactions with the receptor, these drugs reduce the depolarization and contraction evoked by nerve stimulation or agonist administration (*Figure 1.18*).

Iv injection of these agents into birds and amphibia evokes flaccid paralysis of all skeletal muscle.

24

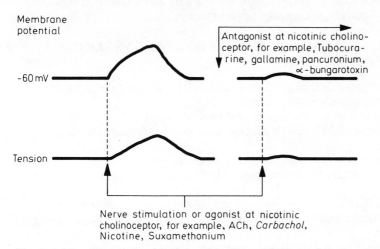

0 mV

Membrane
potential

Antagonist at nicotinic cholinoceptor, for example, Tubocurarine, gallamine, pancuronium,
α - bungarotoxin

-60 mV

Tension

Nerve stimulation or agonist at nicotinic
cholinoceptor, for example, ACh, *Carbachol*,
Nicotine, Suxamethonium

Figure 1.18 *Slow skeletal muscle: the effects of antagonists at*
nicotinic cholinoceptors on the electrical activity and tension
development of a single fibre

The pharmacology of the cholinoceptor of ganglia

The receptor was originally designated 'nicotinic' since Nicotine could readily
mimic the action of ACh at this site. Nicotinic cholinoceptors of ganglia are
characterized by the orders of drug potency shown in *Table 1.4.*

Table 1.4 *Orders of drug potency at the nicotinic cholinoceptor of ganglia*

(1)	*Agonists*		
	ACh	>>	Muscarine
	Carbachol		Methacholine
	Nicotine		
(2)	*Antagonists*		
	Pentolinium	>>	*Atropine*
	Tubocurarine		α-bungarotoxin

Notes:
(1) Compounds to the left of the >> symbol are potent but not equally so,
those to the right are so impotent that they may be regarded as inactive at
this site.
(2) The nicotinic cholinoceptor of ganglia differs from that of skeletal
muscle — particularly with regard to the order of antagonist potency
(*Table 1.2*).

Nicotinic cholinoceptors of ganglia are located over the whole of the cell bodies of sympathetic and parasympathetic ganglia (particularly numerous beneath the terminal boutons of preganglionic fibres). They are also found on axons/axon terminals of postganglionic sympathetic neurones.

NORMAL SEQUENCE OF EVENTS DURING GANGLIONIC TRANSMISSION

(1)   Simultaneous arrival of action potentials in a sufficient number (*see below*) of preganglionic nerve terminals.

(2)   Release of ACh into synaptic cleft (width 20 nm).

(3)   Diffusion of ACh down a concentration gradient towards the ganglion cell body.

(4)   Association of ACh with nicotinic cholinoceptors.

(5)   Depolarization of the ganglion cell body (excitatory post-synaptic potential, epsp).

(6)   If the epsp crosses the threshold of excitability (*see below*) an action potential is triggered and this moves down the postganglionic axon (*Figure 1.19*).

(7)   Dissociation of ACh/cholinoceptor complex.

(8)   Hydrolysis of ACh.

(9)   Transport of choline back into the preganglionic nerve terminals.

(10) Resynthesis of ACh.

(11) Storage of ACh in vesicles.

Compare and contrast the above sequence of events with those occurring during neuromuscular transmission in twitch muscle fibres (page 19).

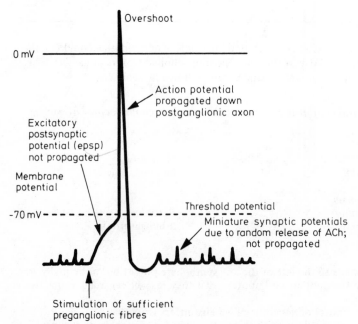

Figure 1.19   *The electrical activity of an autonomic ganglion cell body*

Note that for effective ganglionic transmission (that is, production of an epsp big enough to cross the threshold) an appreciable number of preganglionic terminals must discharge transmitter in a synchronous fashion. Discharge of one terminal bouton would not normally evoke an action potential in the postganglionic cell body.

THE EFFECTS OF AGONISTS (AT NICOTINIC CHOLINOCEPTORS) ON GANGLIONIC TRANSMISSION

ACh, *Carbachol*, Nicotine

These activate nicotinic receptors of the ganglion cell body and evoke depolarization. If this depolarization is sufficiently rapid and sufficiently intense to cross the threshold of excitability, the ganglion cell body generates an action potential. Since these drugs are not readily inactivated by AChE (even ACh, if in great excess) the ganglion cell body generally generates a burst of action potentials and then enters a state where its membrane potential is less −ve than the threshold of excitability. This is the stage of depolarizing blockade of ganglionic transmission (*Figure 1.20*). Under such circumstances the ganglion cell body becomes refractory (as regards action potential generation) to stimulation of the pre-ganglionic neurones. Blockade of transmission persists until such time as the membrane of the ganglion cell body has repolarized to a level more −ve than the threshold of excitability.

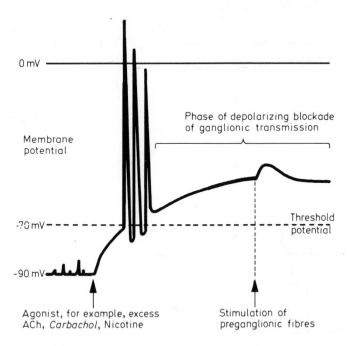

Figure 1.20 *The effects of agonists at nicotinic cholino-ceptors on the electrical activity of an autonomic ganglion cell body*

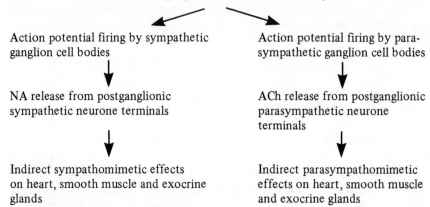

Activation of ganglionic nicotinic cholinoceptors

Action potential firing by sympathetic
ganglion cell bodies

↓

NA release from postganglionic
sympathetic neurone terminals

↓

Indirect sympathomimetic effects
on heart, smooth muscle and exocrine
glands

Action potential firing by parasympathetic ganglion cell bodies

↓

ACh release from postganglionic
parasympathetic neurone
terminals

↓

Indirect parasympathomimetic
effects on heart, smooth muscle
and exocrine glands

Figure 1.21

Note the analogy with the actions of these drugs on neuromuscular transmission
in twitch skeletal muscle fibres (page 21).

As a consequence of their triggering a burst of action potential discharge by the
ganglion cell body, agonists at the cholinoceptors of ganglia exert indirect
sympathomimetic and parasympathomimetic effects on smooth muscle, cardiac
muscle and exocrine glands (*Figure 1.21*).

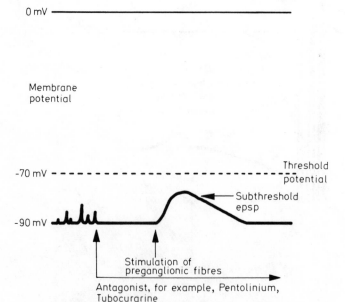

Figure 1.22 *The effects of antagonists at nicotinic
cholinoceptors on the electrical activity of an autonomic
ganglion cell body*

28

The action on heart, smooth muscle or gland is said to be 'indirect' since the nicotinic agonist affects those cells by causing the release of a neurotransmitter.

If an agonist at the nicotinic cholinoceptors of ganglia is administered repeatedly at short intervals, then the indirect sympathomimetic/parasympathomimetic effects described above exhibit tachyphylaxis (that is, response amplitude declines rapidly with successive doses). The explanation is probably that subsequent doses of the agonist reach the ganglion cell body while it is still in the phase of depolarizing blockade.

Since these agents activate all sympathetic and parasympathetic ganglia, their injection into the whole animal has very diverse effects. For this and other reasons, none of these agents is used clinically for its action on ganglion cell bodies.

Table 1.5   *The important effects of ganglion blockade (for example by*
Pentolinium, a competitive antagonist at nicotinic cholinoceptors of ganglia)

Sympathetic interruption	Organ	Parasympathetic interruption
	Eye	
	Ciliary muscle	Relaxed
	Pupil	Dilated
Relaxed	Nictitating membrane	
	Lacrimal and salivary glands	Dry
	Heart	
	SA node	Tachycardia, mild
	Gut, stomach and rectum	
	Propulsive muscle	Reduced motility and constipation
	Gastric and pancreatic exocrine glands	Reduced secretion
	Bladder	Retention of urine
	Genital apparatus	
Failure of ejaculation	Seminal vesicles and vas deferens	
	Blood vessels of erectile tissue of external genitalia	Impotence
Dilated; postural hypotension	*All blood vessels*	
	Skin	
Relaxed	Pilomotor muscles	
Reduced secretion	Eccrine sweat glands	

THE EFFECTS OF ANTAGONISTS AT THE NICOTINIC CHOLINOCEPTORS OF GANGLIA

Pentolinium

These are competitive antagonists at the nicotinic cholinoceptors of ganglia. By reducing the number of transmitter/receptor interactions these agents reduce the epsp until it fails to cross the threshold of excitability. At this point ganglionic transmission fails (*Figure 1.22*).

These drugs block transmission through all ganglia (both parasympathetic and sympathetic) and at the adrenal medulla. They competitively antagonize ACh, Nicotine or *Carbachol* applied to these sites. *Table 1.5* shows their effects in the whole animal from which you can deduce whether an organ is normally dominated by parasympathetic or sympathetic tone.

These agents have little therapeutic application because their effects in the whole body are so diverse. *Pentolinium* (a quarternary ammonium salt) is given by injection to lower BP in emergencies, for example, in hypertensive encephalopathy (brain dysfunction due to excessively high BP), pulmonary oedema (oedema of the lungs due to left-sided heart failure), eclampsia (convulsions associated with high BP in toxaemia of pregnancy) (page 283).

The pharmacology of the cholinoceptor of smooth muscle, cardiac muscle and exocrine glands

The receptor was originally designated 'muscarinic' since Muscarine could readily mimic the action of ACh at these sites. Muscarinic cholinoceptors of smooth muscle, cardiac muscle and exocrine glands are characterized by the orders of drug potency shown in *Table 1.6*.

ANATOMY OF PARASYMPATHETIC NEUROEFFECTOR JUNCTIONS (pages 4, 8)

Those smooth muscle cells, cardiac muscle cells and exocrine gland cells which receive a cholinergic innervation are supplied by postganglionic cholinergic neurones. Most neurones of this type belong anatomically to the parasympathetic division of the autonomic nervous system. In the sympathetic division most postganglionic neurones are noradrenergic — but there are two which are cholinergic: (1) those supplying the eccrine sweat glands; and (2) those which provide a vasodilator pathway to the arterioles of skeletal muscle.

Muscarinic cholinoceptors are probably located over the entire surface of effector cells. They are also found on cells which do not receive a cholinergic innervation, for example, the ventricular myocardium and the smooth muscle of most blood vessels.

Table 1.6   *Orders of drug potency at the muscarinic cholinoceptor*

(1)	*Agonists*		
	ACh		
	Methacholine		
	Carbachol	>>	Nicotine
	Pilocarpine		
	Muscarine		
(2)	*Antagonists*		
	Atropine	>>	Tubocurarine
	Hyoscine [scopolamine]		*Pentolinium*
			α-bungarotoxin

Notes:
(1) Compounds to the left of the >> symbol are potent but not equally so, those to the right are so impotent that they may be regarded as inactive at this site.
(2) The muscarinic cholinoceptor differs from nicotinic cholinoceptors both as regards the order of agonist potency and order of antagonist potency (*Tables 1.2* and *1.4*).

NORMAL SEQUENCE OF EVENTS DURING CHOLINERGIC TRANSMISSION TO AUTONOMIC EFFECTOR CELLS

(1) Arrival of action potential in the postganglionic nerve terminal.
(2) Release of ACh into the junctional cleft (width 20–1000 nm).
(3) Diffusion of ACh down a concentration gradient towards the effector cell.
(4) Association of ACh with muscarinic cholinoceptor.
(5) (*a*) In cells where ACh has excitatory action (*Table 1.7*) – transmitter/ muscarinic cholinoceptor interaction evokes a non-specific increase in membrane permeability to hydrated ions of both large and small diameter which causes depolarization (excitatory postjunctional potential) with an increase in action potential frequency of the effector cell membrane.
(*b*) In cells where ACh has inhibitory action – transmitter/muscarinic cholinoceptor interaction evokes a selective increase in membrane permeability to hydrated ions of small diameter (for example, K^+) which causes hyperpolarization (inhibitory postjunctional potential) with a decrease in action potential frequency of the effector cell membrane.
Note that since many autonomic effector cells exhibit spontaneous electrical activity, the interaction of ACh with the muscarinic cholinoceptor tends not to initiate but rather to modify ongoing electrical activity.
(6) Dissociation of the ACh/cholinoceptor complex.
(7) Hydrolysis of ACh by neural AChE and diffusion of ACh away from the site of action.
(8) Transport of choline back into the nerve terminal.
(9) Resynthesis of ACh.
(10) Storage of ACh in vesicles.

Table 1.7   *The muscarinic effects of* ACh

Eye	
Ciliary muscle	Contracted
Circular muscle of iris	Contracted
Lacrimal and salivary glands	Secretion
Heart	
SA node (rate)	Inhibited
AV node and conducting tissue (rhythm and excitability)	Depressed
Ventricular myocardium (force)	Depressed*
Lungs	
Bronchioles	Constricted
Bronchial glands	Secretion
Gut, stomach to rectum	
Propulsive muscle	Contracted
Gastric and pancreatic exocrine glands	Secretion
Bladder	
Detrusor	Contracted
Genital apparatus	
Vessels of erectile tissue	Dilated
All blood vessels throughout the body	Dilated*
Skeletal muscle	
Blood vessels involved in fainting and exercise	Dilated
Skin	
Eccrine sweat glands	Secretion

* Two effects of administered ACh which cannot be mimicked by autonomic nerve stimulation.
Muscarinic receptors are not restricted to cells receiving a cholinergic nerve supply.

THE EFFECTS OF AGONISTS AT MUSCARINIC CHOLINOCEPTORS

ACh, methacholine, *Carbachol* (*Figure 1.23*), *Pilocarpine* and Muscarine activate muscarinic cholinoceptors and cause either depolarization or hyperpolarization of autonomic effector cells analogous to the physiological excitatory or inhibitory postjunctional potentials (page 31) but lasting much longer. They give rise to the excitatory and inhibitory effects listed in *Table 1.7.*

These effects are called (rather imprecisely) parasympathomimetic effects. Hence, agonists at muscarinic cholinoceptors can also be called directly acting parasympathomimetics. (Contrast these agents with other drugs which can cause the same effects but by different mechanisms — the indirectly acting

parasympathomimetics. Examples include the agonists at the nicotinic cholinoceptors of ganglia (page 25) and anticholinesterases (page 36).

ACh and Muscarine are not used clinically.

Carbachol is used to stimulate the activity of the smooth muscle of the gut,
bladder and ureters (for example, to expel gas from intestine prior to radiography,
to reverse postoperative atony of the gut and bladder, to accelerate the passage
of ureteric stones).

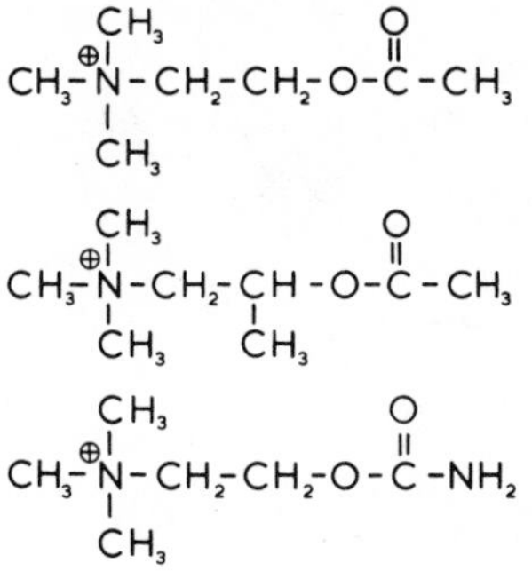

$$CH_3-\overset{\overset{\displaystyle CH_3}{|}}{\underset{\underset{\displaystyle CH_3}{|}}{\overset{\oplus}{N}}}-CH_2-CH_2-O-\overset{\overset{\displaystyle O}{\|}}{C}-CH_3 \quad \text{ACh}$$

$$CH_3-\overset{\overset{\displaystyle CH_3}{|}}{\underset{\underset{\displaystyle CH_3}{|}}{\overset{\oplus}{N}}}-CH_2-\underset{\underset{\displaystyle CH_3}{|}}{CH}-O-\overset{\overset{\displaystyle O}{\|}}{C}-CH_3 \quad \text{Methacholine}$$

$$CH_3-\overset{\overset{\displaystyle CH_3}{|}}{\underset{\underset{\displaystyle CH_3}{|}}{\overset{\oplus}{N}}}-CH_2-CH_2-O-\overset{\overset{\displaystyle O}{\|}}{C}-NH_2 \quad \textit{Carbachol}$$

Figure 1.23   *Structures of some agonists at
the muscarinic cholinoceptor*

Pilocarpine is used to counteract mydriatic drugs and also to lower intraocular
pressure in acute attacks of narrow angle glaucoma (long-term relief from attacks
may require surgery) and in long-term control of open angle glaucoma.

THE EFFECTS OF COMPETITIVE ANTAGONISTS AT
MUSCARINIC CHOLINOCEPTORS

Atropine, Dicyclomine, hyoscine, *Tropicamide, Homatropine, Mebeverine.*

Quaternary ammonium derivatives — atropine methonitrate, ipratropium,
Propantheline

Antiparkinsonism drugs, for example, *Benzhexol* (trihexyphenidyl HCl)

Tricyclic antidepressants, for example, *Imipramine.*

The anti-arrhythmics, *Procainamide* and *Quinidine.*

These agents all produce a competitive (surmountable) antagonism of ACh at the
muscarinic cholinoceptor. Injection of these agents results in the effects shown in
Table 1.8.

Atropine is the type substance of the muscarinic blocking agents. It has two
actions which cannot be explained in terms of blockade of cholinergic
transmission in the periphery: (1) it causes histamine release, by virtue of its
basicity (*Table 2.14*), which results in dilatation of cutaneous vessels; and
(2) it stimulates the CNS. In therapeutic doses *Atropine* stimulates the vagal
centre to evoke a transient bradycardia. This precedes the tachycardia due
to occupation of myocardial muscarinic receptors by *Atropine.* In toxic doses it
causes restlessness, excitement, hallucinations, delirium and convulsions. Therapeutic uses are as follows:

33

Table 1.8   *The important effects of competitive antagonists at muscarinic cholinoceptors*

Eye	
Ciliary muscle	Relaxed (cycloplegia)
Circular muscle of iris	Relaxed (mydriasis)
Lacrimal and salivary glands	Dry
Heart	
SA node (rate)	Tachycardia
AV node	Increased conduction
Lungs	
Bronchial glands	Dry
Gut, stomach to rectum	
Propulsive muscle	Reduced motility
Exocrine glands	Reduced secretion
Bladder	Difficulty of micturition
Skin	
Eccrine sweat glands	Dry

Notes:
(1)   *In vivo*, muscarinic blockade is more readily produced in some organs than in others. The susceptibility to blockade of sweat, bronchial and salivary glands > heart and muscles of eye > smooth muscle of bladder and GI tract > gastric glands.
(2)   It is easier to block the effects of exogenous (injected) ACh than those of endogenous (released from nerve terminals) ACh. (The concentration of ACh in a narrow cleft during neuroeffector transmission can be high enough to surmount the blockade produced by relatively large doses of atropine-like drugs.)

(1)   Routine mydriasis (diagnostic retinoscopy) carries a risk of precipitating glaucoma, particularly in the elderly, so choose a short-acting mydriatic, for example, *Tropicamide.*
(2)   Iritis/iridocyclitis are inflammatory conditions in which the iris tends to adhere to the anterior surface of the lens. A mydriatic with a long action is preferred, for example, *Homatropine,* hyoscine.
(3)   Anaesthetic premedication for effects on bronchial secretions and heart: hyoscine (sedative) is often preferred to *Atropine* (CNS stimulant).
(4)   Protection against undesired effects of anticholinesterases during anti-cholinesterase therapy and poisoning (page 38).
(5)   Parkinsonism (page 131). Atropine-like drugs, for example, *Benzhexol* are used to control tremor and excessive salivation.
(6)   Muscarinic (rapid-type mushroom) poisoning results from ingestion of toadstools which contain appreciable amounts of Muscarine, for example, the red-staining inocybe (*Inocybe patouillardii*). *Atropine* is a specific antidote.

(7) Travel sickness — hyoscine useful (page 300).
(8) Bronchial asthma — ipratropium useful (page 291).

Cholinesterases and their inhibitors

ACETYLCHOLINESTERASE (AChE)

AChE is found in and near the endings of all cholinergic axons and in erythrocytes. It is the activity of AChE which is primarily responsible for transmitter inactivation during cholinergic transmission (*Figure 1.11*).

AChE exhibits relatively high substrate specificity — it hydrolyses certain of the esters of choline (*Table 1.9*).

Table 1.9   *Hydrolysis of choline esters by AChE and ChE*

Substrate	Rate of hydrolysis	
	AChE	ChE
ACh	+++	++
Carbamoylesters of choline, for example, *Carbachol*	0	0
Suxamethonium	0	+

+ = hydrolysis; 0 = no hydrolysis

Substrate attachment occurs both at the anionic and esteratic sites of the active centre of AChE (*Figure 1.24*).

CHOLINESTERASE (pseudocholinesterase, ChE)

ChE is found in blood serum, in the liver and in certain effector cells.

The substrate specificity of ChE is low (compare with AChE). It not only hydrolyses certain choline esters (compare and contrast with AChE, *Table 1.9*) but will also hydrolyse esters unrelated to choline (for example, *Procaine*).

Roughly 1 in 3000 individuals is a homozygote with an abnormal gene pair which directs the synthesis of an atypical form of ChE. The atypical enzyme hydrolyses Suxamethonium exceedingly slowly so that a homozygote producing the atypical enzyme stays paralysed for some hours when given this drug (page 257).

The atypical form of ChE is relatively resistant to inhibition by cinchocaine [dibucaine]. Measurement of the 'dibucaine number' (percentage inhibition of serum ChE activity produced by a standard concentration of dibucaine) gives an indication of whether the subject possesses abnormal genes as regards ChE synthesis.

CHOLINESTERASE INHIBITORS

Competitive inhibitors

Neostigmine, Physostigmine (eserine), *Pyridostigmine, Edrophonium*

The inhibition of AChE produced by these agents can be overcome by increasing the substrate (for example, ACh) concentration; that is, the inhibition is surmountable. The inhibited enzyme can readily be reactivated by subjecting it to dialysis — the inhibition is reversible. With the exception of *Physostigmine*, all agents in this group have molecular structures which contain a quaternized N atom, and hence are fully ionized over a wide pH range. The +ve charge on the quaternized N atom facilitates attachment of these agents to the anionic site of the active centre of AChE (*Figure 1.24*).

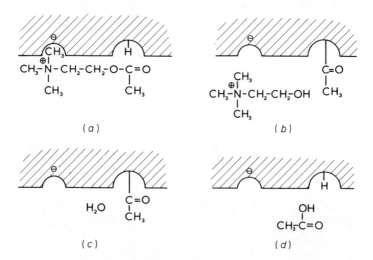

Figure 1.24   *Hydrolysis of ACh by acetylcholinesterase. (a) Attachment of ACh to anionic and esteratic sites. (b) Acetylation of esteratic site with liberation of choline. (c) and (d) Hydrolytic reactivation of esteratic site with liberation of acetic acid*

Since *Physostigmine* is a tertiary amine its inhibition of AChE is pH-dependent. Attachment of *Physostigmine* to the anionic site of AChE only occurs when the N atom of the amine group is +vely charged.

Edrophonium is unique among the competitive inhibitors of AChE in that it is not an ester. *Edrophonium* cannot therefore combine with the esteratic site of AChE. This may explain the very brief duration of *Edrophonium*'s action *in vivo*.

AChE and ChE are equally sensitive to the actions of the competitive inhibitors.

Non-competitive inhibitors

Ecothiopate [echothiophate], malaoxon from *Malathion*

The inhibition of AChE produced by these agents cannot be overcome by increasing the substrate (for example, ACh) concentration — the inhibition is insurmountable. The inhibited enzyme cannot be reactivated by dialysis — the inhibition is irreversible.

The non-competitive inhibitors of AChE are organophosphorus esters and all can bind firmly to (phosphorylate) the esteratic site of AChE (*Figure 1.25*).

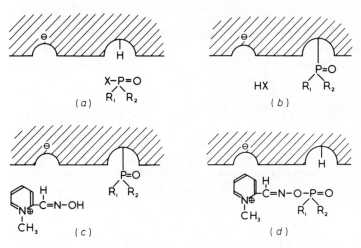

Figure 1.25   *Organophosphorus inhibition of acetylcholinesterase. (a) and (b) Phosphorylation of esteratic site with liberation of acid (HX). (c) and (d) Reactivation of esteratic site by pralidoxime*

Ecothiopate is the only member of the group possessing a quaternized N atom and therefore the only member of the group which also attaches to the anionic site of AChE.

ChE is more susceptible to the actions of the non-competitive inhibitors than AChE.

CONSEQUENCES OF CHOLINESTERASE INHIBITION

Inhibition of AChE delays the biotransformation of ACh. The resulting accumulation of endogenous ACh evokes parasympathomimetic effects (page 32 and *Table 1.1*) including excessive sweating, salivation and bronchial secretion, miosis, bradycardia and diarrhoea. These effects can be minimized by the administration of an antagonist at muscarinic cholinoceptors, for example, *Atropine.*

When AChE is inhibited by about 80 per cent, the accumulation of ACh at the skeletal neuromuscular junction evokes depolarizing blockade of neuromuscular

37

transmission (page 21 and *Figure 1.15*). At this point death may ensue from respiratory paralysis — effectively due to ACh poisoning.

USES OF CHOLINESTERASE INHIBITORS

Competitive inhibitors of AChE are used in the diagnosis and treatment of myasthenia gravis (a disease characterized by weakness and rapid tiring of skeletal muscle). *Edrophonium* is a diagnostic agent — a +ve result is indicated by a brief increase in muscular power following its injection. *Neostigmine* and *Pyridostigmine* are used in the symptomatic treatment of myasthenia usually in conjunction with *Atropine* to minimize the effects of ACh at muscarinic cholinoceptors. Over-dosage with *Neostigmine* or *Pyridostigmine* can itself precipitate muscle weakness due to depolarizing blockade of neuromuscular transmission — a 'cholinergic crisis'. *Edrophonium* can be used to distinguish between a cholinergic crisis and the effects of under-treatment or increased disease severity. An injection of *Edrophonium* will briefly exacerbate a cholinergic crisis but will briefly increase muscle power in the case of under-dosage with an AChE inhibitor.

Neostigmine is used to reverse the neuromuscular blockade evoked by Tubocurarine or gallamine (*Table 1.3*). The injection of *Neostigmine* is preceded by an injection of *Atropine* in order to minimize the effects of ACh at muscarinic cholinoceptors.

Physostigmine and *Ecothiopate* are used as miotics — the former to counteract the actions of mydiatric drugs — both to lower intraocular pressure in congestive (narrow angle) glaucoma. The use of these agents in the eye carries a risk of systemic toxicity since they are both well absorbed from the conjunctival sac.

Malathion is used as an insecticide in the treatment of pediculosis (page 180) Other organophosphorus anticholinesterases are used as agricultural insecticides or military nerve gases.

REACTIVATION OF CHOLINESTERASES INHIBITED BY ORGANOPHOSPHORUS COMPOUNDS

The inhibition of esterases evoked by organophosphorus compounds is irreversible in the sense that the phosphorylated esteratic site cannot spontaneously hydrolyse. If, and only if, the phosphorylation is recent, the enzyme can be reactivated by agents which are more nucleophilic than water, for example, Pralidoxime (*Figure 1.25*).

Industrial, agricultural or military poisoning with organophosphorus anticholinesterases is treated by injection of both *Atropine* and Pralidoxime.

The pharmacology of noradrenergic neuroeffector transmission

Revise

- The anatomy of the sympathetic nervous system (pages 2 and 5).
- The effects of stimulating sympathetic neurones (*Table 1.1*).
  (Noradrenergic neurones synthesize, store, and release as their transmitter NA.

They include:

- Most postganglionic sympathetic neurones (exceptions are those neurones supplying the eccrine sweat glands and those providing a vasodilator pathway to the arterioles of skeletal muscle. Although anatomically sympathetic, these fibres transmit by means of ACh).
- Some neurones lying entirely within the CNS.

ANATOMY OF SYMPATHETIC NEUROEFFECTOR JUNCTIONS (page 8)

Compare parasympathetic neuroeffector junctions (page 30). Those smooth muscle, cardiac muscle and exocrine gland cells which receive a noradrenergic innervation are supplied by postganglionic sympathetic neurones. The receptor

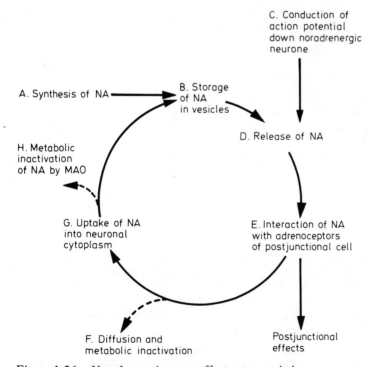

Figure 1.26   *Noradrenergic neuroeffector transmission*

sites for NA (α- and β-adrenoceptors, page 44) are located over the entire surface of the effector cells. They can also be found on cells which do not receive a noradrenergic innervation (*Table 1.13*).

NORADRENERGIC TRANSMISSION

The process of noradrenergic neuroeffector transmission (*Figure 1.26*) is basically similar at all sites in the body.

Synthesis of NA

The synthesis of NA may arbitrarily be regarded as the first stage in the process of noradrenergic transmission. The starting material in NA biosynthesis is dietary L-phenylalanine. This aminoacid is actively absorbed from the gut and oxidized by hepatic phenylalanine hydroxylase to form L-tyrosine. The L-tyrosine circulates in the bloodstream and is actively transported into the cytoplasm of noradrenergic neurones. Its conversion to NA (*Figure 1.27*) follows.

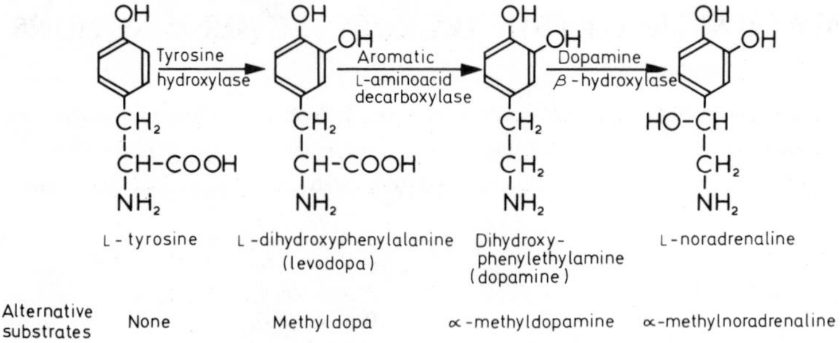

Figure 1.27   *Synthesis of NA*

Within the neuronal cytoplasm, L-tyrosine is hydroxylated to form L-dihydroxy-phenylalanine (L-DOPA, *Levodopa*). This reaction is catalysed by cytoplasmic tyrosine hydroxylase and is the rate limiting step in the biosynthesis of NA. The activity of tyrosine hydroxylase is governed by the cytoplasmic concentration of NA, high NA concentration inhibiting enzyme activity. This is an example of feedback (product) inhibition.

In contrast to other enzymes involved in the synthesis of NA, tyrosine hydroxylase exhibits high substrate specificity. This stage in NA synthesis is therefore less susceptible to drug (alternative substrate) attack.

Aromatic L-aminoacid decarboxylase is a cytoplasmic enzyme of low substrate specificity and converts L-DOPA to dopamine. It can be inhibited by *Benserazide* and by *Carbidopa* (methyldopa hydrazine). These agents are relatively large, hydrophilic molecules and do not enter the brain (page 231). They can therefore provide a selective inhibition of peripherally located enzyme. This phenomenon is exploited in order to reduce the adverse peripheral effects of *Levodopa* in the treatment of Parkinsonism (page 131).

Dopamine, synthesized within the neuronal cytoplasm, is actively transported into the transmitter storage vesicles of the axon terminals. Here, the dopamine is

40

oxidized by dopamine β-hydroxylase (an enzyme of low substrate specificity) to form NA. Dopamine β-hydroxylase requires trace amounts of copper and is therefore inhibited by copper-chelators (for example, diethyldithiocarbamate, a metabolite of disulphiram, a drug used in the aversion therapy of alcoholism).

Storage of NA in vesicles

Endogenous NA is stored in membrane-limited vesicles which are formed in the neuronal cell body and transported to the varicosities of the axon terminal by axoplasmic flow. Within the vesicles NA is stored as a complex with ATP and a soluble protein called chromogranin. The retention of NA by the vesicles is aided both by the formation of this storage complex and also by the continued operation of the amine uptake process in the vesicle membrane (a process requiring the breakdown of ATP by Mg^{2+}-dependent ATPase).

Drugs which interfere with vesicular retention of NA   *Reserpine* inhibits the amine uptake process in the vesicle membrane and thereby allows the leakage of NA into the cytoplasm where it is largely metabolized by neuronal monoamine oxidase (page 52). Furthermore, since vesicular dopamine uptake is inhibited, NA synthesis is impaired. For these two reasons the storage vesicles become depleted of NA (chromaffin cells of the adrenal medulla and central noradrenergic, dopaminergic and tryptaminergic neurones are also susceptible to this action of *Reserpine,* pages 56 and 139).

NA depletion is accelerated by action potential activity in the neurone. Noradrenergic neuroeffector transmission fails when NA content is reduced to about 25 percent of normal. When large doses of *Reserpine* are used, recovery of neurone function depends upon the synthesis of new vesicles and their transport to the axon terminals (about 10 days).

Pretreatment with Reserpine

(1)   Abolishes the effects of noradrenergic neurone activity.
(2)   Abolishes the effects of agents which act by causing the release of NA from axon terminals – the indirectly acting sympathomimetics (page 48).
(3)   Does not reduce responses of effector cells to exogenous NA or other directly acting sympathomimetics (page 46).

Guanethidine (but not other noradrenergic neurone blocking agents, page 42) also causes *Reserpine*-like depletion of axonal NA stores.

Reserpine is used to treat hypertension (page 282). Its adverse effects include severe (suicidal) depression.

Drugs which compete with NA for vesicular storage   Certain drugs, on gaining access to the neuronal cytoplasm, can compete with dopamine or NA for uptake into the vesicles. They may then stoichiometrically displace NA from its storage site. Drugs in this group include α-methyldopamine formed from *Methyldopa* and certain indirectly acting sympathomimetics (for example, Tyramine, *Ephedrine,* amphetamine).

Consequences of NA displacement

(1) Less NA is available for release during neuroeffector transmission.
(2) The displacing drug may be released in place of NA during neuroeffector transmission (false transmission).
(3) The response of the effector cell to the displacing drug may result from the pharmacological effects of displaced NA (*see* indirectly acting sympathomimetics, page 48).

Methyldopa (compare triethylcholine acting on cholinergic transmission, page 16) can act as a substrate of aromatic L-aminoacid decarboxylase and hence be converted to α-methyldopamine. Since α-methyldopamine is not a substrate for neuronal MAO, it competes very successfully with dopamine for transport into the storage vesicles. Vesicular dopamine β-hydroxylase then oxidizes α-methyldopamine to yield α-methylnoradrenaline which functions as a false transmitter since it can be stored in the vesicles and subsequently be released into the junctional cleft on arrival of the nerve action potential. Since α-methylnoradrenaline is approximately equipotent with NA in evoking a response from effector cells in the periphery (that is, the heart and blood vessels), the process of neuroeffector transmission is little affected. α-Methylnoradrenaline is reported to be more potent than NA at presynaptic (release-inhibiting) receptors and seems to exert its effects by reducing the amount of transmitter released from central noradrenergic neurones involved in the control of BP.

Pretreatment with Methyldopa

(1) Reduces the effects of noradrenergic and dopaminergic neurone activity in the CNS.
(2) Does not reduce the responses of effector cells to exogenous NA or other directly acting sympathomimetics, page 46.

Methyldopa is used in the treatment of hypertension (page 282). Adverse effects include drowsiness, depression and fluid retention.

Neuronal action potential conduction

Compare with action potential conduction in cholinergic neurones, page 16. Action potential conduction down the noradrenergic axon can be prevented (and hence transmission will be prevented) by local anaesthetics (for example, *Lignocaine*) and by Tetrodotoxin. These agents prevent action potential conduction by membrane stabilization (page 57). They are not selective for noradrenergic neurones (pages 16 and 57).

In contrast, the noradrenergic neurone blocking agents (*Guanethidine*, *Bethanidine* and *Debrisoquine*) selectively impair transmission at noradrenergic neuroeffector junctions. These agents are weak local anaesthetics but are selectively accumulated by noradrenergic neurones. They are transported into the cytoplasm of noradrenergic axon terminals by the same mechanism (page 53) which transports NA into the cell.

The intraneuronal mechanism of action of the adrenergic neurone blocking agents is poorly understood. *Guanethidine* (but not *Bethanidine* or *Debrisoquine*) causes a *Reserpine*-like transmitter depletion on prolonged administration (page 41). However, the noradrenergic neurone blocking agents prevent neuroeffector transmission long before measurable depletion of neural NA content occurs. Hence, unless these agents cause depletion of an immeasurably small but essential pool of transmitter, an alternative explanation of their actions must be sought.

The most popular hypothesis is that, as substrates for the neuronal NA uptake process, the noradrenergic neurone blocking agents are accumulated within noradrenergic neurones to local anaesthetic concentrations. By stabilization of membranes, these agents may prevent NA release either by preventing nerve action potential conduction in terminal neuronal branches or by interfering with exocytosis.

The noradrenergic neurone blocking agents

(1) Prevent the effects of noradrenergic neurone activity.
(2) Prevent the effects of those indirectly acting sympathomimetics which utilize the neuronal NA uptake mechanism to gain access to the neuronal cytoplasm (for example, Tyramine, *Ephedrine,* amphetamine; page 48) and of those which generate nerve action potentials (for example, Nicotine; pages 28 and 48).
(3) Do not reduce the effects of exogenous NA or other directly acting sympathomimetics (page 46). Indeed, if the directly acting sympatho-mimetic is a substrate for the neuronal NA uptake process its effects will be potentiated.

The selectivity of the noradrenergic neurone blocking agents and their ability to modify the actions of some indirectly and directly acting sympathomimetics all depend on their being substrates for the neuronal NA uptake process. The actions of adrenergic neurone blocking agents are impaired by other drugs which compete with them for uptake into the neurone (for example, Tyramine) or which block the uptake process (for example, *Cocaine* and *Imipramine*, page 54).

The adrenergic neurone blocking agents are useful in the treatment of hypertension (page 282). Unwanted effects include postural and exercise hypotension, diarrhoea and failure of ejaculation.

Guanethidine eyedrops can lower intraocular pressure in chronic, simple, open angle glaucoma and can reduce the exophthalmos and eyelid retraction of hyperthyroidism.

Release of NA from axon terminals

Compare with the release of ACh from cholinergic axons (page 16). Two physiological mechanisms for NA release exist.

Action potential-evoked release. As an action potential invades the terminal axon, membrane permeability changes occur. Na^+, Cl^- and Ca^{2+} enter the cell and K^+ emerges. The influx of Ca^{2+} triggers many storage vesicles to release NA, ATP, chromogranin and dopamine β-hydroxylase into the junctional cleft (exocytosis). The empty vesicles are probably retained within the cell and subsequently refilled with transmitter.

Since transmitter release by this mechanism requires the nerve action potential, it will be prevented by local anaesthetics, Tetrodotoxin and adrenergic neurone blocking agents.

Transmitter release by this mechanism requires the influx of Ca^{2+}, and is reduced if the ECF is deficient in this ion or contains a high concentration of Mg^{2+}.

After treatment of tissues with *Methyldopa,* action potentials release α-methyl-noradrenaline (false transmission, page 42) from the terminals of noradrenergic axons.

Spontaneous release   The random migration of storage vesicles to the cell surface can result in the spontaneous discharge of their contents into the junctional cleft. Although the amount of NA released is small, it can still influence the membrane of the postjunctional cell if the cleft width is narrow, for example, spontaneous postjunctional potentials are seen in some noradrenergically innervated smooth muscles (compare with the miniature epps seen at the motor end plate of skeletal muscle – *Figure 1.13*).

Since this release mechanism does not require the arrival of nerve action potentials, it is unaffected by Tetrodotoxin. *Reserpine*, by depleting the vesicles of stored NA (page 41), prevents both the spontaneous and action potential-evoked release of NA.

The interaction of NA with postjunctional adrenoceptors

Compare the interaction of ACh with muscarinic cholinoceptors (page 31).

NA which has been released into the junctional cleft diffuses down its concentration gradient and reversibly forms complexes with receptors (adreno-ceptors) on the surface of the membrane of the effector cell. Some function of this interaction (page 69) determines the nature and size of the change in ionic permeability of the postjunctional cell membrane.

(1)   In cells where NA has an excitatory action, the NA–adrenoceptor inter-action evokes a non-specific increase in membrane permeability to hydrated ions of both large and small diameter, and this causes depolarization (excitatory postjunctional potential) with an increase in action potential frequency of the effector cell membrane.

(2)   In cells where NA has an inhibitory action, the NA–adrenoceptor inter-action evokes a selective increase in membrane permeability to hydrated ions of small diameter (for example, K^+) – and this causes hyperpolariza-tion (inhibitory postjunctional potential) with a decrease in the action potential frequency of the effector cell membrane.

Since many autonomic effector cells exhibit spontaneous electrical activity, the interaction of NA with the adrenoceptor tends not to initiate but rather to modify ongoing electrical activity.

There are two types of adrenoceptor which may be distinguished by character-istic relative orders of potencies for both agonists and antagonists: the α-adrenoceptor (*Table 1.10*) and the β-adrenoceptor (*Table 1.12*).

Table 1.10   *The α-adrenoceptor*

Relative order of agonist potency
NA≅*Adrenaline* [epinephrine] > *Phenylephrine* > Methoxamine >>
Isoprenaline [isoproterenol]
Relative order of antagonist potency

Phentolamine	>>	*Propranolol*
Ergotamine		*Oxprenolol*
Chlorpromazine		Practolol
Phenoxybenzamine		

Note: Compounds to the left of the >> symbol are potent but not equally so,
those to the right are so impotent that they may be regarded as inactive at the
α-adrenoceptor.

The effects mediated by α-adrenoceptors are listed in *Table 1.11.*

Table 1.11   *The effects mediated by α-adrenoceptors*

Eye	
Radial muscle of iris	Contracted
Eyelids and nictitating membrane	Contracted
Gut	
Propulsive smooth muscle	Relaxed
Bladder	
Bladder neck and trigone	Contracted
Genitalia	
Seminal vesicles and vas deferens	Contracted
All blood vessels	Constricted
Pilomotor muscles	Contracted

Table 1.12   *The β-adrenoceptor*

Relative order of agonist potency
Isoprenaline > *Adrenaline* > NA >> *Phenylephrine* > Methoxamine
Relative order of antagonist potency

Propranolol	>>	Phentolamine
Oxprenolol		*Ergotamine*
Practolol		*Chlorpromazine*
		Phenoxybenzamine

Notes:
(1)   Compounds to the left of the >> symbol are potent but not equally so,
those to the right are so impotent that they may be regarded as inactive at
the β-adrenoceptor.
(2)   There is some evidence for a subdivision of β-adrenoceptors, for example,
cardiac β-adrenoceptors (β_1 receptors) differ from those found in the
smooth muscle of the respiratory tract (β_2 receptors).

The effects mediated by β-adrenoceptors are listed in *Table 1.13*.

Table 1.13   *The effects mediated by β-adrenoceptors*

Heart	
SA node	Increased firing rate
AV node	Reduced refractory period
Purkinje fibres	Reduced refractory period
	Increased automaticity
Ventricular myocardium	Increased force of contraction
Gut	
Propulsive smooth muscle	Relaxed
Respiratory tract	
Smooth muscle	Relaxed
Uterine smooth muscle	Relaxed
Arterioles of skeletal muscle †	Dilated
Adipocytes *	Lipolysis
Liver cells *	Gluconeogenesis
Skeletal muscle cells *	Glycolysis

* Note that β-adrenoceptors can be found on cells which do not receive a noradrenergic innervation (cf muscarinic cholinoceptors, *Table 1.7*). Note also that, in many effectors, the activation of β-adrenoceptors is accompanied by stimulation of adenylate cyclase and therefore an increase in cellular content of cAMP.
† Receive noradrenergic innervation but NA released activates only α-adrenoceptors (*Table 1.11*). β-adrenoceptors here activated by circulating agonists.

The effects of agonists at adrenoceptors

Adrenaline, Isoprenaline, Methoxamine, NA, *Orciprenaline, Phenylephrine, Salbutamol.*

These drugs activate one or both types of adrenoceptor (*Tables 1.10* and *1.12*) thereby causing either depolarization or hyperpolarization of autonomic effector cells analogous to the physiological excitatory or inhibitory junctional potentials but lasting much longer.

These effects are called (rather imprecisely) sympathomimetic effects. Hence, agonists at adrenoceptors can also be called directly acting sympathomimetics. (Contrast these agents with other drugs which cause the same effects but by different mechanisms – the indirectly acting sympathomimetics. Examples include Tyramine-like agents which displace NA from axon terminals (page 48) and the agonists at the nicotinic cholinoceptors of ganglia (pages 27 and 48).

Structure/activity relationships for agonists at adrenoceptors   Most directly acting sympathomimetics are structural analogues of *Adrenaline.* This agent is a potent agonist at both the α- and β-adrenoceptors. Slight changes in the structure of the *Adrenaline* molecule can yield compounds which selectively activate either the α- or β-adrenoceptor.

Table 1.14

Ratio of potency at α- to potency at β-adrenoceptor	Agonist classification
High value ($\gg$ 1)	Selective agonist at the α-adrenoceptor
Intermediate value of (about 1)	Non-selective agonist
Low value ($\ll$ 1)	Selective agonist at the β-adrenoceptor

Figure 1.28 shows a classification of agonists at the adrenoceptor according to their selectivity of action.

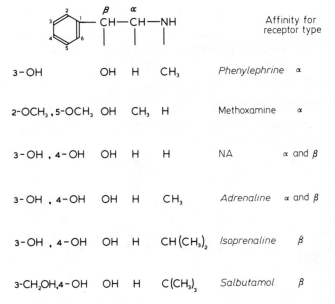

3−OH	OH	H	CH$_3$	*Phenylephrine*	α
2-OCH$_3$, 5-OCH$_3$	OH	CH$_3$	H	Methoxamine	α
3−OH , 4−OH	OH	H	H	NA	α and β
3−OH , 4−OH	OH	H	CH$_3$	*Adrenaline*	α and β
3−OH , 4−OH	OH	H	CH(CH$_3$)$_2$	*Isoprenaline*	β
3-CH$_2$OH,4−OH	OH	H	C(CH$_3$)$_3$	*Salbutamol*	β

Figure 1.28   *Classification of directly acting sympathomimetic drugs*

Notes
(1) An alternative name for 1,2-dihydroxybenzene is catechol therefore 3,4-dihydroxyphenylethylamines are catecholamines.
(2) The β-carbon atom of phenylethanolamines is optically active. The biosynthesis of the physiological compounds NA and *Adrenaline* yields the ℓ-isomer (in which the greater biological activity resides).
(3) The physiological compounds NA and *Adrenaline* have relatively low selectivity of action and can therefore elicit effects mediated by both α- and β-adrenoceptors.
(4) Provided that excessive drug concentrations are avoided, the synthetic drugs Methoxamine and *Phenylephrine* elicit only the effects mediated by α-adrenoceptors (*Table 1.11*). The synthetic drugs *Isoprenaline, Salbutamol*

and *Orciprenaline* elicit only the effects mediated by β-adrenoceptors (*Table 1.13*).

(5) In general, increasing the size of the substituent on the nitrogen atom of the phenylethylamine molecule increases selectivity for β-adrenoceptors.

Eyedrops containing *Phenylephrine* or *Adrenaline* produce brief periods of mydriasis during diagnostic retinoscopy. Such eyedrops are also effective in lowering intraocular pressure (possibly by reducing the production of aqueous humour) in primary open angle glaucoma.

Adrenaline and NA are included in the formulation of some local anaesthetic injections. By causing vasoconstriction at the injection site these agents prolong the local anaesthesia.

Adrenaline is given iv to evoke vasoconstriction, bronchodilatation and a reduction in capillary permeability in the control of anaphylactic shock (page 107) and other severe forms of urticaria.

Adrenaline and selective agonists at the β-adrenoceptor (*Isoprenaline, Orciprenaline* and *Salbutamol*) are used to reduce airways resistance in bronchial asthma (page 290). The associated risk of tachycardia, ectopic beats and dangerous arrhythmias is least with *Salbutamol*, since this drug can relax bronchial smooth muscle at doses which have little or no cardiac stimulant activity.

Indirectly acting sympathomimetics

An indirectly acting sympathomimetic does not itself activate adrenoceptors. It evokes sympathomimetic effects either by promoting the release of neuronal NA (for example, Tyramine, Nicotine) or by preventing the inactivation of NA (for example, *Cocaine*).

Tyramine-like indirectly acting sympathomimetics Certain chemical modifications of the *Adrenaline* molecule (for example, loss of catechol-OH groups; loss of the β-OH group; methylation of the α-C atom) yield agents which cannot themselves activate adrenoceptors. Examples include Tyramine, *Ephedrine* and amphetamine (*Figure 1.29*).

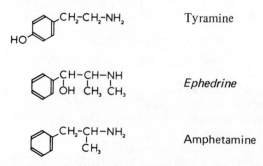

Figure 1.29 *The structures of some indirectly acting sympathomimetic drugs*

However, these drugs act as substrates for the NA uptake process in the neuronal membrane (page 53) and gain access to the neuronal cytoplasm by that route. They are then transported into the transmitter storage vesicles where they

48

stoichiometrically displace NA. A high proportion of the displaced NA escapes from the neurone and subsequently activates postjunctional adrenoceptors.

Agonists at the nicotinic cholinoceptors of ganglia ACh, Nicotine and *Carbachol* can evoke release of neural NA (*Figure 1.21*) and thereby induce sympathomimetic effects.

Inhibitors of the neuronal uptake of NA Cocaine and *Imipramine* inhibit the neuronal uptake of NA. Endogenous NA (spontaneously released or released

Table 1.15 *Comparison of directly acting and indirectly acting sympathomimetics*

Directly acting, for example, NA	*Indirectly acting, for example,* Tyramine, *Ephedrine* and Amphetamine	*Explanation for property of indirectly acting drug*
Chemically unstable	Chemically more stable	Drug molecule lacks catechol OH groups
Pharmacological effects are brief	Pharmacological effects are prolonged	Drug molecule relatively resistant to transformation
Poorly absorbed from gut	Better absorption from gut	Drug molecule lacks catechol OH groups and is relatively less polar
Poor penetration of CNS and thus weak CNS effects	Better penetration of CNS and thus stronger CNS effects	Drug molecule lacks catechol OH groups and is relatively less polar
Postganglionic denervation potentiates	Postganglionic denervation prevents action	Drug must enter neurone to be active; neurones absent
Cocaine and *Imipramine* potentiate	*Cocaine* and *Imipramine* prevent action	Drug must enter neurone to be active; entry into neurone prevented
Summates with NA	Potentiates NA	Drug competes with NA for neuronal uptake
Reserpine does not prevent action	*Reserpine* prevents action	Drug cannot displace neural NA when transmitter stores are depleted
Phenelzine does not modify action	*Phenelzine* potentiates	MAO inhibition delays biotransformation of drug or of NA released by drug
Repeated equal doses have equal effects	Tachyphylaxis occurs	Neuronal NA stores become depleted by repeated drug challenge

by neuronal action potentials) therefore accumulates in the junctional cleft and evokes sympathomimetic effects.

The properties of the tyramine-like group of indirectly acting sympathomimetics are compared with those of directly acting sympathomimetics in *Table 1.15.*

Ephedrine is effective as a bronchodilator in bronchial asthma and as a nasal vasoconstrictor. Unwanted effects include wakefulness and (in elderly males) urinary retention.

Antagonists at adrenoceptors

These drugs, to a certain extent, resemble NA structurally. They are therefore able to combine with adrenoceptors but, unlike NA, the antagonists are unable to activate the adrenoceptor. Thus, they do not evoke an active biological response from the effector cell.

Antagonists at the α-adrenoceptor

Phentolamine, Phenoxybenzamine, *Chlorpromazine, Ergotamine, prazosin*

By combining with the α-adrenoceptor, these antagonists reduce the access of agonists. They thereby reduce those effects of sympathetic nerve activity or sympathomimetic drug action (both direct and indirect) which are mediated by α-adrenoceptors (*Table 1.11*).

Phentolamine, *Prazosin, Chlorpromazine* and *Ergotamine* each act as competitive (surmountable, reversible) antagonists (page 69) at the α-adrenoceptor.

In contrast, Phenoxybenzamine acts as a non-competitive (insurmountable, irreversible) antagonist (page 70) at the α-adrenoceptor. Phenoxybenzamine is a β-haloalkylamine (related to the nitrogen mustards, page 175). In neutral or alkaline solution it forms the highly reactive ethyleniminium ion. This ion either alkylates reactive groups of the cell membrane (for example, the α-adrenoceptor) or spontaneously condenses with water to form an inactive alcohol (*Figure 1.30*).

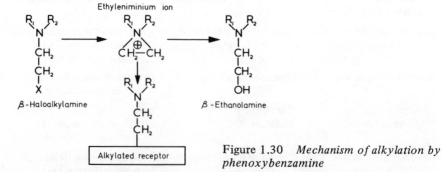

Figure 1.30   *Mechanism of alkylation by phenoxybenzamine*

Note that low concentration or short exposure time enables Phenoxybenzamine selectively to alkylate α-adrenoceptors. Higher concentration or longer exposure time leads to the alkylation of other receptors, for example, H_1 histamine receptors, D 5-HT receptors and muscarinic cholinoceptors.

The blockade of α-adrenoceptors has relatively little application in therapeutics.

50

Phentolamine is a useful aid in the diagnosis of phaeochromocytoma (a tumour of the adrenal medullary chromaffin cells). A +ve result is indicated when an iv injection of **Phentolamine** produces a dramatic but brief fall in BP to near or below normal.

Phenoxybenzamine protects vascular smooth muscle from high circulating concentrations of catecholamines produced by phaeochromocytoma. Its irreversible action affords prolonged protection.

Other antagonists at α-adrenoceptors have useful properties unrelated to α-adrenoceptor blockade. *Chlorpromazine* (a phenothiazine) is a neuroleptic which is used to treat schizophrenia and can suppress vomiting. These actions of *Chlorpromazine* on the CNS may result from the drug's interaction with receptors for dopamine and 5-HT in addition to central α-adrenoceptors (page 140). The α-adrenoceptor blockade evoked by **Chlorpromazine** is responsible for some of the drug's unwanted effects, for example, hypotension.

Ergotamine (an ergot alkaloid) is effective against migraine because it has direct vasoconstrictor properties.

Antagonists at the β-adrenoceptor

Propranolol, Oxprenolol, Practolol

By combining with the β-adrenoceptor, these antagonists reduce the access of agonists. They thereby reduce those effects of sympathetic nerve activity or sympathomimetic drug action (both direct and indirect) which are mediated by β-adrenoceptors (*Table 1.13*).

Propranolol, Oxprenolol and practolol each act as competitive (surmountable, reversible) antagonists (page 69) at the β-adrenoceptor. In concentrations higher than those required for blockade of β-adrenoceptors, *Propranolol* and *Oxprenolol* directly stabilize the membranes of excitable cells (page 63). Practolol exhibits selectivity as an antagonist at cardiac β-adrenoceptors. It can antagonize NA on the heart at doses which have little or no effect on the relaxant action of NA on respiratory tract smooth muscle.

Propranolol and *Oxprenolol* lower the heart rate by blockade of cardiac β-adrenoceptors. This prolongs diastole and reduces myocardial oxygen demand. The exercise tolerance of patients with angina pectoris is thereby increased. *Propranolol* and *Oxprenolol* can be used to lower the BP of hypertensive patients (page 281) and are effective in the correction of certain cardiac arrhythmias, especially those due to *Digoxin* toxicity or thyrotoxicosis. *Propranolol* and *Oxprenolol* may be used to protect cardiac β-adrenoceptors from high circulating concentrations of catecholamines prior to, or during, the surgical removal of a phaeochromocytoma.

Unwanted effects of *Propranolol* include the precipitation of cardiac failure in patients with a small cardiac reserve and aggravation of bronchoconstriction in asthmatic patients. It is claimed that the risk of these unwanted effects is smaller in the case of *Oxprenolol* as a consequence of intrinsic sympathomimetic (partial agonist) activity. The risk of precipitating bronchoconstriction is minimal with practolol. Unfortunately, severe lesions of the cornea and peritoneum developed in a number of patients being treated chronically with practolol, causing it to be withdrawn from general use. Practolol is still available for acute use, under supervision, in hospitals.

Metabolic inactivation of NA

Enzymic degradation is not an important mechanism for the inactivation of NA released during neuroeffector transmission. The NA in the junctional cleft is largely inactivated by neuronal uptake (page 53).

Sympathomimetic amines circulating in the bloodstream (for example, amines from the diet, injected drugs, *Adrenaline* released from the adrenal medulla) are inactivated by enzymic destruction to a variable extent. Metabolic inactivation assumes greatest importance if the circulating catecholamines are present in large amounts and are not substrates for neuronal uptake.

Circulating sympathomimetic amines may be metabolized by catechol O-methyl transferase (COMT), MAO or by both enzymes (*Figure 1.31*).

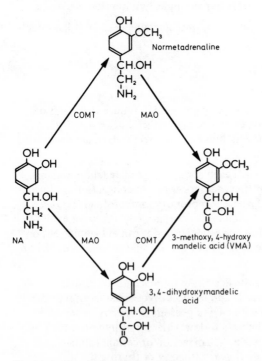

Figure 1.31   *Metabolism of NA*

COMT is found in the liver and certain effector cells but not in noradrenergic neurones. This enzyme can utilize any catechol as substrate. The O-methylated product may undergo conjugation (page 224) to form a sulphate or glucuronide, or may be oxidized by MAO to form the corresponding acid.

MAO is found in the intestine, in the liver and in the cytoplasm of noradrenergic neurones. MAO can utilize many aryl- and alkyl-amines (for example, NA, *Adrenaline,* Tyramine, 5-HT) as substrates but not those with a large N-substituent (for example, *Isoprenaline*) nor those with an α-methyl substituent (for example,

Ephedrine, amphetamine, α-methyldopamine). The product is the corresponding acid or glycol (*Figure 1.31*).

The major product of biotransformation of NA and *Adrenaline* is 3-methoxy-4-hydroxymandelic acid (vanillylmandelic acid, VMA). The urinary excretion of VMA is raised in phaeochromocytoma and can be measured as a diagnostic test.

Drugs which interfere with biotransformation of NA All catechols can act as competitive inhibitors of COMT but COMT inhibition is not therapeutically exploited.

MAO inhibitors (page 136) of which there are two major types: (1) competitive, for example, Tranylcypromine; and (2) non-competitive, the hydrazine group, for example, *Phenelzine.* By inhibiting MAO, these agents potentiate dietary Tyramine. Significant amounts of Tyramine are found in cheese, beef extracts (Bovril), yeast extracts (Marmite), pickled herrings and some alcoholic drinks. Some sympathomimetics administered as therapeutic agents, for example, *Adrenaline, Ephedrine, Levodopa* and phenylpropanolamine (a common ingredient of proprietary cold remedies) are also potentiated. Potentiation of sympathomimetics can result in dangerous hypertensive crises.

MAO inhibition can potentiate a sympathomimetic drug by: (1) delaying the biotransformation of the drug itself (for example, *Adrenaline,* Tyramine); or by (2) delaying the biotransformation of any NA released by the drug (for example, Tyramine, *Ephedrine*).

MAO inhibitors lack selectivity for they can also inhibit the mixed function oxidase enzymes (page 222) of the liver. They can therefore delay the biotransformation of (and thus potentiate) many drugs which are not substrates for MAO (for example, *Ephedrine,* Amphetamine, *Pethidine* [meperidine] and *Morphine*).

The multiplicity of their drug interactions limits the usefulness of MAO inhibitors in the treatment of endogenous depression (page 138).

Neuronal uptake of NA

Uptake into the cytoplasm of noradrenergic neurones is the major mechanism of inactivation for NA released during neuroeffector transmission or NA injected as a small iv dose. Blockade of uptake therefore causes potentiation of exogenous NA or that released by a nerve impulse.

The uptake process is located in the axonal membrane and has the following properties.

(1)   Operates against a concentration gradient.
(2)   Requires an energy supply.
(3)   Requires Na^+.
(4)   Is saturable.
(5)   Is moderately substrate specific.

Substrates for the neuronal NA uptake process include:
(1) Certain directly acting sympathomimetics, that is, NA and *Adrenaline* (note that the synthetic drugs, Methoxamine, *Phenylephrine, Isoprenaline, Orciprenaline* and *Salbutamol* are not substrates); (2) certain indirectly acting sympathomimetics,

53

that is, Tyramine, Amphetamine, *Ephedrine;* and (3) the adrenergic neurone blocking agents *Guanethidine, Bethanidine, Debrisoquine.*

Drug interactions among the substrates for neuronal NA uptake:
(1) By competing for neuronal uptake, the Tyramine-like indirectly acting sympathomimetics and the adrenergic neurone blocking agents potentiate NA and *Adrenaline;* (2) The Tyramine-like indirectly acting sympathomimetics and the adrenergic neurone blocking agents are mutually antagonistic since they compete for the uptake process (and thus for access to their sites of action).

Non-transported inhibitors of neuronal NA uptake

Cocaine inhibits the NA uptake process at concentrations less than those required to produce local anaesthesia. *Cocaine* can thus potentiate endogenous NA released either spontaneously or in response to an action potential from the axon terminal (for example, the mydriasis evoked by *Cocaine* eyedrops).

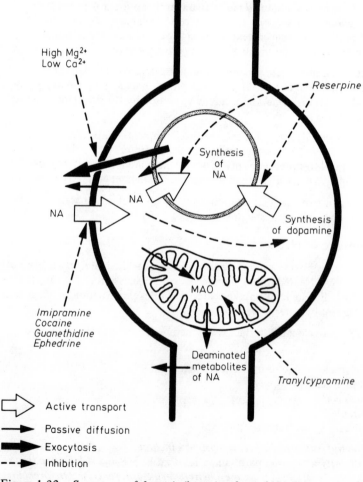

Figure 1.32   *Summary of drugs influencing fate of NA in a noradrenergic neurone*

54

The antidepressant actions of the tricyclic agents (for example, *Imipramine* and *Amitryptyline* may be attributed to their blockade of amine uptake in the CNS (page 135).

Drug interactions with non-transported inhibitors of NA uptake   By blocking neuronal uptake *Cocaine* and tricyclic antidepressants: (1) potentiate NA and *Adrenaline* (by delaying their inactivation); and (2) antagonize the Tyramine-like indirectly acting sympathomimetics and the adrenergic neurone blocking agents (by preventing access to their sites of action).

Fate of NA transported into the neuronal cytoplasm

A small proportion of the NA entering the cytoplasm by way of the membrane uptake process is metabolized by mitochondrial MAO (page 52). The majority of the NA entering the neurone by this route is transported into the storage vesicles for subsequent transmitter use (compare with the uptake of choline and use in ACh synthesis, (page 17).

See Figure 1.32 for a summary of the mechanisms of NA uptake and release from noradrenergic neurones.

The adrenal medulla

The chromaffin cells which comprise the adrenal medulla arise embryologically from the same cells which give rise to postganglionic noradrenergic neurones. However, the embryonic medullary cells do not develop long axons or threshold electrical characteristics. Instead they develop a high capacity for the storage and release of catecholamines.

The medullary chromaffin cells synthesize NA (*Figure 1.27*) but also possess an additional enzyme for conversion of NA to *Adrenaline* (*Figure 1.33*).

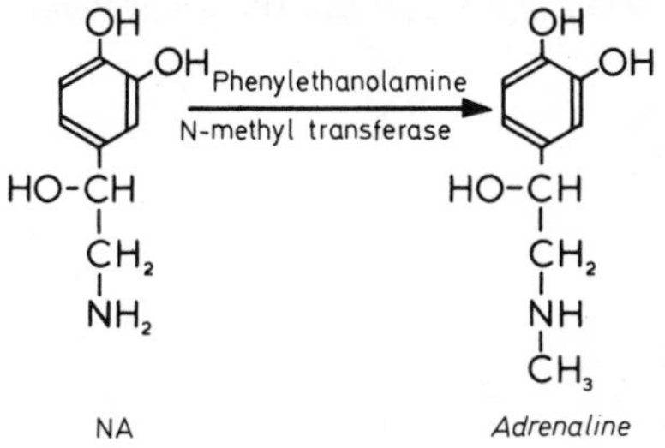

Figure 1.33   *The synthesis of adrenaline by the adrenal medulla*

Medullary chromaffin cells are innervated by preganglionic cholinergic neurones. ACh released from these fibres activates nicotinic cholinoceptors (page 25) on the chromaffin cells. Receptor activation causes a small, non-propagated depolarization (analogous to an epsp, page 26 and *Figure 1.19*) and the subsequent Ca^{2+}-dependent exocytotic release of *Adrenaline* into the bloodstream.

The released *Adrenaline* can activate α- and β-adrenoceptors at all sites in the body. The effects of circulating *Adrenaline* are thus all those of stimulating noradrenergic neurones together with the following.

(1) Arteriolar dilatation in skeletal muscle.
(2) Reduced capillary permeability.
(3) Lipolysis (adipose tissue).
(4) Gluconeogenesis (liver).
(5) Glycolysis (skeletal muscle).
(6) Restlessness and anxiety (CNS).

DRUG ACTION ON THE ADRENAL MEDULLA

Secretion of *Adrenaline* is stimulated by agonists at nicotinic cholinoceptors (page 27) and inhibited by antagonists at nicotinic cholinoceptors (page 30).

The chromaffin cells are susceptible to the amine-depleting actions of *Reserpine* and *Guanethidine* (page 41).

Local anaesthetics

Local anaesthesia is a drug-induced reversible blockade of nerve impulses in a restricted region of the body. Examples of the drugs used for this purpose are *Amethocaine* [tetracaine] , *Cocaine, Lignocaine, Procaine* and *Proxymetacaine* [proparacaine].

ACTIVE FORM OF MOLECULE

Local anaesthetics are weak bases (pK_a = 8–9) and consist of an amino-group (hydrophilic) connected by an intermediate group (usually a carbon chain) to an aromatic residue (lipophilic). The linkage between the intermediate group and the aromatic group may be an amide (*Lignocaine*) or an ester (all the other local anaesthetic drugs above) (*Figure 1.34*).

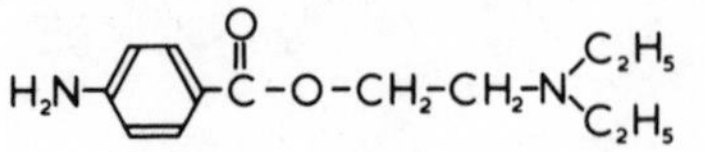

Procaine

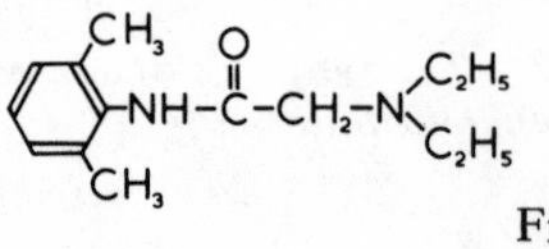

Lignocaine

Figure 1.34

The active form of the molecule is the cation, which at pH 7.4 forms about 90 per cent of the drug in solution. However, it is only the unionized form of the drug which is able to cross the various membranous barriers before the site of action is reached (page 249).

56

SITE OF ACTION

Most local anaesthetics are relatively non-specific — they exert stabilizing effects on the membranes of all types of excitable cells and even non-excitable cells (for example, red blood cells). Their principal site of action is the outer part of the cell membrane (outer protein monolayer and the phospholipid monolayer lying immediately below), since this is where regulation of membrane permeability to Na^+ and K^+ occurs.

MECHANISM OF ACTION

Local anaesthetics reduce the membrane permeability changes to Na^+ and K^+ which occur in response to an excitatory stimulus. If these membrane permeability changes are sufficiently suppressed, the cell fails to support the propagation of action potentials, but its resting membrane potential is unaltered.

EFFECTS OF APPLICATION TO A SINGLE NEURONE

There is a safety factor for the conduction of the neuronal action potential. The action potential propagates because it acts as a suprathreshold stimulus (local circuit currents) for adjacent inactive regions of the neuronal membrane. Local anaesthetics can have graded effects on the neuronal action potential and its propagation. A low concentration of local anaesthetic increases the stimulus strength required to elicit an action potential. The rate of rise, amplitude, rate of fall and conduction velocity of that action potential are all reduced.

If sufficient local anaesthetic is applied, the action potential becomes so reduced in amplitude that it ceases to act as a suprathreshold stimulus for adjacent, inactive regions of the neuronal membrane. Hence, conduction ceases and propagated action potentials can no longer be initiated or recorded no matter what stimulus strength is employed.

APPLICATION OF LOCAL ANAESTHETICS TO RESTRICTED REGIONS OF NEURONES

The local circuit currents responsible for action potential propagation can jump over a section of neurone in which permeability changes have been prevented by local anaesthetic application. For a non-myelinated neurone about 5 mm of neurone must be stabilized to prevent jumping by the action potential. In myelinated neurones three successive nodes must be stabilized.

EFFECTS OF LOCAL ANAESTHETICS ON BUNDLES OF NEURONES

In general, neurones of small diameter are more susceptible to blockade than those of large diameter. This may result from their larger surface area : volume ratio. Since afferent neurones of differing diameter subserve different sensory modalities a local anaesthetic injection may result in the loss of the various sensations in a distinct order (sharp pain before warmth before pressure).

EFFECTS OF IONS ON LOCAL ANAESTHETIC ACTION

A raised ECF Na^+ concentration antagonizes local anaesthetic action, because the Na^+ concentration gradient across the cell membrane is increased and this ensures a greater Na^+ influx for a given permeability change. Conversely, a lowered ECF Na^+ concentration augments local anaesthetic action.

Ca^{2+} plays an important part in regulating the permeability of the cell membrane to Na^+ and K^+. An increase in ECF Ca^{2+} concentration reduces membrane permeability to Na^+ and K^+, makes the membrane less excitable and hence augments local anaesthetic action. A reduction in ECF Ca^{2+} concentration has the converse effects.

EFFECTS OF LOCAL ANAESTHETICS ON THE CNS

All nitrogenous local anaesthetics cause stimulation of the CNS, resulting in restlessness, tremor, convulsions and respiratory stimulation. The stimulant effects may result from a selective depressant action on inhibitory neurones. Central stimulation is followed by depression; death following overdosage results from respiratory failure.

METHODS OF ADMINISTRATION

Topical or surface anaesthesia

The drug is applied directly to mucous membranes. To be effective as a topical anaesthetic a drug must: (1) in its non-ionized form, be relatively lipid soluble; (2) at pH 7.4, exist in appreciable amounts as its non-ionized form (that is, have a pK_a of 8.7 or less; page 249).

Infiltration anaesthesia

The drug is injected sc to anaesthetize fine sensory nerve branches.

Nerve block anaesthesia

The drug is injected near a nerve trunk and, in consequence, the transmission of both afferent and efferent impulses is prevented. This results in loss of sensation and muscle paralysis in the area supplied by the nerve trunk.

Spinal anaesthesia — subarachnoid block

The drug is injected into the subarachnoid space (*Figure 1.35*) usually in the lower spine. The dispersion of the injected fluid and hence the locus and extent of local anaesthesia depends on: (1) the site of the injection; (2) the volume and speed of the injection; (3) the post-injection position of the patient; and (4) the specific gravity (SG) of the injected solution. The SG of the cerebrospinal fluid (CSF) varies from 1.003 to 1.009. A hypobaric solution (SG < 1.003) tends to rise through the CSF whilst a hyperbaric solution (SG > 1.009) tends to sink through the CSF. An isobaric solution tends to remain at the level of the injection site.

Spinal anaesthesia produces analgesia (loss of pain sensation) and muscle relaxation without the patient losing consciousness. However, the level of anaesthesia within the spinal cord cannot be precisely controlled. Unwanted effects may include reduced cardiac output, hypotension and neurological complications.

Epidural block

The drug is injected into the fatty material in the epidural space (*Figure 1.35*) where the spinal nerves are covered by a thick layer of dura. The drug may have to diffuse into the subarachnoid space or outside the spinal canal before its

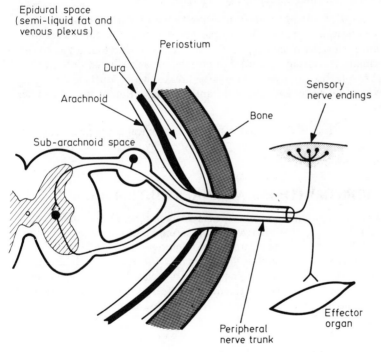

Figure 1.35   *Sites for the production of local anaesthesia*

effects can be mediated. However, the drug cannot penetrate to the brain, since the epidural space terminates at the foramen magnum.

Iv administration

Lignocaine iv is effective in the suppression of serious cardiac ventricular arrhythmias (page 63).

PROPERTIES OF INDIVIDUAL LOCAL ANAESTHETICS

Amethocaine has a pK_a = 8.0 and is suitable for all types of local anaesthesia.

Cocaine has a pK_a = 8.0. Its use is restricted to the topical anaesthesia of the eye, nose and throat.

In concentrations less than those required to produce local anaesthesia, *Cocaine* inhibits the uptake of NA into noradrenergic neurones (*see* page 54 for the consequences of the uptake-inhibiting properties of *Cocaine*).

Cocaine is unique among the local anaesthetics in having a powerful stimulant action on the cerebral cortex. It evokes euphoria, indifference to pain and fatigue, appetite suppression (anorexia) and an elevation of body temperature (pyrexia). Cortical stimulation is the basis of *Cocaine*'s liability to abuse. Tolerance develops to the stimulant effects but not to the CNS depression which follows.

Lignocaine has a pK_a = 8.7 and is suitable for all types of local anaesthesia. It is effective in the control of cardiac arrhythmias (page 63).

Procaine has a pK_a = 8.9 and cannot therefore be used for topical anaesthesia. It is used for infiltration, nerve block and spinal anaesthesia only. Since *Procaine* has some direct vasodilator activity, its formulations often include a vasoconstrictor (for example, *Adrenaline*) in order to prolong the anaesthesia. *Procaine* is hydrolysed by plasma ChE (page 35) and the breakdown products include aminobenzoate which can antagonize the antibacterial action of sulphonamides (page 173).

Proxymetacaine has a pK_a = 8.0 and is suitable for topical anaesthesia. It is non-irritant, has a short duration of action and is especially suitable for topical anaesthesia of the eye.

OTHER AGENTS WITH LOCAL ANAESTHETIC-LIKE ACTIONS

The noradrenergic neurone blocking agents (*Guanethidine, Debrisoquine* and *Bethanidine*) selectively anaesthetize the fine terminals of noradrenergic neurones (page 42). They are used in the treatment of hypertension (page 282). Tetrodotoxin is used as a research tool in animal experiments only. It selectively abolishes action potentials whose rising phase is associated with the influx of Na^+. It is effective when applied to the outer surfaces of neurones but ineffective when applied only to the inner surface of the neuronal membrane (pages 16 and 42).

Anti-arrhythmic drugs

***

Revise

- The physiological mechanisms underlying the initiation and spread of the cardiac excitation wave.

- The innervation of the heart and the effects of ACh and NA on cardiac cells (page 10).

Some arrhythmias may be attributed to defects in the transmission of the cardiac action potential. Such transmission defects can lead to a reduction in the rate of ventricular contraction, for example, the heart block resulting from reduced transmission through the AV node.

Transmission defects can also lead to an increase in the frequency of ventricular contraction due to the phenomenon of re-entry (*Figure 1.36*). In the normal heart (*Figure 1.36a*) impulses from the AV node travel down both branches of the bundle of His to excite the ventricles. After cellular damage in one of the

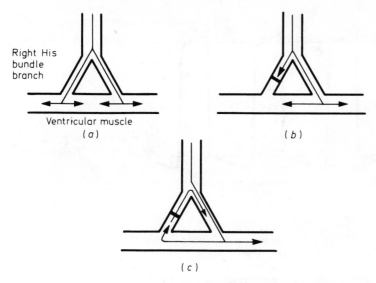

Figure 1.36 *Establishment of a re-entry type of cardiac arrhythmia (a) Normal conduction. (b) Uni-directional block in right His bundle branch. (c) Retrograde transmission through right His bundle branch*

bundle branches (*Figure 1.36b*) the normograde transmission of impulses in that branch may be prevented (unidirectional block). However, by travelling through the cells of the ventricular myocardium, a cardiac impulse may retrogradely pass through that bundle branch (*Figure 1.36c*) to cause premature re-excitation of the ventricles.

Other arrhythmias may be attributed to the development of pacemaker sites remote from the SA node. Such a site is known as an ectopic focus. Ectopic foci may be induced by cellular damage or the actions of drugs (for example, catecholamines, cardiac glycosides). The cells of an ectopic focus exhibit an exaggerated tendency to depolarize during diastole, that is, increased automaticity (*Figure 1.37*).

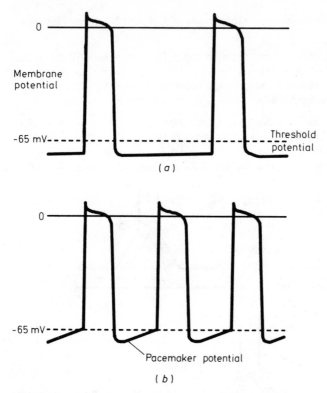

Figure 1.37 *Electrical activity of Purkinje cells. (a) Normal cell under influence of impulses arriving from AV node. (b) Cell acting as an ectopic pacemaker*

CORRECTION OF ARRHYTHMIAS

Some mild arrhythmias (for example, occasional ectopic beats) require little treatment beyond reassurance of the patient. Others (such as atrial paroxysmal tachycardia) may revert to normal rhythm spontaneously or can be induced to revert by reflex vagal stimulation (for example, pressure applied to the eyeballs or one carotid sinus). Direct current shock is effective in inducing the reversion of several types of tachyarrhythmia.

The anti-arrhythmic drugs may be used as alternatives to or supplements of the above means of achieving cardioversion. The anti-arrhythmic drugs may be divided into several major groups based on electrophysiological observations in animals.

GROUP 1: MEMBRANE STABILISERS

This group includes *Procainamide, Quinidine, Lignocaine* and *Phenytoin*. These drugs reduce both the slope of the pacemaker potential and the rate of rise of the cardiac action potential. Thus the automaticity of ectopic foci is reduced, especially in damaged cells.

Procainamide and *Quinidine* also prolong cardiac action potential duration and lengthen the effective refractory period. This worsens conduction in damaged cells of the bundle of His and the probability of re-entry arrhythmias (*Figure 1.36*) is reduced (bi-directional block).

Lignocaine and *Phenytoin* reduce action potential duration and shorten the effective refractory period. This tends to improve conduction in damaged cells of the bundle of His, reducing the likelihood of re-entry arrhythmias.

Procainamide and *Quinidine* are principally used in the prophylaxis of ectopic beats, but they have low therapeutic indices. Both drugs depress the force of myocardial contraction at concentrations close to those required for the suppression of arrhythmias. They may therefore precipitate cardiac failure in patients with low cardiac reserve. The −ve inotropic effects of *Procainamide* and *Quinidine* extend also to skeletal muscle (aggravation of myasthenia gravis) and vascular smooth muscle (hypotension).

Procainamide and *Quinidine* are antagonists at muscarinic cholinoceptors (page 33). By removing the effects of vagal tone at the SA node, these drugs induce a mild tachycardia. By removing the effects of vagal tone at the AV node, these agents may precipitate a hazardous 'paradoxical' tachycardia in patients with atrial flutter or fibrillation.

Cardiotoxic doses of *Procainamide* and *Quinidine* directly depolarize Purkinje fibres and increase their automaticity (an effect opposite to that seen at therapeutic concentrations). Toxic doses of these agents can thereby induce hazardous ventricular arrhythmias.

Additional unwanted effects associated with *Quinidine* include tinnitus (ringing in the ears), dizziness and other symptoms collectively known as 'cinchonism'.

Lignocaine is effective in the suppression of ventricular arrhythmias − particularly those observed after myocardial infarction. *Phenytoin* is also used to suppress ventricular arrhythmias − particularly those attributable to digitalis toxicity.

Lignocaine (but not *Phenytoin*) is an antagonist at muscarinic cholinoceptors. It may, therefore, evoke mild tachycardia by removing the effects of vagal tone at the SA node. Other unwanted effects of *Lignocaine* may be attributed to actions on the CNS and include confusion, fits, sweating and drowsiness.

Unwanted effects of *Phenytoin* include hypotension and hyperplasia of the gums.

GROUP 2: ANTIADRENERGIC

Propranolol and *Oxprenolol* are antagonists at β-adrenoceptors (page 51). By removing the effects of sympathetic tone and circulating adrenaline throughout the heart, these agents reduce automaticity, increase effective refractory period and decrease the conduction velocity of the action potential. This is the principal mechanism by which these agents suppress arrhythmias.

In addition, in high doses these agents suppress the automaticity of ectopic foci and suppress re-entry type arrhythmias by mechanisms similar to those described for *Procainamide*.

Propranolol and *Oxprenolol* have a limited role in the management of arrhythmias. They are effective in the treatment of arrhythmias induced by catecholamines (phaeochromocytoma and thyrotoxicosis) and those attributed to digitalis toxicity.

In concentrations close to those required for suppression of arrhythmias, *Propranolol* depresses the force of cardiac contraction. *Propranolol* may thus precipitate cardiac failure. It may also precipitate bronchial asthma (page 288). It is claimed that the risk of these unwanted effects is smaller with *Oxprenolol.*

GROUP 3: DRUGS WHICH PROLONG REFRACTORY PERIOD

Amiodarone prolongs the refractory period of most cardiac muscle cells possibly by reducing K^+ conductance. It is currently being evaluated for use in supraventricular arrhythmias.

GROUP 4: INHIBITORS OF CALCIUM TRANSPORT

Verapamil blocks the movement of calcium across the myocardial cell membrane and is useful in the treatment of supraventricular arrhythmias which depend on slow calcium-dependent action potentials. Verapamil reduces the slope of the pacemaker potential in SA nodal cells. It exerts a –ve inotropic action and is thus contraindicated in patients receiving antagonists at β-adrenoceptors.

Calcium transport inhibitors also act on smooth muscle and vasodilatation may result.

OTHER ANTI-ARRHYTHMIC DRUGS

Isoprenaline and *Orciprenaline* (page 46) are agonists at β-adrenoceptors. They are sometimes used to alleviate heart block which complicates myocardial infarction. By activating β-adrenoceptors these drugs improve conduction through the AV node and stimulate pacemaker activity in Purkinje fibres. A hazard associated with their use is the precipitation of dangerous ventricular arrhythmias. Electrical pacemaking is used to evoke ventricular contraction in established complete heart block, for example, Stokes–Adams syndrome (severe bradycardia with attacks of unconsciousness).

Digoxin, by reducing the conduction through the AV node, can reduce the frequency of ventricular contraction in atrial tachycardia, flutter or fibrillation (page 275).

Appendix

THE RELATIONSHIP BETWEEN DRUG CONCENTRATION AND EFFECT

The effects of many drugs are related to their concentration (within certain limits) in a smoothly graded manner, for example, a piece of intestinal smooth muscle may shorten progressively as the concentration of a spasmogenic drug is increased. The relationship between the drug concentration and effect is generally hyperbolic (*Figure 1.38a*). For convenience, pharmacologists generally

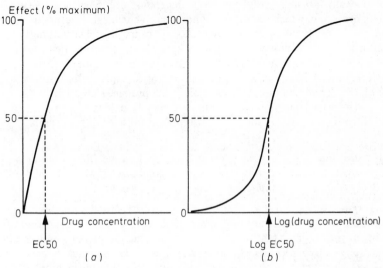

Figure 1.38   *Concentration-effect and log-concentration effect curves*

relate effect to the log of the drug concentration (*Figure 1.38b*). The resulting log concentration / effect curve is sigmoid and contains a useful central portion (between about 20 and 80 per cent of the maximal effect) where effect is linearly related to the log of the drug concentration.

EC'N' NOTATION

The concentration (or dose) of a drug which evokes a biological effect equivalent to N per cent of the maximal effect is known as the EC 'N' (ED 'N'), for example, EC50 means the concentration of drug evoking a half-maximal effect (*Figure 1.38a*).

POTENCY

The potency of a drug is a measure of the dilution in which it evokes a specified effect, thus a drug which evokes the specified effect when present in great dilution is said to be highly potent.

Most commonly the specified effect used in assessment or comparison of drug potencies is the half-maximal effect, thus potency = 1/EC50. The relative order of potency within a series of drugs is therefore the inverse of the rank order of their EC50 values and is independent of the absolute magnitude of their maximal effects.

THEORIES OF DRUG ACTION

Drug actions may be divided into two general classes: (1) structurally non-specific actions; and (2) structurally specific actions.

Structurally non-specific actions and Ferguson's principle

Certain chemically dissimilar drugs can evoke depression of biological activity. Their common action, which seems to be unrelated to chemical structure is known as a structurally non-specific action. A good example of a structurally non-specific action is the induction of general anaesthesia. This may be brought about by a wide variety of chemically dissimilar compounds including inert gases (for example, xenon), halogenated hydrocarbons (for example, chloroform, Halothane), cyclic hydrocarbons (for example, cyclopropane), ethers (for example, diethylether), alcohols (for example, Ethanol), oxides of nitrogen (for example, Nitrous oxide, N_2O) and derivatives of barbituric acid (for example, Thiopentone).

It is highly probable that drugs can exert structurally non-specific actions on a biological system without entering into chemical combination with any component of that system (for example, the chemically inert gas argon).

In 1935, Ferguson suggested that an agent acting by a structurally non-specific mechanism produces a depressant biological effect when a critical proportion of the volume of the biophase (the phase in which the drug produces its biological effect) is occupied by molecules of that agent. Thus, equal biological effects are produced when agents achieve the same relative saturation of the biophase.

This 'relative saturation' can sometimes be measured even when the nature of the biophase is unknown. In the case of gases or volatile liquids at equilibrium it is the ratio of their partial pressure (P) to the maximal pressure possible under the given conditions, that is, the saturated vapour pressure (P_s). A function of this ratio is known as the thermodynamic activity of the drug.

$$\text{Thermodynamic activity} = \text{constant} \times P/P_s.$$

Ferguson reasoned that the measurement of thermodynamic activity will distinguish between drugs acting by structurally non-specific or structurally specific mechanisms. The thermodynamic activities of drugs acting by a structurally non-specific mechanism in a defined biological system should be the same — the activities of drugs acting by structurally specific mechanisms should differ from this value and from each other. *Table 1.16* shows the threshold toxic concentration of a variety of vapours on wireworms.

The second column of *Table 1.16* shows the toxic concentration expressed as P/P_s. Note how, over a 450-fold range of concentration, the P/P_s values of most of the listed agents are approximately equal. Most agents in the list seem, therefore, to be exerting a common structurally non-specific action. In contrast,

66

Table 1.16 *The ability of various volatile agents to kill wireworms*

Compound	Threshold toxic concentration (μmol/ℓ)	P/P_s at threshold toxic concentration
Dimethylaniline	7	0.4
Ammonia	23	0.00008
Bromoform	94	0.5
Tetrachloroethane	141	0.6
Chlorobenzene	200	0.5
Toluene	420	0.4
Heptane	800	0.5
Hexane	3000	0.6

ammonia has a much smaller P/P_s value, indicating that its action is structurally specific.

It is possible that a particular drug may be able to exert a structurally non-specific action in one biological system and a structurally specific action in a second system.

Structurally specific drug actions and receptor theory

Most drugs exert structurally specific actions. Such actions: (1) result in selective interference with biological activity, that is, they affect some biological functions but not others; (2) may result either in stimulation or in depression of biological activity.

Actions of this sort are very dependent on the chemical structure of the drug — so much so, in some cases, that one stereoisomer may be active whilst the other stereoisomer may be totally inactive. We deduce that the drug produces its effects by an interaction with some chemical component of the living cell. This component is called a receptor. The structure of the receptor is complementary to that of the drug. It can be pictured as the three-dimensional mirror image of the drug (lock and key analogy).

A drug receptor has two fundamental properties: (1) the ability to bind or associate with certain structurally similar drug molecules; and (2) the ability to

Table 1.17 *Comparison of drug receptors with other biological binding sites*

Biological binding site	Interaction	End effect
Drug receptor	Attachment of drug	Triggering of response
Active centre of enzyme	Attachment of substrate	Chemical alteration of substrate
Carrier molecule of transport mechanism	Attachment of substrate	Transport of substrate

initiate a biological response when an appropriate drug molecule is associated with it.

Drug receptors are in some ways analogous to the active centres of enzymes and biological transport mechanisms (*Table 1.17*).

The binding of drugs to receptor sites

The binding of drugs to their receptor sites can be described in terms of the Law of Mass Action:

$$\text{Drug} + \text{receptor} \underset{k_2}{\overset{k_1}{\rightleftharpoons}} \text{Drug–receptor complex}$$

Let initial molar concentration of drug = [D]
Let initial molar concentration of receptor = [P]
The initial molar concentration of the drug–receptor complex will be zero. What is the molar concentration of each of the reactants when the reaction is at equilibrium?

Let us assume: (1) that the drug is present in such excess that its concentration is not significantly altered by maximal formation of drug–receptor complex; (2) that one molecule of drug combines with one molecule of receptor; and (3) that the fraction of receptor molecules combined with the drug at equilibrium is r
Then, at equilibrium

Molar concentration of free drug = [D]
Molar concentration of drug–receptor complex = r [P]
Molar concentration of unoccupied receptor = $(1-r)$ [P]
The rate of the forward reaction = k_1 [D] $(1-r)$ [P]

where k_1 = association rate constant.

The rate of the back reaction = $k_2 r$ [P]

where k_2 = dissociation rate constant. Since equilibrium conditions prevail, these two rates may be equated:

$$k_1 \text{ [D] } (1\text{-}r) \text{ [P]} = k_2 r \text{ [P]}.$$

Rearranging:

$$\frac{k_1}{k_2} = \frac{r}{(1\text{-}r) \text{ [D]}} = K_a$$

where K_a is known as the equilibrium affinity constant.

Active and passive biological responses: agonists and antagonists

A drug-induced response from a living cell is active if a change in ongoing activity occurs even when the cell is isolated from all external biological control factors (for example, neurotransmitters and hormones). Active responses may be either excitatory (for example, depolarization of the membranes of excitable cells, muscle contraction, increased glandular secretion) or inhibitory (for example, hyperpolarization of the membranes of excitable cells, muscle relaxation, reduced glandular secretion).

In contrast, passive responses are observed when a drug acts to remove the effects of some external biological factor regulating cellular function.

Of the drugs which attach to a particular receptor site: Agonists form a drug—receptor complex which is capable of triggering an active response from the cell. Antagonists form a drug—receptor complex which cannot evoke an active response from the cell. Antagonists simply prevent attachment of agonists to the receptor. The response to the antagonist is therefore passive — blockade of the effects of an agonist.

The triggering of responses by agonists: modern receptor occupancy theory

Relatively little is known about the mechanism by which an agonist triggers an active biological response. Modern receptor occupancy theories propose that drugs have a property known as 'efficacy' or 'intrinsic activity' which governs their ability to trigger an active biological response once they have combined with a receptor.

It is envisaged that drugs with high efficacy can evoke the maximal effect which the biological system is capable of producing. Such drugs are known as full agonists and, in some circumstances, may be able to elicit the maximum possible effect without occupying all the receptors. In such circumstances the receptors not occupied by the drug are known as 'spare receptors'.

A drug with low efficacy cannot evoke the maximal response of which the biological system is capable, despite occupancy of all available receptors. A drug of this type is known as a 'partial agonist'. By competing for the same receptors, a partial agonist can antagonize a full agonist. Partial agonists which are therapeutically exploited include those acting at the opiate receptor (page 145).

Pure antagonists have zero efficacy.

Antagonism

Antagonism is the name given to the interaction between two drugs when the biological effect of the two drugs together is smaller than the expected sum of their individual effects.

The many mechanisms by which antagonism can occur may be divided into two principal kinds: (1) where the concentration of agonist at its site of action is reduced by the antagonist (it alters agonist disposition, page 264); and (2) where the concentration of agonist at its site of action is not reduced by the antagonist. This may be due to one of several mechanisms:

Direct mechanisms

The agonist and antagonist have the same receptors.

Competitive antagonism
The agonist and antagonist compete for occupancy of the same receptors. Since both agents combine with the receptor in a readily reversible fashion, the

proportion of receptors occupied by each agent at any instant is related to their relative concentration and affinities for the receptor. The proportion of receptors occupied by the competitive antagonist at any instant can be reduced by increasing the concentration of agonist; that is, the antagonism is surmountable.

The effects of a competitive antagonist on the shape and position of the curve of log concentration against effect of an agonist are shown in *Figure 1.39*. Increasing the concentration of antagonist causes progressive parallel shift of the curve of log concentration against effect of the agonist to the right along the log concentration axis. The slope of the curve is unchanged and the maximal effect is undiminished.

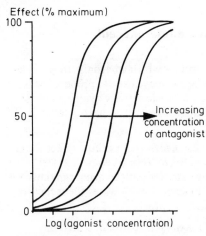

Figure 1.39   *Competitive antagonism*

A competitive antagonist binds only weakly to the receptors, so that its effects are readily dissipated by washing; that is, the antagonism is reversible. Examples of competitive antagonism include the following: *Atropine* antagonism of ACh at muscarinic cholinoceptors; Phentolamine antagonism of NA at α-adrenoceptors.

Non-competitive antagonism

The agonist and antagonist occupy the same receptors. However, the antagonist forms a strong chemical (for example, covalent) bond with the receptor, which is not easily disrupted. As time passes, more and more of the receptors become inactivated in this fashion. Increasing the concentration of the agonist may delay the onset of the antagonism but cannot prevent the eventual outcome; that is, the total inactivation of all the receptors. The effects of a non-competitive antagonist on the shape and position of the curves of log concentration against effect of agonists are shown in *Figure 1.40*.

Figure 1.40a shows a biological system where no spare receptors exist. Increasing the concentration of the antagonist (or increasing exposure time to a single concentration of the antagonist) results in a progressive proportional depression of the agonist log concentration against effect curve, without change in its position on the log concentration axis.

Figure 1.40b illustrates the effects of a non-competitive antagonist in a biological system where spare receptors exist. In this circumstance, the antagonist causes a rightwards shift of the agonist log concentration against effect curve until the spare receptors are inactivated. Thereafter no further rightward shift occurs — the agonist log concentration against effect curve becomes depressed.

70

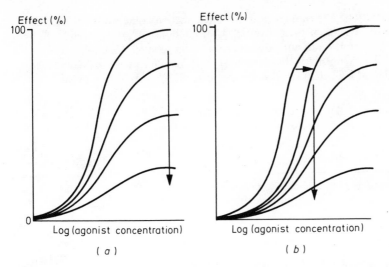

Figure 1.40 *Non-competitive antagonism. (a) Biological system with no spare receptors. (b) Biological system having spare receptors*

Providing no spare receptors are available, a non-competitive antagonist reduces the maximal response that can be attained, no matter what agonist concentration is used. The antagonism is therefore said to be insurmountable. The reversibility of non-competitive antagonism depends on the type of chemical bond which is formed between the receptor and the antagonist. Some non-competitive antagonists can be removed from the receptor by prolonged washing or the use of a chemical reactivator. Other non-competitive antagonists have truly irreversible reactions, for example: α-bungarotoxin antagonism of ACh at the nicotinic cholinoceptors of skeletal muscle; Phenoxybenzamine antagonism of NA at α-adrenoceptors.

Indirect mechanisms of antagonism

The agonist acts indirectly to cause the release of or to potentiate a second agonist — this second agonist acting as the final mediator of the observed response. The antagonist (which can be of the competitive or non-competitive type) occupies the same receptor as the mediator agonist.

Examples of this kind of antagonism include: *Atropine* antagonism of the contractile effect of Nicotine (mediated by ACh released from postganglionic parasympathetic nerves) on the guinea-pig ileum; *Propranolol* antagonism of the stimulant effect of Tyramine (mediated by NA released from postganglionic sympathetic nerves) on the isolated heart.

Functional antagonism

Consider the situation where two different agonists, by activating different receptors, evoke opposing responses from a single biological system, for example, one agonist causing active contraction of a piece of smooth muscle and a second agonist causing relaxation. If two such agonists are administered together then the net response will be smaller than either of their individual effects. This phenomenon has been termed 'functional antagonism'.

71

This term may be a misnomer since the phenomenon could well represent the algebraic summation of the individual agonist actions and, if so, would fall outside the definition of antagonism provided on page 69. Examples of 'functional antagonism' include: reversal by *Adrenaline* of histamine-induced contraction of bronchial smooth muscle; reversal by ACh of vasoconstriction induced by NA.

Table 1.18   *Drug receptors*

Receptor designation	Page reference
Skeletal muscle nicotinic cholinoceptor	*(Table 1.2)*
Neural tissue nicotinic cholinoceptor	*(Table 1.4)*
Muscarinic cholinoceptor	*(Table 1.6)*
α-adrenoceptor	*(Table 1.10)*
β-adrenoceptor	*(Table 1.12)*
H₁ histamine receptor	*(Table 2.15)*
H₂ histamine receptor	*(Table 2.15)*
M 5-HT receptor	111
D 5-HT receptor	111
Opioid receptor	145

Identification and classification of drug receptors

A drug receptor can only be identified by challenging the biological system with a range of drugs and then noting the narrow spectrum of structurally related drugs (both agonists and antagonists) which will enter into combination with the receptor.

Examples of drug receptors which have been identified in this way are presented in *Table 1.18.*

2
Endocrine pharmacology

INTRODUCTION

In the mammalian body chemical messengers are often employed to transmit information from one cell to another. The peripheral (page 1) and CNS (page 125) sections deal with the theme of drugs which interact with one class of chemical messengers — the neurotransmitters. The theme of this section is interaction with chemical messengers other than neurotransmitters (*Table 2.1*).

Table 2.1

	Cell type of origin	*Transport medium*
Neurotransmitter	Nerve	Interstitial fluid
Local hormone	Non-nerve	Interstitial fluid
Neurohumour	Nerve	Blood
Hormone	Non-nerve	Blood

The hypothalamus is considered first since this is an important example of neural tissue which secretes neurohumours. By this means it controls the anterior pituitary gland which in turn controls many of the other endocrine systems to be discussed. Also included in this section are some less obvious examples of this theme — anticoagulants and diuretics.

Hypothalamo-pituitary axis

The pituitary gland is situated at the base of the brain and is connected by the pituitary stalk to the hypothalamus. The posterior pituitary gland secretes antidiuretic hormone (ADH, page 103) and oxytocin (page 114) from nerve endings. These nerves have their cell bodies in the hypothalamus. The anterior pituitary gland comprises non-innervated endocrine gland cells which synthesize, store and secrete the pituitary trophins which include the following:

Follicle-stimulating hormone (FSH)
Luteinizing hormone (LH)
Thyroid-stimulating hormone (thyrotrophin, TSH)
Adrenocorticotrophic hormone (corticotrophin, ACTH)
Growth hormone (GH)
Prolactin

Their secretion is controlled by neurohumours synthesized in neurones in the hypothalamus. The neurohumours are released into the blood of capillaries which unite to form the sole blood supply of the anterior pituitary gland (a portal system).

HYPOTHALAMO–PITUITARY NEUROHUMOURS

These are substances which promote or inhibit the synthesis and secretion of an anterior pituitary hormone. They are also called hypothalamic releasing or release inhibiting hormones.

The word 'factor' replaces the word 'hormone' where the structure has not been identified. Generally, there is one neurohumour for each anterior pituitary hormone. Supra-physiological doses of the neurohumours may affect the secretion of other anterior pituitary hormones.

(1) There is only one neurohumour controlling FSH and LH secretion, FSH/LH releasing hormone, which is a decapeptide. The mechanism of differential release of FSH and LH is poorly understood.
(2) Prolactin secretion is inhibited by prolactin release inhibiting factor. Its structure is unknown but it probably acts upon receptors in the pituitary which are also sensitive to dopamine.
(3) TSH secretion is promoted by TSH releasing hormone which is a tripeptide. This is not entirely specific as it can also release prolactin.
(4) Somatostatin or GH release inhibiting hormone is a tetradecapeptide which inhibits GH secretion.
(5) The neurohumour which controls ACTH secretion has not been identified.

These neurohumours are not exclusively localized in the hypothalamus and may possess other actions both centrally and peripherally; for example, somatostatin is found in the pancreas and may inhibit both insulin and glucagon secretion (page 93). The plasma half-lives of the neurohumours are very short (< 5 minutes) therefore clinical applications are presently limited to diagnostic procedures which require tests of pituitary integrity.

FEEDBACK MECHANISMS

Feedback in the control of pituitary hormone secretions involves the central (hypothalamus and/or anterior pituitary) monitoring of the plasma concentration of a peripherally produced hormone and the consequent alteration of anterior pituitary hormone secretions to maintain a predetermined concentration. Feedbacks may be overridden by higher physiological processes; for example, stress will increase ACTH and hence adrenal steroid secretion so that normal physiological plasma concentrations are exceeded. A unique transient +ve feedback operates to promote gonadotrophin secretion above the set point in pubertal and adult females and is usually seen where high plasma concentrations of oestrogen follow low priming concentrations — as occur preceding ovulation.

DRUG INTERACTIONS

Drugs which disturb central neurotransmitter processes can produce disturbances in anterior pituitary secretion; for example, *Reserpine*, barbiturates, phenothiazines and *Morphine* inhibit gonadotrophin secretion which leads to decreased libido and infertility. *Phenytoin* increases GH secretion which produces hyperplasia of the gums. High serum prolactin concentrations associated with gynaecomastia (increased breast size), galactorrhoea (inappropriate breast secretion), impotence and infertility can result from the use of *Reserpine* and *Chlorpromazine* which act centrally by decreasing prolactin release inhibiting factor activity of the brain. *Metoclopramide* (an anti-emetic, page 301) can produce similar effects by antagonizing prolactin release inhibiting factor at its pituitary (dopamine) receptor. An agonist at dopamine receptors bromocriptine, an ergot derivative, is useful therapeutically to decrease prolactin secretion. *Bromocriptine* will suppress lactation. It will also promote fertility in both sexes where raised prolactin plasma concentrations are associated with disturbances of gonadal activity and/or impotence. Bromocriptine will suppress GH release in acromegalic patients. In normal subjects GH release is paradoxically increased after *bromocriptine*.

The feedback mechanisms are also exploited for therapeutic purposes. The combined type of oral contraceptive inhibits gonadotrophin release and therefore ovulation does not occur. Oestrogens and progestogens are administered to men to reduce LH and hence androgen secretion in an attempt to influence androgen-dependent prostatic cancer. *Clomiphene* (an oestrogen antagonist) will prevent the —ve feedback action of oestrogens leading to a surge of gonadotrophin secretion and ovulation. Therefore it is useful in infertility associated with high plasma oestrogen concentration such as in the Stein—Leventhal syndrome (polycystic ovaries, anovulation, oligomenorrhoea).

Gonadotrophins

A gonadotrophin is a substance producing growth and development of the gonads.

The gonadotrophins, except Prolactin, are high MW (25,000—70,000) glycoproteins (*Table 2.2*).

Table 2.2

Name	Symbol	Synthesis site	Extraction site
Follicle-stimulating hormone	FSH	Anterior pituitary	Anterior pituitary
Luteinizing hormone	LH	Anterior pituitary	Anterior pituitary
Prolactin	PRL	Anterior pituitary	Anterior pituitary
Human chorionic gonadotrophin	HCG	Trophoblast	Urine
Human menopausal gonadotrophin	HMG	Anterior pituitary	Urine
Pregnant mares' serum gonadotrophin	PMSG	Endometrial cups	Serum

Prolactin is a protein (MW about 25,000). FSH, LH, *human chorionic gonadotrophin* (HCG) and TSH consist of a common α-chain and different β-chains. The β-chain provides specificity of action. *Human menopausal gonadotrophin* (HMG) is a mixture of gonadotrophins, mainly FSH.

GONADOTROPHIC ACTIONS IN THE FEMALE

It is cyclical changes in the pituitary gonadotrophin secretions which produce corresponding ovarian changes and hence the changes characteristic of the human menstrual cycle.

At birth each human ovary contains about 200,000 oocytes, each enclosed in follicular cells to form primordial follicles. Oocytes have partially undergone first meiotic division. FSH (co-operating with a low concentration of LH as during the follicular phase of the menstrual cycle) promotes growth of a few oocytes and their follicular cells. It also promotes 17-β-oestradiol secretion by the thecal cells of these follicles (*Figure 2.1*) which leads to a surge of LH secretion (+ve feedback, page 75).

The LH induces final maturation of one (usually) oocyte and completion of first meiotic division. Ovulation and conversion of the remaining follicle to a corpus luteum occurs about 10 hours later. This corpus luteum secretes 17-β-oestradiol and progesterone under the influence of LH.

If the oocyte is fertilized the resulting blastocyst implants into the endometrium of the uterus about 7 days after ovulation. The trophoblast soon secretes HCG which maintains the steroidogenic activity of the corpus luteum. Immunoassay of HCG may be used for the diagnosis of pregnancy. In a menstrual cycle in which the ovum is not fertilized, the corpus luteum regresses, due to lack of gonadotrophins and steroid secretion declines. This withdrawal of steroid hormones produces loss of endometrium (menstruation).

STEROID SYNTHESIS

Steroid synthesis to the progesterone stage is common for the adrenal cortex, testis and ovary (*Figure 2.2*).

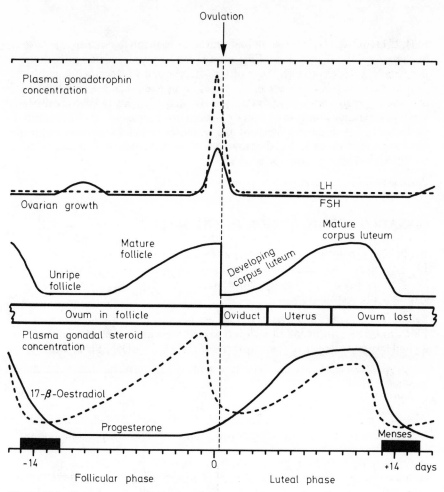

Figure 2.1 *Events occurring during the human menstrual cycle*

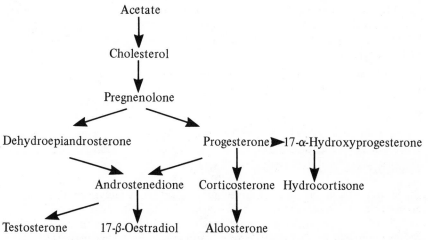

Figure 2.2 *Simplified pathways of steroid synthesis in adrenal cortex, testis and ovary*

FSH, LH (and ACTH) increase steroid synthesis, probably by increasing conversion of cholesterol to pregnenolone. FSH and LH selectively stimulate synthesis in the gonads. This selective synthesis of testosterone and 17-β-oestradiol derives from the presence of receptors and enzymes in the gonads and the relative absence of enzymes capable of forming corticosteroids. Similarly, only the thecal cell of the ovary possess large amounts of enzymes converting precursors to 17-β-oestradiol. In the testis, LH stimulates synthesis and secretion of mainly testosterone (plus some androstenedione and 17-β-oestradiol). Note, testosterone secretion in the female derives mainly from the adrenals.

Prostaglandin $F_{2\alpha}$ can reduce progesterone synthesis.

GONADOTROPHIC ACTION IN THE MALE

In the male gametogenesis is mainly controlled by FSH and steroidogenesis by LH. Sites of sperm production are the seminiferous tubules of the testes. Between the tubules are Leydig cells which are the major site of testosterone synthesis and secretion.

Before puberty, the seminiferous tubules are lined by diploid spermatogonia. FSH stimulates continued cell divisions so that there are increased numbers of diploid spermatogonia and spermatocytes (*Figure 2.3*). Also, FSH induces

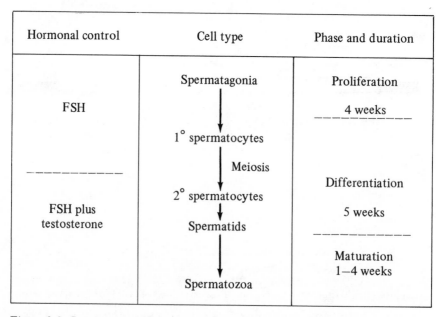

Hormonal control	Cell type	Phase and duration
FSH	Spermatagonia ↓ 1° spermatocytes	Proliferation 4 weeks
FSH plus testosterone	Meiosis ↓ 2° spermatocytes ↓ Spermatids ↓ Spermatozoa	Differentiation 5 weeks — Maturation 1—4 weeks

Figure 2.3 *Spermatogenesis in man*

the Sertoli cells to secrete an androgen-binding protein which maintains a high androgen concentration in the tubule lumen. Meiosis is stimulated by FSH and testosterone. Spermatozoa pass to the epididymides where final maturation occurs and it can be 1—3 weeks before sperm appear in the ejaculate. The total duration of spermatogenesis and sperm transport into the ejaculate in man is 12–15 weeks. Gametogenesis is a continuous process in the male in contrast to a cyclical process in female.

GONADOTROPHIC ACTIVITY

Gonadotrophins can be subdivided and defined by actions they produce (*Table 2.3*). HCG has mainly LH-like actions while HMG and pregnant mares' serum gonadotrophin have mainly FSH-like actions.

Table 2.3   *Classification of gonadotrophic activity*

FSH-like activity	LH-like activity
In the female	
Oocyte growth	Oval maturation
Follicular growth	Ovulation
Mainly 17-β-oestradiol secretion	Structural integrity of corpus luteum
	17-β-oestradiol and progesterone secretion
In the male	
Spermatogenesis	Testosterone secretion

THERAPEUTIC USE

One cause of female infertility is irregular and insufficient endogenous gonadotrophin secretion and therefore absence of ovulation. Replacement therapy with HMG (which possesses follicle-stimulating activity) followed by HCG (which possesses luteinizing activity) can lead to ovulation and pregnancy if the ovaries are capable of responding. Excessive response leads to ovarian enlargement and haemorrhage, multiple ovulations and multiple pregnancy. This can be prevented by monitoring the rise in plasma oestrogens as a measure of the response to HMG. If this is excessive then HCG is not given. Human FSH and LH are little used (shortage of material), as are FSH and LH from other species (antibody formation).

Immunization against the β-chain of HCG may provide a possible means of reducing fertility.

Exogenous gonadotrophins have proved of little value in the treatment of male infertility where that is due to reduced secretion of endogenous gonadotrophin In part this may be due to the long time (10–13 weeks) between the first spermatogonial division and final maturation.

Replacement therapy for steroid hormone deficiencies usually involves the use of steroids rather than gonadotrophins.

Oestrogens, progestogens and androgens

An oestrogen, progestogen or androgen is a compound which produces a similar range of effects to those produced by 17-β-oestradiol, progesterone or testosterone respectively. Most such compounds show specificity of action but some possess properties of the other types of steroid at higher doses (for example, a progestogen could possess oestrogenic activity due to an inherent property of the compound or due to a metabolite possessing oestrogenic activity).

Most reproductive and non-reproductive steroid hormones have a similar molecular mechanism of action. Tissue selectivity is achieved by the presence of specific soluble protein receptors which are found in the cytoplasm of the target cell (for example, oestrogen specific in the uterus, androgen specific in the prostate). Steroids pass from the blood into the cell, combine with the receptor and the complex moves into the nucleus (*Figure 2.4*). Here an interaction with the chromatin produces the metabolic events unique to that target tissue.

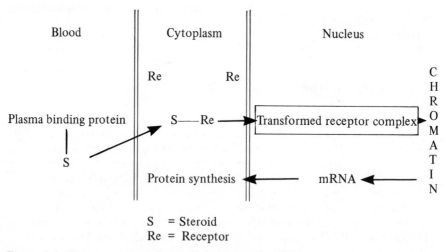

S = Steroid
Re = Receptor

Figure 2.4 *The interaction of steroids with target cells*

All naturally occurring steroid hormones have a very short $t_{1/2}$ ($<$ 4 hours) and are inactive orally. Simple structural alterations of the steroid molecule produce dramatic changes in biological activity (*Figure 2.5*). Modification of the basic structure by esterification or alkylation (at positions 1 or 17) will extend the $t_{1/2}$ into the therapeutically useful range.

The steroids are metabolized by the liver and conjugated to form the sulphate and glucuronide. Excretion of the metabolite is mainly in the urine but some is excreted in the bile. Once in the gut, bacteria act on the conjugates to release free steroid which is then reabsorbed — enterohepatic circulation.

OESTROGENS

The major secretory product of the ovarian follicles is 17-β-oestradiol which is rapidly metabolized to less potent oestrogens — oestriol and oestrone. *Figure 2.1* shows the steroid secretion pattern during the menstrual cycle.

Table 2.4   *Effects of oestrogens*

System affected	Consequence
Female reproductive organs	
Fallopian tubes, uterus, vagina	Growth and development
Mammary glands	Growth and development of ducts
Uterine endometrium	Proliferation (irregular menstruation)
Cervical epithelium	Thin and copious mucus (good sperm penetration)
CNS	
FSH and LH secretion	+ve and −ve feedback
Prolactin secretion	Increases
Libido	Indispensable in lower mammals; role in humans not clear
Chemosensitive trigger zone (CTZ)	Nausea and vomiting
Blood	
Coagulation factors	Predisposition to thromboembolic phenomena
Sex hormone binding globulin	Increases plasma concentration
Lipid metabolism	Increases plasma triglycerides
	Decreases plasma cholesterol
Metabolic actions	
General	Weak net anabolic action
Carbohydrate metabolism	Weak diabetogenic action
Fluid mobilization	Salt and water retention exacerbates possible hypertension
Other actions	
Long bones	Growth
Epiphyses	Closure
Axillary and pubic hair	Growth in female pattern
Oestrogen-dependent cancers	Growth after low doses
Carcinogenesis	In general, no conclusive evidence, however, endometrial carcinoma may be induced in postmenopausal women

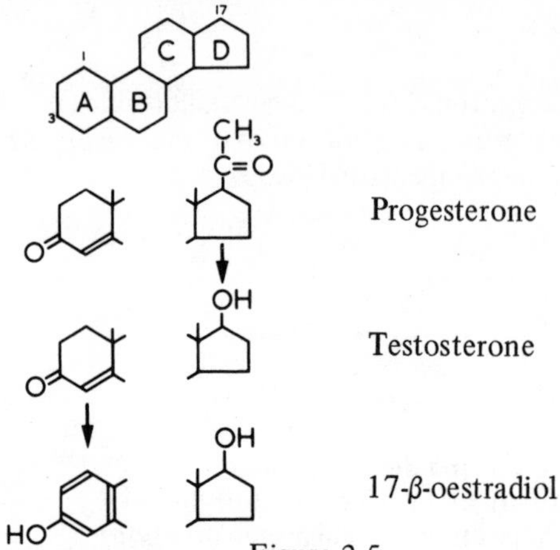

Progesterone

Testosterone

17-β-oestradiol

Figure 2.5

Preparations

(1) Steroidal, for example, *Ethinyloestradiol*, orally active. Mestranol is the 3 methyl ether of ethinyloestradiol and is an inactive prodrug converted to ethinyloestradiol by the liver.
(2) Non-steroidal — orally active, for example, *Stilboestrol* [diethylstilbestrol] and *Dienoestrol*. This group of oestrogens is suspected of carcinogenic activity, therefore their use is restricted to topical applications or post-menopausal breast cancer.

Therapeutic use

Oestrogens are used for either their direct actions or indirect hypothalamus/pituitary feedback actions. Oestrogen therapy alone is not recommended due to the high incidence of side-effects, for example, uterine endometrial hyperplasia leading to bleeding from the vagina. Progestogens are usually administered concurrently to obtain the desired effect (combination therapy, page 85).

Replacement therapy (small doses)

(1) Relief of menopausal symptoms (natural or premature) which include vasomotor instability, anxiety, depression, atrophy of secondary sexual organs. Oestrogens will not relieve osteoporosis but may prevent its development.
Note: Senile vaginitis or vulvitis is the only indication for topical application.
(2) Primary ovarian failure. Oestrogens will initiate pubertal changes which are maintained with combination therapy.

Neoplastic disease (large doses)

(1) Androgen-dependent prostatic tumours.
(2) Advanced breast cancer (page 88).

Suppression of lactation

Large doses are administered immediately postpartum. *Bromocriptine* is now preferred (page 75).

Postcoital contraception

Large doses are administered for up to five days. The action occurs after fertilization and possible mechanisms are the expulsion of the blastocyst from the uterus or the prevention of implantation.

Contraindications are pregnancy, oestrogen-dependent breast carcinoma, cardiovascular disease, liver disease.

OESTROGEN ANTAGONISTS

These compete with oestrogens for their cytoplasmic receptors (*Figure 2.4*). *Clomiphene* and tamoxifen are non-steroidal orally active compounds which antagonize all the specific oestrogenic actions.

Therapeutic use

(1)   Infertility in a patient with an intact hypothalamus-pituitary-ovarian axis and raised plasma oestrogen concentration, for example, Stein–Leventhal syndrome (page 75), amenorrhoea on discontinuing contraceptive tablets. A short period of administration will induce ovulation and initiate menstrual cycles by preventing oestrogen's inhibitory (−ve feedback) action at the hypothalamus allowing gonadotrophin secretion and therefore follicular development.
(2)   Advanced breast cancer (page 88). Clinical experience has only been obtained with tamoxifen postmenopausally. Regression can only be obtained during continuous therapy which is relatively free of side-effects.

PROGESTOGENS

The major progestogen, progesterone is secreted by the corpus luteum of the ovary as well as the placenta during pregnancy. Most progestational effects are only seen after previous priming of the target organs with oestrogens.

Preparations

(1)   Progesterone derivatives. Medroxyprogesterone acetate and *Hydroxyprogesterone* hexanoate [caproate], are not orally active, the latter has no detectable effect on gonadotrophin secretion.
(2)   19-Nortestosterone derivatives. All this group of steroids have an ethinyl substitution at the 17-α-position which makes them orally active and extends the $t_{1/2}$, for example, *Norethisterone* [norethindrone], lynestrenol, ethynodiol and norgestrel. As well as the progestational effects (*Table 2.5*) this group may possess androgenic, oestrogenic or anti-oestrogenic activity because of intrinsic activity in the molecule or metabolism to active compounds.

Table 2.5   *Effects of progestogens*

System affected	Consequence
Female reproductive organs	
Fallopian tubes, uterus, vagina	Growth and development
Mammary glands	Growth and development of the lobular-alveolar system
Uterine endometrium	Increased secretion. Withdrawal leads to menstruation
Cervical epithelium	Viscous and scanty mucus (poor sperm penetration)
CNS	
FSH and LH secretion	−ve feedback
Libido	Synergistic with oestrogens in lower mammals
Consciousness	Sedative (large doses)
Body temperature	Thermogenic
Pregnancy	
Uterus, placenta, foetus	Necessary for normal course of pregnancy
Metabolic actions	
General	Net catabolic action
Fluid mobilization	Salt and water loss

Therapeutic use

Progestogens are usually used in combination with oestrogens. However, the following list indicates where a progestogen has been found useful alone.

Contraception

(1)   Continuous oral administration (19-nortestosterone derivatives) as in the 'mini-pill', the dose is lower than in the combined oral contraceptives. The action is a combination of effects on the CNS, pituitary, ovary, Fallopian tube, endometrium and the cervical mucus. Ovulation is suppressed in about 50 per cent of women and menstrual cycles occur normally. The pregnancy rate is similar to that occurring after IUDs, namely, 2 per hundred women years (HWY). The incidence of ectopic pregnancies is increased.

(2)   Three-monthly im depot injections of the progesterone derivatives. Gonadotrophin secretion is suppressed so ovulation does not occur. Amenorrhoea may occur after 12 months. Continued patient compliance is not required therefore it is useful when pregnancy is contraindicated, for example, rubella vaccination. The pregnancy rate is low, about 0.5/HWY.

Both approaches are useful during lactation and in women who suffer from oestrogen-related side-effects.

Threatened and habitual abortion

Progestogens (large doses) are widely used during the first trimester in spite of little evidence of efficacy. 19-nor-testosterone derivatives are contraindicated as they may virilize the foetus.

84

Endometriosis (ectopic endometrial growth)

Continuous long term use is aimed at producing regression of tissue mass.

Inoperable endometrial carcinoma

Large doses produce remission which is maintained for about 15 months.

OESTROGEN PLUS PROGESTOGEN

Oral combination therapy (one oestrogen plus one progestogen) is used at lower doses than single drug therapy as the constituents are synergistic.

Therapeutic use

The oestrogens (synthetic steroidal) are combined with the progestogens derived from 19-nortestosterone. The combination is usually administered as a 21-day course followed by a 7-day tablet-free interval during which bleeding from the endometrium occurs (not true menstruation). Practically any cycle length can be produced by continuing administration of these drugs. Prediction of the potencies of the combinations is difficult due to the variable amounts of oestrogenic, androgenic and anti-oestrogenic activity. The combination can be tailored to the patient response.

Replacement therapy

Treatment of menopausal symptoms and primary ovarian failure. The combination provides better cycle control than oestrogens alone and avoids continuous therapy.

Menstrual irregularities

Treatment of dysmenorrhoea (painful menses) and dysfunctional uterine bleeding (abnormal menstrual pattern). The therapeutic aim is to impose regular drug-induced cycles by inhibiting the endogenous sexual rhythm.

Contraception

The combined type of oral contraceptive tablet produces almost complete suppression of gonadal activity and therefore no ovulation. Other progestational effects contribute to the contraceptive action (page 84). The pregnancy rate is low, about 0.1/HWY.

Adverse effects

Adverse effects which tend to disappear after the first months of administration

(1) Oestrogenic — nausea, vomiting, headache, weight gain, enlarged and tender breasts, decreased libido.
(2) Progestogenic — increased appetite, weight gain, decreased libido, depression, cramps, acne.

Less transient adverse effects

(1) Thromboembolic disorders. The mortality rate due to deep vein thromboses is increased 5—10 times and the incidence of cerebrovascular disease is increased 3—9 times. These increases are greater with age (> 35 years), length of medication and dose of oestrogenic and possibly progestogenic component. Contraceptive tablets contain 50 μg or less of ethinyloestradiol or mestranol.

(2) Hypertension. The incidence is reversibly increased about 3 times and is greater with age, cigarette smoking, obesity, family history of hypertension and dose of the oestrogenic component.

(3) Urinary tract infections. The incidence is increased by about 1.5 times, probably by altering vaginal pH.

(4) Glucose tolerance is decreased but the incidence of diabetes is not increased.

(5) Thyroid function tests are impaired.

(6) Amenorrhoea may follow cessation of use; however, fertility is not significantly different from that in non-users 18 months after ceasing treatment.

Contraindications

Breastfeeding and diabetes (not absolute), cardiovascular disease including hypertension and thromboembolism, liver disease, pregnancy, young oligomenorrhoeic girls, elective surgery, immobilization.

Drug interactions

Drugs which increase the metabolic activity of the liver, for example, *Rifampicin* [rifampin] , *Phenytoin* or the barbiturates decrease the plasma concentrations of the steroids and hence the efficacy of the contraceptive tablet — recognized by breakthrough bleeding or later by pregnancy. Antibiotics which affect the gut bacteria may also produce these effects by decreasing the enterohepatic circulation of the steroids.

ANDROGENS

Androgens are substances which cause masculinization. Testosterone is the most important androgen and is secreted by the Leydig cells of the testis and to a smaller extent by the adrenal cortex of both sexes. Testosterone is converted to the more potent derivative 5-α-dihydrotestosterone in some target tissues of the body.

Preparations

(1) *Testosterone propionate* is given by injection in oil im weekly. It is hydrolysed to testosterone. The dosage interval can be extended by administering a mixture of *Testosterone esters* which are hydrolysed at different rates.

Table 2.6   *Effects of androgens*

System affected	Consequence
Reproductive organs	
Internal and external genitalia	Sexual differentiation in the foetus. Growth and development
Spermatogenesis	Low concentrations stimulate
	High concentrations inhibit via −ve feedback on gonadotrophins
CNS	
LH secretion	−ve feedback
FSH secretion	−ve feedback but probably not as important as the unidentified testicular factor inhibin
Foetal hypothalamus	Suppression of cyclic control of gonadotrophins
Libido	Augments in both sexes
Metabolic actions	
General	Marked net anabolic action (nitrogen retention)
Fluid mobilization	Salt and water retention
Other actions	
Long bone	Growth
Epiphyses	Closure
Muscle	Growth
Hair	Growth in male pattern. Paradoxically responsible for male pattern baldness
Skin	Thickening. Increased secretion from sebaceous glands (acne)
Vocal cords	Growth
Blood	Increased erythropoiesis
Liver	17-α-alkylated derivatives cause cholestatic jaundice

(2)   *Fluoxymesterone.* Alkylation at the 17-α-position reduces the rate of metabolism of steroids. This results in orally active preparations but also some hepatoxicity (cholestatic jaundice).

(3)   Mesterolone is alkylated in position 1. This results in oral activity and a low incidence of hepatotoxicity. This weak androgen has primarily peripheral actions.

(4)   Anabolic steroids, for example, *Methandienone* [methandrostenolone] and *Nandrolone.* Androgens have useful anabolic actions and synthetic derivatives show some separation between the anabolic and androgenic actions but the ratio of anabolic to androgenic potency is only 2–3 times that of testosterone which militates against their use, particularly in women and children. Abuse of these drugs is common among athletes.

Therapeutic use

Replacement therapy

Initiation or maintenance of the growth of the male secondary sexual characteristics, for example, after castration or gonadal failure with delayed puberty.

Treatment of infertility

Male infertility is usually resistant to treatment. Spermatogenesis requires gonadotrophins plus androgens. The latter usually suppress gonadotrophin secretion by —ve feedback. Mesterolone is useful as it acts peripherally and does not decrease gonadotrophin secretion.

Contraception

High doses are required for complete suppression of spermatogenesis. The onset and offset time of their action (14 weeks) is the sperm transit time between spermatogenesis and appearance in the ejaculate. Continuous therapy is required. Presently at an experimental stage.

Growth stimulation

Human GH is not freely available. Androgens have been useful in children with hypothalamic, pituitary or gonadal failure or malfunction. (They tend to increase stature by increasing the rate of linear growth but also increase the rate of ossification so the mature height may be reduced by early closure of the epiphyses). In girls and prepubertal boys masculinization will occur.

Advanced breast cancer

Thirty per cent of breast tumours will regress in response to hormone manipulations, that is, empirical treatment which may involve the removal of the hormone-producing gland, for example, ovary or adrenal (premenopause) or the administration of large doses of androgens, oestrogens or the antagonist oestrogen — tamoxifen. Androgens are the drug treatment of choice at and around the menopause. The action may be exerted via the —ve feedback at the pituitary or directly on the tissue. The side-effects are virilization, that is, growth of facial hair, hoarseness of voice plus an increase in libido.

Stimulation of erythropoiesis

Large doses are administered for at least two months in aplastic anaemia, leukaemia and refractory anaemia. The response is variable and said to be mediated by increased production of erythropoietin by the kidney.

ANDROGEN ANTAGONISTS

Cyproterone competes with androgen for the steroid receptor (page 80) and antagonizes the specific actions of androgens; however, it is also a very potent progestogen.

Therapeutic use

It decreases sexual drive in sexual offenders but does not alter the direction of the desire. It may find a use in androgen-dependent syndromes, for example, precocious puberty, acne, prostatic hyperplasia.

Antispermatogenic chemicals

There are a variety of drugs and chemicals which will modify spermatogenesis although none is currently suitable as a male contraceptive. Such compounds either inhibit spermatogenesis or modify the sperm such that fertilization does not ensue. There are two major mechanisms of drug action as follows:

Direct action on sperm cells

Many alkylating agents and antimetabolites when used in cancer chemotherapy (page 205) inhibit spermatogenesis at specific stages leading to infertility. The time from commencement of drug administration to sterility is dependent on the stage of spermatogenesis affected. For example, *Busulphan* selectively kills spermatogonia. The stages from spermatocytes onward continue at the normal rate and therefore sterility will not occur for upwards of 14 weeks. Animal studies with the compound α-chlorohydrin has shown it is possible to produce rapid and reversible sterility by preventing sperm maturation in the epididymides.

Indirect action via suppression of secretion of gonadotrophins

As the gonadotrophins are necessary for spermatogenesis, so any drug which suppresses their secretion sufficiently and for a prolonged period will eventually produce sterility. Therefore, oestrogens, progestogens and androgens can all produce sterility via their −ve feedback actions at the hypothalamus or anterior pituitary. The time to the onset of sterility is usually at least 14 weeks. Most drugs do not affect the stem cells within the seminiferous tubules so that fertility usually returns after cessation of drug treatment. This may take several months.

The thyroid gland and drugs used in thyroid abnormalities

The function of the thyroid gland is the synthesis, storage and release of the thyroid hormones L-thyroxine and L-tri-iodothyronine.

SYNTHESIS AND RELEASE

Ingested iodine is converted to I^- and absorbed from the alimentary canal. The thyroid concentrates I^- 20–200 times with respect to the plasma concentration by active transport (the I^- pump) from the circulation to the colloid of the gland. The I^- is oxidized to free iodine under the influence of peroxidase enzyme and reacts with tyrosine molecules attached to thyroglobulin to give mono-iodotyrosine (MIT) then di-iodotyrosine (DIT). Two DIT molecules undergo an oxidative condensation, with the elimination of alanine, to form thyroxine.

Some tri-iodothyronine is also formed from MIT + DIT. At this stage MIT, DIT, thyroxine and tri-iodothyronine are in peptide linkage to the thyroglobulin. Release involves the proteolytic breakdown of the peptide bonds between iodinated compounds and thyroglobulin. Thyroxine and tri-iodothyronine pass out of the thyroid cells into the circulation. MIT and DIT are de-iodinated by microsomal iodotyrosine dehalogenase to I^- and tyrosine which are reused in synthesis. Ninety-nine per cent of the plasma thyroid hormones are protein bound, particularly to an α-globulin called thyroxine binding globulin. Ninety per cent of the circulating hormone is thyroxine, the remainder is tri-iodothyronine. Thyroxine is only slowly eliminated from the body ($t_{1/2}$ 6—7 days), tri-iodothyronine more rapidly ($t_{1/2}$ 2 days). Both compounds are conjugated in the liver with glucuronic and sulphuric acids. There is an entero-hepatic circulation of the hormones.

An important route of metabolism for thyroxine is to tri-iodothyronine (about 20 per cent converted). Tri-iodothyronine is about four times as active as thyroxine so that this conversion may account for most of the observed activity of thyroxine.

CONTROL OF SYNTHESIS AND RELEASE

This involves the hypothalamus and anterior pituitary gland as discussed on page 73. TSH releasing hormone from the hypothalamus influences the release

Table 2.7

Effect	Hypothyroid state (myxoedema or Gull's disease, cretinism)	Hyperthyroid state (thyrotoxicosis, exophthalmic goitre, Graves' disease)
Oxygen consumption Heat production Basal metabolic rate	Decreased	Increased
CNS	Impaired mentality Poor memory and concentration Drowsiness	Excitability, restlessness, apprehension, insomnia
Somatic motor nervous system	Decreased activity	Increased activity
Sympathetic nervous system	Decreased activity	Increased activity
Cardiovascular system	Bradycardia, fall in cardiac output and BP	Tachycardia, increase in cardiac output and BP
Gastrointestinal tract	Activity diminished, constipation	Activity increased, diarrhoea
Sensitivity to catecholamines	Decreased	Increased

of TSH from the anterior pituitary gland. Via a primary action involving increased concentration of cAMP within the thyroid cell, TSH stimulates all stages of synthesis and release of the thyroid hormones. A −ve feedback system exists such that increased blood thyroid hormone concentration reduces the output of TSH from the anterior pituitary.

EFFECTS OF THYROID HORMONE

In general, thyroid hormones increase the O_2 consumption of most metabolically active tissues (exceptions are brain, testes, uterus, spleen and anterior pituitary). They stimulate lipid catabolism, protein synthesis and intestinal carbohydrate absorption. The effect on body systems can best be illustrated by comparison between the hypothyroid and hyperthyroid states (*Table 2.7*).

USE OF THYROID HORMONE

Thyroxine sodium [levothyroxine] and *Liothyronine* sodium (L-tri-iodothyronine) are only used as replacement therapy to treat hypothyroid states. *Thyroxine* is normally the drug of choice for maintenance therapy but *Liothyronine* may be preferred when a rapid onset of action (hypothyroid coma) or shorter duration of action (hypothyroidism with ischaemic heart disease) is required.

Thyrotoxicosis

In thyrotoxicosis there is excess circulating thyroid hormone. This may be due to the following:

(1) Diffusely enlarged gland producing excess hormone. This is Graves' disease and is associated with a circulating immunoglobulin, long acting thyroid stimulator (LATS) which is not subject to feedback control.
(2) A multinodular goitre (Plummer's disease)
(3) Stimulation by excess TSH from a tumour
(4) An autonomously functioning nodule (toxic adenoma)

Drugs used in thyrotoxicosis

(1) Thioamide derivatives: *Carbimazole* and *Propylthiouracil.* These probably interfere with tyrosine iodination but evidence is also available that these compounds block the coupling of iodotyrosines to form iodothyronines. The drugs are well absorbed from the intestine and widely distributed in tissues. Response to treatment takes several weeks with the euthyroid state produced in 1−2 months. To avoid relapse prolonged treatment may be necessary (1.5−2 years), even then relapse is common: up to 50 per cent, many within 3 months of stopping treatment. Thioamides may also be used before thyroid surgery and to hasten euthyroidism after radiation therapy. Side-effects include skin rashes, lymphadenopathy and fever (3−5 per cent of patients treated) and agranulocytosis (0.5 per cent). *Propylthiouracil* is useful when rashes develop to *Carbimazole* as there is not usually cross-sensitivity.

(2)   Monovalent ions. (a) Potassium perchlorate competes with I^- for the active uptake process and blocks I^- access to the gland. It is used only infrequently when toxic reactions prevent the use of the thioamides. Its most serious toxic effect is aplastic anaemia. (b) Iodide. A paradoxical effect of high I^- intake is to control hyperthyroidism. The mechanism of action is unclear but I^- promotes involution of the hypertrophied tissue with an increase in colloid storage and a decreased release of thyroid hormone. The effects are rapid in onset (10–15 days for maximal effect) but not sustained. I^- is useful before surgery to prepare the gland for subtotal thyroidectomy but only after prior treatment with antithyroid drugs and together with other antithyroid drugs and supportive measures in thyrotoxic crisis. It is prescribed as *Iodine aqueous* [strong iodine] *solution.*

(3)   Radioactive iodine. Radioactive iodine is treated exactly as unlabelled iodine by the body and is rapidly and efficiently trapped by the thyroid gland, incorporated into the iodo-aminoacids and deposited into the colloid of the follicles. Several isotopes of iodine are available (*Table 2.8*). ^{131}I is the most

Table 2.8

Isotope	$t_{1/2}$	Radiation emitted	Application
^{125}I	57 days	Gamma rays	Diagnostic aid
^{131}I	8 days	Beta particles	Diagnostic aid and treatment
		Gamma rays	of hyperthyroidism
^{132}I	2.3 hours	Beta particles	Diagnostic aid
		Gamma rays	

widely used although the ultra-short $t_{1/2}$ of ^{132}I has the advantage of delivering much lower radiation doses than either ^{131}I or ^{125}I and is therefore preferred in diagnostic tests in infants and young children, during pregnancy and whenever sequential tests of thyroid function are planned.

There are two basic uses of radioactive iodine. (a) Diagnostic: the dose is measured in μCi. It is an invaluable aid to the diagnosis of myxoedema and hyperthyroid states and the classification of goitre. (b) Treatment of hyper-thyroidism: ^{131}I is normally employed and the dose is measured in mCi. The radioactive iodine is deposited in the colloid of the follicles from where the destructive β-particles originate. The average depth of penetration of the particles is 0.5 mm which means in practice that damage is confined exclusively to the parenchymal cells lining the follicles of the thyroid gland with little or no damage to surrounding tissue. The response is slow (this is overcome by administering antithyroid drugs postoperatively) and there is a high incidence of myxoedema (up to 50 per cent of cases in eight years postoperative) due to the difficulty in estimating the effective dose.

(4)   Antagonists at β-adrenoceptors (page 51) have been observed to reduce many of the symptoms and signs of thyrotoxicosis, for example, nervousness, atrial fibrillation, myocardial contractility and cardiac output. There is no effect on basal metabolic rate or I^- utilization (as measured with ^{131}I). *Propranolol* is valuable prior to thyroidectomy, after irradiation and in thyrotoxic crisis (in

conjunction with antithyroid drugs and supportive measures). As sole treatment for thyrotoxicosis the success rate differs little from the spontaneous remission rate and the patient remains biochemically hyperthyroid throughout the treatment.

Insulin and glucagon

Terminology used in glucose metabolism

Glycogenesis: the synthesis of glycogen from glucose.
Glycogenolysis: the conversion of glycogen to glucose, mainly in the liver.
Glycolysis: the oxidation of glucose or glycogen to pyruvate and lactate by the Embden—Meyerhof pathway.
The citric acid cycle (Krebs' cycle, tricarboxylic acid cycle): final common pathway of oxidation of carbohydrate, fat and protein, through which acetyl-CoA is completely oxidized to CO_2 and water.
Hexose monophosphate shunt (pentose phosphate pathway): an alternative route (to glycolysis and the citric acid cycle) from glucose to CO_2 and water.
Gluconeogenesis: the formation of glucose or glycogen from non-carbohydrate sources. The principal substrates for gluconeogenesis are aminoacids, lactate and glycerol.
Lipolysis: breakdown of fats to smaller molecules — usually to fatty acids and glycerol.
Lipogenesis: the reverse process to lipolysis.
Ketosis: excessive ketone body production.

Pancreatic cell types

For the recent nomenclature regarding cell types in the islets of Langerhans, *see Table 2.9.*

Table 2.9

Old name	Secretory product	New name
α_2	Glucagon	A
β	Insulin	B
α_1	Somatostatin	D

INSULIN

The fine control of metabolism of foodstuffs depends on the precise response of the B-cells to stimuli activating or inhibiting secretion of insulin which is ejected from the B-cell by storage granule rupture. Insulin is a polypeptide of two chains joined by disulphide bridges (MW about 6,000) and can exist as a monomer, dimer or hexamer (3 dimers). Two molecules of zinc are co-ordinated in the hexamer which is presumably the form stored in the B-cell. The biologically active form of the hormone is thought to be the monomer. Main stimulants to insulin secretion are likely to be blood glucose concentration perfused through pancreas, intestinal releasing factors (glucagon may be one), aminoacid concentrations, ketone concentration and other extraneous factors such as GH and glucocorticoids. Normal insulin secretion by a pancreas is about 30—60 Units/day.

The more important effects of insulin on carbohydrate, fat and protein metabolism are:

(1) Carbohydrate metabolism. Blood glucose concentration is decreased by:
     (*a*) an increase in glycogen synthesis in liver and muscle; (*b*) an increase in
     cellular glucose utilization; (*c*) a decrease in gluconeogenesis from protein.
(2) Fat metabolism. Storage fat in adipose tissue increases, plasma-free fatty
     acid (FFA) concentrations are reduced by: (*a*) an increase in lipogenesis;
     (*b*) a decrease in lipolysis.
(3) Protein metabolism. Protein content is increased by: (*a*) an increase in
     aminoacid utilization; (*b*) a decrease in protein breakdown.

Diabetes mellitus

The causes of diabetes mellitus are not fully understood. The disease is manifested by raised concentrations of blood sugar (hyperglycaemia) and glucose in the urine (glycosuria).

Biochemistry

The biochemical effects of diabetes are complex and interrelated. The more important ones may be deduced by considering the effects of insulin on carbohydrate, fat and protein metabolism outlined above. Since diabetes mellitus is associated with a lack (relative or absolute) of insulin its manifestations are the opposite of insulin's effects.

Other factors

Many other factors, mainly hormonal, have been shown to be capable of producing a diabetic syndrome in man and animals. The more important ones are the following:

(1) Glucagon. A polypeptide secreted by the A-cells of the islets of Langerhans.
     It is a very potent hormone which raises blood sugar concentration and
     increases FFA release.
(2) GH promotes growth in the immature animal by laying down protein but
     in adults has been shown to be diabetogenic.
(3) Glucocorticoids have many actions which are opposite to those of insulin
     and when given therapeutically for other purposes over prolonged periods
     are diabetogenic.

(4)   Adrenaline inhibits insulin release (via α-adrenoceptors) and promotes glycogenolysis.

Types of diabetes mellitus are shown in *Table 2.10.*

Table 2.10

| Typical features | Type | |
	Growth onset (juvenile)	Maturity onset
Age group (onset)	Younger, about 12 years on	Older, > 25 years
Plasma insulin	Very low or absent	Normal or reduced (delayed secretion to glucose stimulus)
B-cell function	Very low or absent	Normal or reduced
Ketosis	Yes (if treatment delayed)	No
Treatment	Insulin	Diet ± oral hypoglycaemics
Others	Insulin responsive	Tendency to insulin resistance

Treatment

Diabetic patients may be divided into about one-third treatable by diet alone, one-third by diet plus oral hypoglycaemics and one-third by diet plus insulin.

Diet alone: patient usually maturity onset, overweight, therefore initial weight reduction and careful diet sufficient to maintain normal or near normal blood sugar and prevent glycosuria.

Diet plus oral hypoglycaemic agents: this category falls within maturity onset group and may respond indefinitely to oral therapy except during periods of stress such as surgery or acute illness when insulin may be necessary.

Sulphonylureas, for example, *Tolbutamide, Chlorpropamide, Glibenclamide.* Certain sulphonamides, being tested for potential antibacterial activity were also found to possess blood glucose lowering properties. Attached to the benzene ring of the sulphonamide is an amino group which although essential for anti-bacterial activity is not necessary for the hypoglycaemic activity and can therefore be substituted. Substitution resulted in the sulphonylurea compounds used presently as oral hypoglycaemic agents (*Table 2.11*). The prime action of

Table 2.11

Drug	$t_{1/2}$ hours	Frequency per day	Effective daily dosage range
Tolbutamide	4	2	0.5–2 g
Chlorpropamide	35–40	1	100–500 mg
Glibenclamide	12	1–2	2.5–20 mg

all sulphonylurea compounds is stimulation of the B-cells of the islets of Langerhans to secrete insulin, therefore there is an absolute requirement for functioning islet cell tissue. The more potent sulphonylurea compounds such as *Glibenclamide,* are thought to have additional action stimulating synthesis of insulin. Side-effects of the sulphonylurea compounds include hypoglycaemia, skin rashes, mild jaundice and diarrhoea.

Biguanides, for example, *Phenformin* and *Metformin* do not act like the sulphonylureas. The exact mechanism by which glucose concentration is lowered is unknown. The islets of Langerhans are not stimulated but, nevertheless, biguanides are inactive in the absence of insulin. The biguanides may: promote uptake of glucose into muscle; increase insulin sensitivity; impair glucose uptake from the gut. Side-effects of the biguanide compounds include anorexia and lactic acidosis.

Insulin plus diet: this regimen is necessary in virtually all cases of growth onset diabetes and in adults who are ketotic when first seen. All insulin for the treatment of diabetics is extracted from the pancreas of cows (bovine) or pigs (porcine).

Use of unmodified, soluble, rapidly acting, insulin preparations has certain disadvantages the main one being the frequency of administration. Insulin injection can be painful as a result of the low pH of the preparation and cause fibrosis at the site of injection (which reduces absorption of insulin). Modifications of the insulin preparations (*Table 2.12*) have helped to overcome these problems: for example (1) combination with proteins — protamine — precipitating the insulin and delaying its release; (2) combination with zinc — zinc delays the onset and prolongs the action of insulin by crystallizing the insulin and delaying its release.

Table 2.12

Insulin	Other names	Time of onset (hours)	Duration of effect
Insulin injection	Soluble	1	S
Neutral insulin injection		1	S
Insulin zinc suspension (Amorphous) [prompt]	Semilente	1	I
Isophane insulin	Isophane	2	I
Insulin zinc suspension	Lente	2–7	L
Insulin zinc suspension (Crystalline) [extended]	Ultralente	4–7	L
Protamine zinc insulin		4–7	L

S = short, I = intermediate, L = long. All from mixed bovine and porcine sources.

Although both pork and beef insulin are immunogenic in man, immunological resistance to insulin action is uncommon. When this does occur, antibodies are mainly directed against the beef component and impurities and may be overcome by changing to a pure pork preparation. Other problems associated with insulin therapy include minor allergic reactions and lipoatrophy at the site of injection. These effects can be significantly reduced by using the newer highly purified or monocomponent (either bovine or porcine) preparations.

Use of somatostatin (page 74)

Mounting evidence suggests that all the metabolic derangements that characterize diabetes mellitus (in particular juvenile) cannot be explained by the traditional concept of insulin lack. The hyperglycaemia of juvenile diabetes may require, in addition to insulin deficiency, a relative excess of glucagon. The polypeptide somatostatin, secreted by the D-cells of the pancreas inhibits secretion of glucagon from the A-cells. Analogues of somatostatin may prove to be potentially useful therapeutic agents in the treatment of juvenile diabetes mellitus.

Use of kallikrein

Bradykinin and kallikrein (which releases bradykinin, page 114) have been shown to increase the uptake of glucose into insulin-dependent tissues. Treatment of mature diabetics with kallikrein may prove a useful adjunct to present therapeutic regimens.

Many pharmacological agents can also produce or unmask diabetes and these are listed in *Table 2.13*.

Table 2.13

Agent	Mechanism of action
Streptozocin and alloxan	B-cell cytotoxic
Immunosuppressives	Inhibit insulin synthesis
α-adrenoceptor agonists, β-adrenoceptor antagonists, thiazide diuretics, *Diazoxide, Phenytoin*	Inhibit insulin secretion
Corticosteroids, ACTH, GH, oestrogen/progestogen oral contraceptives	Gluconeogenesis, lipolysis (or tissue resistance to insulin)

Hypoglycaemia

Normal fasting blood glucose concentrations average $3.3-5.6$ mmol/ℓ; < 2.6 mmol/ℓ is termed hypoglycaemia. The symptoms and signs of hypoglycaemia fall into the following two groups:

(1)   Those due to adrenaline release. These include hunger, pallor, sweating, apprehension and tachycardia. The adrenaline response is sometimes sufficient to raise blood glucose concentration by eventual mobilization of liver glycogen (mediated by β-adrenoceptors).

(2) Those due to neuroglycopoenia. If the adrenaline response is insufficient then the symptoms and signs due to neuroglycopoenia occur and include mental confusion, incoherent speech, retrograde amnesia and delirium. The main causes of hypoglycaemia are insulin administration and sulphonylurea drugs.

Treatment

Glucose
Glucagon increases the liver's output of glucose and the response produced is proportional to the glycogen reserve of the liver.

Diazoxide is related to the thiazide diuretics (pages 104 and 281). It is reserved for treating the chronic hypoglycaemia of excess insulin secretion. It may cause an increase in circulating catecholamine concentration which indirectly alters glucose concentration, or it may directly block insulin release from the pancreas.

The adrenal cortex and the corticosteroids

The function of the adrenal cortex is the synthesis and release of the adrenal steroids hydrocortisone, corticosterone and aldosterone (minor amounts of 11-deoxycorticosterone and androgens are also produced).

Synthesis is from cholesterol (*Figure 2.2*)

CONTROL OF SYNTHESIS AND RELEASE

There is no storage of hormones within the adrenal cortex, thus the rate of release is virtually identical to the rate of synthesis. The synthesis and release of hydrocortisone and corticosterone involves the hypothalamus and anterior pituitary gland as discussed on page 74. ACTH releasing factor from the hypo-thalamus increases the release of ACTH from the anterior pituitary. This polypeptide stimulates the synthesis of hydrocortisone and corticosterone from cholesterol, probably through a mechanism involving cAMP. A −ve feedback exists, increased plasma concentration of hydrocortisone reduces the output of ACTH releasing factor and ACTH. Some evidence has been presented suggesting that the hypothalamus is also influenced by the concentration of ACTH. Higher centres of the brain, such as those involved in the response to stress are also able to influence the hypothalamus.

Aldosterone synthesis and release is stimulated by angiotensin formed in the blood from an inactive precursor (angiotensinogen) by renin. Renin is released from the juxtaglomerular apparatus in the kidney in response to a fall in blood volume, renal perfusion pressure or plasma Na^+ concentration. The action of the released aldosterone to promote Na^+ retention and of the angiotensin to constrict blood vessels (page 101) tends to raise these parameters and reduce further renin release.

In the plasma the corticosteroid hormones are largely protein bound (hydro-cortisone > 90 per cent) mainly to an α-globulin (transcortin). Metabolism occurs in the liver giving water-soluble metabolites with little or no activity which are excreted by the kidney.

PHYSIOLOGICAL AND PHARMACOLOGICAL ACTIONS OF THE ADRENAL STEROIDS

The adrenal cortex functions as an organ of homeostasis, enabling the body to cope with a changing environment, and the adrenal steroids exert the following effects:

(1) Carbohydrate metabolism — decreased glucose uptake and increased gluconeogenesis.
(2) Fat metabolism — mobilization of fatty acids from adipose tissue.
(3) Protein metabolism — induced peripheral aminoacid mobilization.
(4) Electrolyte balance — increased Na^+ retention and K^+ loss by the kidney.

These effects are believed to be exerted by interaction of the steroids with specific steroid receptors within cells leading to altered protein and enzyme synthesis. The steroids are also necessary for the maintenance of the normal functional capacities of the skeletal muscle, cardiovascular and central nervous systems. Supra-physiological doses of steroids reduce inflammatory responses (page 119), allergic reactions (through suppression of the inflammatory response following antigen-antibody reaction) and the immune response. The formation and activity of lympoid tissue is reduced.

The effects on electrolyte balance are labelled mineralocorticoid, all the others including the anti-inflammatory action are labelled glucocorticoid. Aldosterone exerts exclusively mineralocorticoid effects, hydrocortisone exerts mainly glucocorticoid activity but large doses also influence electrolyte balance.

USE OF ACTH AND THE ADRENAL STEROIDS

Preparations

ACTH (*Corticotrophin*) and *Tetracosactrin* (a synthetic analogue of ACTH consisting of the adrenocorticotrophic component of ACTH, that is, its first 24 aminoacid sequence).

(1) Diagnostically to determine if adrenal insufficiency is due to pituitary or adrenal failure. If the adrenal cortex is capable of response there will be increased urinary steroid metabolites.
(2) Treatment of anterior pituitary failure (replacement therapy with steroids may be preferred).
(3) Treatment of non-endocrine disorders, for example, rheumatic and collagen diseases, status asthmaticus, anaphylactic shock.

The major problem with the use of ACTH is the necessity for parenteral admin-istration to avoid proteolytic destruction of the polypeptide structure. Hyper-sensitivity reactions do occur but rarely.

Modification of the structures of the natural adrenal steroids has produced compounds which have the following properties:

(1) Mainly glucocorticoid activity but with significant mineralocorticoid activity, *Prednisolone, Prednisone, Cortisone.*
(2) Glucocorticoid activity with no significant effect on salt and water metabolism, *Betamethasone, Dexamethasone, Fluocinolone.* Some separation of the anti-inflammatory action from the metabolic glucocorticoid activities has been achieved with *Beclomethasone.*
(3) Mineralocorticoid activity with no significant glucocorticoid actions, *Fludrocortisone.*

Alteration in structure also changes plasma $t_{1/2}$ by influencing protein binding and metabolism. Compounds may be shorter acting, $t_{1/2} < 1.5$ days (for example, *Prednisolone*); or longer acting, $t_{1/2} > 2$ days (for example, *Dexamethasone*). Uses are divided into the following two categories:

Replacement therapy

Note that there is little risk of adverse effects when adrenal steroids are used for replacement therapy as plasma concentrations are in the physiological range. The type of analogue (mineralocorticoid or glucocorticoid) chosen will depend on the condition treated. Anterior pituitary failure and acute adrenal failure usually require only a glucocorticoid compound, chronic adrenal failure may require either or both types and congenital hyperplasia usually requires a glucocorticoid although on occasions both types may be required.

Treatment

Treatment with glucocorticoids is palliative, not curative. Compounds are needed with a high glucocorticoid and low mineralocorticoid activity.

Among conditions treated with glucocorticoids are rheumatic carditis, systemic lupus erythematosus (a generalized vascular disorder involving skin, joints, pleura, kidney, CNS and blood cells in which immunological abnormalities play a central pathogenic role), ocular inflammation, many inflammatory conditions of the skin and rheumatoid arthritis (page 316). Glucocorticoids may also be used in allergic states, for example, chronic asthma (page 290) and hay fever (as depot injection). The ability of glucocorticoids to cause involution of lymphoid tissue may be employed to give temporary remission in leukaemia, and their action on the immune response may be used in an attempt to prevent rejection in transplant operations.

Treatment with glucocorticoids presents two main risks: (1) abrupt withdrawal after prolonged high dosage may result in acute adrenal insufficiency due to suppression of ACTH and atrophy of the gland; (2) prolonged treatment always carries risks, which must be weighed against benefits in serious conditions. Many of the adverse effects are clearly extensions of the physiological actions including hyperglycaemia, Na^+ and water retention, increased susceptibility to infection, muscle wasting, osteoporosis and a state resembling Cushing's syndrome. Other adverse reactions include perforating peptic ulcers, hypercoagulability of blood, lens cataract formation, increase in intraocular pressure and psychoses.

Interference with synthesis or action

Metyrapone decreases the synthesis of hydrocortisone, corticosterone and aldosterone by inhibiting the enzyme which converts 11-deoxyhydrocortisone to hydrocortisone and 11-deoxycorticosterone to corticosterone and aldosterone.

It may be used as a diuretic in cases of resistant oedema associated with excess aldosterone secretion and also as a test of pituitary function. In this case as plasma hydrocortisone concentration falls ACTH will be released to stimulate the adrenal cortex and large quantities of 11-deoxysteroids will appear in the urine. Hypersecretion of adrenal steroids from adrenal neoplasms or due to ectopic ACTH will also be reduced by *Metyrapone.* Aminoglutethimide inhibits the first reaction in steroidogenesis and reduces the production of all three steroid hormones. It may prove to be useful to reduce hypersecretion due to autonomously functioning adrenal tumours and ectopic ACTH production.

Spironolactone acts as a competitive antagonist to aldosterone, thereby reducing Na^+ and water retention by the kidney (page 105).

TESTING OF THE HYPOTHALAMIC–PITUITARY–ADRENAL SYSTEM

(1) ACTH or *Tetracosactrin:* increased urinary steroid metabolites demonstrates the ability of the adrenal cortex to respond to stimulation.
(2) *Metyrapone:* increased urinary 11-deoxymetabolites demonstrates the ability of the anterior pituitary to respond to decreased plasma steroids.
(3) *Dexamethasone:* decreased urinary steroid metabolites demonstrates suppression of ACTH by the −ve feedback. There will be no effect on elevated steroids from adrenal neoplasms or due to ectopic ACTH.
(4) *Lypressin* (lysine-vasopressin): this behaves like ACTH releasing factor, causing the anterior pituitary to release ACTH − increased urinary steroid metabolites will result.
(5) Insulin: hypoglycaemic stress increases urinary steroid metabolites.

Angiotensin

OCCURRENCE, BIOSYNTHESIS AND METABOLISM

Angiotensin (angiotensin II) is an octapeptide formed by the action of the kidney enzyme, renin, on an inactive plasma α_2 globulin angiotensinogen. An intermediate, relatively inert, decapeptide angiotensin I is formed initially and this is converted to angiotensin II by angiotensin converting enzymes located in the lungs. This enzyme is the same as one of the enzymes responsible for the breakdown of bradykinin.

Angiotensin is rapidly destroyed in man (plasma $t_{1/2}$ = 1–2 minutes) by angiotensinases (mainly aminopeptidases) to give inactive peptides.

ACTIONS OF ANGIOTENSIN

The adrenal cortex is stimulated to release aldosterone.

Angiotensin is the most potent pressor agent known (equipotent molar dose ratio angiotensin : NA = 1:40) causing arteriolar constriction and a rise in diastolic and systolic BP. This action is mainly direct but facilitation of NA release from sympathetic nerves may contribute.

Angiotensin contracts the smooth muscle of the intestine, bronchioles and uterus and stimulates the adrenal medulla (to release catecholamines), parasympathetic and sympathetic ganglia.

ROLE IN PHYSIOLOGY AND PATHOPHYSIOLOGY

The renin-angiotensin system is important in the maintenance of cardiovascular homeostasis and the control of electrolyte balance (page 98). It is also suggested to play a modulatory role in the control of small blood vessel tone by virtue of its facilitatory effects on sympathetic nerve activity. A high renin concentration and hence high angiotensin concentration is a common finding in malignant (but not benign) hypertension (page 279).

PHARMACOLOGICAL AND THERAPEUTIC EXPLOITATION

Angiotensin is marketed as a vasopressor agent. Its use is restricted to raising BP while preparations are being made for more rational therapy such as transfusion with blood or plasma expanders or administration of cardiac glycosides. Use of converting enzyme inhibitors may prove beneficial in certain hypertensive disorders.

Diuretics

Diuretics increase the urine output of ions and fluid from the kidney. They do this by interfering with one or more of the reabsorptive processes occurring in the kidney tubules between the glomerular capsule and junction of the collecting ducts with the ureter. To understand the actions of the diuretics it is necessary to understand the normal reabsorptive processes which take place after filtration at the glomerular capsule. These processes reduce the filtrate from

12.5 ℓ to a volume of urine of about 100 ml in 100 minutes, as well as drastically changing the ionic composition. The regions involved in these processes and the functions performed in each are as follows:

Proximal convoluted tubule

(1) Active reabsorption of the major portion of the filtered Na^+, accompanied passively by Cl^- and water to maintain electrochemical and osmotic balance.
(2) Active reabsorption of all filtered K^+ accompanied passively by Cl^- and water.
(3) The reabsorption of filtered HCO_3^-. This involves the production of HCO_3^- and H^+ within the tubular epithelial cells under the influence of carbonic anhydrase, the transfer of the HCO_3^- to the peritubular vessels and the exchange of the H^+ with Na^+ in the filtrate. This Na^+ is transferred to the peritubular fluid, the H^+ interacts with HCO_3^- in the filtrate, producing water and CO_2 (which may diffuse into the epithelial cells and be used in the production of more HCO_3^-). This HCO_3^- reabsorption can take place throughout the nephron but the major site appears to be the proximal tubule.

Ascending limb of the loop of Henle

Active reabsorption of Cl^- accompanied by Na^+, the rate of reabsorption exceeds that of the reabsorption of water leaving a tubule fluid which is hypotonic as it enters the distal tubule.

Distal convoluted tubule and collecting ducts

(1) Active reabsorption of Na^+, accompanied by Cl^- and water.
(2) Active reabsorption of Na^+ in connection with secretion of K^+, this 'exchange' is increased by aldosterone and by increased delivery of Na^+ to the tubule.
(3) Reabsorption of water, increased by ADH released from the posterior pituitary gland. ADH, via increased formation of cAMP, increases the permeability of the tubule cells and normally results in a tubule fluid which is isotonic in the distal tubule and hypertonic in the collecting duct. Changes in plasma tonicity influence the release of ADH such that more, or less, water is reabsorbed to restore the tonicity to normal. Replacement therapy with *Lypressin* or desmopressin is needed in diabetes insipidus (low secretion of ADH by the posterior pituitary gland).

Compounds reducing or blocking these reabsorptive processes will result in the production of an increased volume of urine with increased concentration of one or more ions.

Benzothiadiazides ('thiazides')

A large group of compounds which are structurally related, have the same mechanism of action and the same maximum effect on urine production. Included in the group are *Bendrofluazide* [bendroflumethiazide], *Chlorothiazide, Hydrochlorothiazide* and *Hydroflumethiazide. Chlorthalidone* is not structurally a thiazide but has identical pharmacological properties. Members of the group vary in their onset and duration of action; the duration appears to depend on the degree of protein binding, the longer acting compounds being more highly bound. The drugs enter the kidney tubule partly by filtration at the glomerulus, partly by active secretion into the proximal tubule. The major action of this group is to block the active reabsorption of Na^+, accompanied by Cl^- and water in the distal tubule (possibly by inhibition of glycolysis). This results in increased volume of urine with increased loss of Na^+ and Cl^-. The increased flow in the distal tubule results in more Na^+-K^+ 'exchange' and increased K^+ loss. Some members of the group also inhibit carbonic anhydrase and thus reduce the reabsorption of HCO_3^- which is lost in the urine. Other renal effects are a reduction in uric acid excretion and a decreased glomerular filtration rate (GFR) (possibly due to a direct action on the renal vasculature).

The increased K^+ secretion may result in hypokalaemia and present problems, particularly in patients receiving *Digoxin* (page 276). This problem may be reduced by the use of K^+ supplements (for example, *Potassium chloride effervescent tablets, Potassium chloride slow tablets*), of thiazide preparations which include a K^+ supplement, or of K^+-sparing diuretics (*see below*). In susceptible patients the hyperuricaemia may induce gout.

Side-effects which are not of renal origin include the induction of hyperglycaemia and aggravation of pre-existing diabetes mellitus, and much less frequently acute pancreatitis, bone marrow depression and hypersensitivity reactions.

In patients with diabetes insipidus the thiazides produce a reduction in the urine volume. This suggests that an increased fraction of the glomerular filtrate is reabsorbed in the proximal tubule leading to a reduction in the Na^+ and water delivered to the distal tubule. Thus, a smaller volume of less dilute urine is produced. This occurs with or without a reduction in GFR.

Thiazide diuretics also possess an antihypertensive effect which is independent of their action on Na^+ and water excretion and probably involves the relaxation of arteriolar smooth muscle. *Diazoxide* (a thiazide analogue) causes profound relaxation of those vessels whilst causing salt and water retention and antagonizing *Bendrofluazide*, thus lending support to the suggestion that the antihypertensive effect of the thiazides is distinct from their diuretic action.

High ceiling or loop diuretics: *Frusemide, Ethacrynic* acid.

Like the thiazides these are absorbed after oral administration, protein bound in the plasma and enter the kidney partly by filtration and partly by active secretion in the proximal tubule. The diuretic action is rapid in onset, short in duration and, as the name suggests, more marked than with other diuretics.

The major action is to reduce active Cl^- reabsorption in the ascending limb of the loop of Henle, although there may be minor actions on Na^+ reabsorption in the proximal tubule and in the case of *Ethacrynic* acid on Na^+ reabsorption in the distal tubule. Na^+–K^+ 'exchange' is increased because of the higher Na^+ load delivered to this region. There is thus an increased urine volume with loss of Na^+, Cl^- and K^+. The Cl^- loss may induce alkalosis and the K^+ loss provoke *Digoxin* intoxication. Uric acid secretion may be reduced resulting in gout in susceptible patients. The very rapid, marked reduction in ECF volume can result in cardiovascular collapse. Other reported side-effects include gastrointestinal upsets, depression of formed elements of the blood and, rarely and with *Ethacrynic* acid only, permanent ototoxicity.

Carbonic anhydrase inhibitors: *Acetazolamide*

Acetazolamide produces a non-competitive inhibition of carbonic anhydrase and therefore reduces the formation of H^+ and HCO_3^- within the epithelial cells of the tubule; this in turn reduces the reabsorption of HCO_3^-. As there is excess enzyme present in the cells a very high degree of inhibition (about 90 per cent) is necessary before there is any effect. This action produces increased urine volume with loss of HCO_3^-. The increased Na^+ load in the distal tubule causes increased Na^+–K^+ 'exchange' and K^+ loss. The loss of HCO_3^- may result in metabolic acidosis as the plasma buffer concentration falls; this is self-limiting – sufficient H^+ is generated from metabolism to exchange with Na^+ in the tubule and thus re-establish HCO_3^- reabsorption from the tubule fluid.

Adverse effects which are infrequent include gastrointestinal upsets (which may be severe), paraesthesiae (tingling and similar sensations) and, even less frequently, bone marrow depression and renal stones. The self-limiting diuresis and the relatively low concentration of HCO_3^- in the filtrate limit the use of *acetazolamide.*

Acetazolamide is useful in the treatment of open angle glaucoma; inhibition of carbonic anhydrase reduces the formation of HCO_3^- and the secretion of aqueous humour; thus, intraocular pressure falls.

Potassium sparing diuretics: *Amiloride, Triamterene*

The major action is to reduce the Na^+–K^+ 'exchange' in the distal tubule (perhaps by reducing membrane permeability) giving a mild diuresis with loss of Na^+. *Triamterene* also has a minor effect on the active Na^+ reabsorption accompanied by Cl^- and water in the distal tubule; *Amiloride* causes some HCO_3^- loss although it appears not to be a carbonic anhydrase inhibitor. The main problem associated with their use is the danger of hyperkalaemia; plasma urea concentration may also be raised. Diuretics of this type are generally used in combinations with thiazide diuretics to reduce the loss of K^+ normally associated with this group.

Aldosterone antagonists: *Spironolactone*

This competitively antagonizes the aldosterone-promoted Na^+ reabsorption with K^+ secretion in the distal tubule, producing a diuresis with loss of Na^+. The magnitude of the effect depends on how much the Na^+–K^+ exchange is influenced by aldosterone. Like *Amiloride* it is useful in combination with the thiazides to reduce the K^+ loss normally associated with their diuretic effect. Again, the main side-effect is the likelihood of raised plasma K^+ concentrations.

Other diuretics of limited use

Xanthines (Theophylline, theobromine, caffeine) all produce a mild diuretic effect but Theophylline is the most potent. The diuresis may partly result from increased renal blood flow and GFR resulting from cardiac stimulation. There is, however, a direct action at the kidney to reduce Na^+ reabsorption which is lost in increased amounts, together with Cl^- and water. The xanthines are of limited use because of the relatively mild effect which is lost on repeated administration, but Theophylline may be used to increase the effectiveness of other diuretics in acute cardiac failure, usually as *Aminophylline* (Theophylline ethylenediamine).

Osmotic diuretics (Mannitol, glycerol [glycerin], urea) are filtered at the glomerulus and are not significantly reabsorbed from the tubules. The presence in the filtrate of these osmotically active solutes limits the reabsorption of water and therefore increases urine output. Osmotic diuretics, by this mechanism, are able to maintain urine volume even when GFR is reduced; they are thus used in the prophylaxis of acute renal failure. Other uses, depending on the same mechanism, are to reduce the volume and pressure of cerebrospinal and intra-ocular fluids.

Ammonium chloride produces both a diuresis and an acidification of the urine. Ammonium chloride dissociates to give NH_3, H^+ and Cl^-. The NH_3 is converted to urea in the liver and the H^+ interacts with HCO_3^- to give water and CO_2, which is lost from the lungs. The net effect is a metabolic acidosis because of the addition of Cl^- to the plasma, with loss of HCO_3^-. Increased Cl^- in the ECF results in more Cl^- being filtered at the glomerulus, escaping reabsorption in the tubules and being excreted with its equivalent cation (Na^+) and water. The metabolic acidosis results in renal compensation, the kidney tubule cells produce NH_4^+ which accompanies the Cl^- (instead of Na^+). The amount of Ammonium chloride excreted in this way becomes equivalent to that originally ingested and the diuretic action ceases. Ammonium chloride was used to correct the self-limiting alkalosis caused by the obsolete mercurial diuretics. It aids elimination of basic drugs (page 247).

Local hormones

HISTAMINE

Occurrence, biosynthesis and metabolism

Histamine is formed from the aminoacid l-histidine by the action of histidine decarboxylase. It is present in many mammalian tissues with especially high concentrations in lung, skin and intestine. Most is stored in the granules of tissue mast cells (basophils in blood) bound electrostatically to the protein carboxyl groups of a heparin-protein complex (*Figure 2.6*).

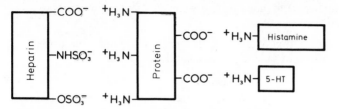

Figure 2.6

The relatively weak carboxyl groups of the protein bind the histamine. The much stronger acidic groups of the heparin molecule are fully neutralized by the basic groups of the protein. This arrangement is significant for the mechanism of histamine release described below. Non-mast cell histamine is located in tissues with a low mast cell content (brain, intestinal mucosa) but the storage sites are unknown. More than 90 per cent of an exogenous histamine load is metabolized either by deamination (enzyme, 'histaminase' = diamine oxidase; product, imidazolyl-acetic acid) or by a combination of N-methylation and deamination (enzymes imidazole-N-methyltransferase and MAO; product, methyl-imidazolyl-acetic acid).

Role in physiology and pathophysiology

Histamine plays a role in the regulation of gastric secretion, in the body's protective mechanism at an injury site (triple response, acute inflammation) and as a mediator in allergic and anaphylactic conditions.

Actions of histamine

On the cardiovascular system histamine dilates small arteries, capillaries and venules. Cerebral vessels are especially sensitive to histamine's dilator action. It also produces increased cerebrospinal fluid pressure and 'histamine headaches'. Histamine increases the permeability of the microcirculation to plasma protein. Thus, the BP falls but the heart rate increases due to reflex baroreceptor nerve stimulation (and a direct stimulant action of histamine on H_2 receptors in the heart, *Table 2.15*).

Lewis's triple response arises from injurious stimuli or can be mimicked by a small quantity of histamine pricked into skin. One sees: (1) a red mark due to capillary dilatation at injury site; (2) a pink flare which is diffuse and surrounds the injury site due to arteriolar dilatation from an axon reflex triggered by sensory nerve stimulation; (3) a wheal (a raised oedematous area close to the injury site) which is due to increased permeability of the microcirculation to protein.

Histamine stimulates the smooth muscle of intestine, bronchioles and uterus directly. It is a powerful stimulant of gastric secretion (mainly direct but also facilitates the secretogogue action of the vagus), both parietal and peptic gland cells are stimulated. It stimulates the adrenal medulla and autonomic ganglia but high concentrations are required. It also stimulates sensory neurones to give itching and sometimes pain.

The antigen-antibody reaction of anaphylaxis releases histamine from tissue stores (mast cells) as do trauma and certain compounds (*Table 2.14*):

Table 2.14

Type of activator	Examples
Tissue damage	Mechanical, chemical heat
Complex macromolecules	Snake and wasp venoms
	Bacterial toxins
	Trypsin and other proteolytic enzymes
High MW polymers	Dextran
	Compound 48:80
Detergents and surface active agents	Bile salts
	Lysolecithin
Basic drugs	*Atropine*
	Morphine
	Codeine
	Tubocurarine
	Antagonists at H_1 receptors

The underlying principle of histamine release is that the heparin-protein complex acts like a weak cation exchange resin. Exposure of the granules to a cation-containing medium results in an instantaneous exchange of histamine with the cation. Basic drugs displace the similarly basic histamine from its binding sites. Detergents, proteolytic enzymes, compound 48:80 and the antigen-antibody reaction of anaphylaxis cause cell disruption, with expulsion of granules into the extracellular cation-containing medium (degranulation), where instantaneous amine release by cation exchange occurs. Since the predominant extracellular cation is Na^+, the mechanism can be represented as in *Figure 2.7.*

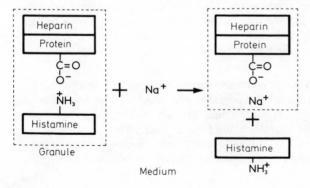

Figure 2.7

Anaphylaxis develops by the following stages:

(1) Exposure of animal or man to a foreign macromolecule (antigen) results in the formation of specific antibodies by the plasma cells.
(2) Circulating antibodies are taken up and firmly bound on the surface of tissue cells.
(3) Re-exposure to antigen results in combination with tissue-bound antibody and tissue damage.
(4) Histamine (and other cell constituents) are released 'explosively'. Other mediators implicated in anaphylaxis include plasma kinins, 5-hydroxytryptamine, prostaglandins and slow-reacting substance of anaphylaxis (SRS—A), which has recently been identified as a chemical relative of the prostaglandins.

Pharmacological and therapeutic exploitation

Histamine itself has no therapeutic value but at one time it was used for the diagnosis of achlorhydria (Pentagastrin is now used). Compounds which are antagonists at histamine receptors or prevent the release of histamine are used therapeutically.

Histamine receptor antagonists

These selectively and competitively antagonize the pharmacological effects of injected or endogenously released histamine. They can be divided into two groups as can histamine receptors (*Table 2.15*).

Table 2.15   *Histamine receptors*

H_1	H_2
Effects mediated	
Contraction of smooth muscle of:	Stimulation of gastric secretion
intestine	Stimulation of the heart
bronchioles	Inhibition of antigenic release of histamine from basophils
Most of depressor effects on BP	Rest of depressor effects on BP
Selective competitive antagonist	
Mepyramine	Cimetidine

Antagonists at H_1 receptors — *Mepyramine* [pyrilamine], *Promethazine, Dimenhydrinate,* Cyproheptadine and Chlorpheniramine. Some cause sedation and have anti-emetic and muscarinic blocking actions, which may not be related to H_1 receptor antagonism. Some are also local anaesthetics. Therapeutically useful in acute urticaria, in seasonal hayfever, against insect bites and stings, in motion sickness and as mild hypnotics. Largely ineffective in asthma or systemic anaphylaxis where other local hormones are involved. Side-effects are frequent but mild and include sedation, anorexia, nausea and vomiting, dizziness and blurred vision.

Antagonists at H_2 receptors Cimetidine. Unlike the antagonists at H_1 histamine receptors this is an imidazole derivative. It inhibits histamine- and Pentagastrin-evoked gastric acid secretion and cardiac stimulation. Cimetidine is currently marketed as an inhibitor of gastric secretion for use in the treatment of gastric and duodenal ulcer (page 271).

Sodium *Cromoglycate* [cromolyn sodium] is a bis-chromone, a derivative of chromone-2-carboxylic acid. It selectively suppresses the release of chemical mediators arising from antigen-antibody reactions or degranulating agents. Precise mode of action unknown but may stabilize the mast cell membrane so that steps between antigen-antibody union and the release of chemical mediators are prevented. It does not affect the course of the response if given after the antigen-antibody interaction and has no anti-inflammatory activity.

Sodium *Cromoglycate* is a very effective drug in hay fever, asthma and milk allergies in babies. It is poorly absorbed from the gut and is administered by inhalation as an insufflation into the nose and respiratory tract, or is applied topically (for example, to the conjunctiva).

5-HYDROXYTRYPTAMINE (SEROTONIN)

Occurrence, biosynthesis and metabolism

5-Hydroxytryptamine (5-HT) is present in many mammalian tissues with highest concentrations in the enterochromaffin cells of the gastrointestinal tract. 5-HT is complexed with heparin and protein within mast cells of rats and mice and although it is not present in normal human mast cells, it has been found in mast cell tumours of man. Elsewhere, 5-HT is stored in association with ATP in intracellular storage particles within the intestinal chromaffin cells, platelets and the specific 5-HT-containing (serotonergic) neurones of the brain (page 127).

The aminoacid tryptophan is hydroxylated to 5-hydroxytryptophan by trypto-phan-5-hydroxylase which is then decarboxylated to 5-HT by aromatic-aminoacid decarboxylase.

The degradation of 5-HT involves its conversion to 5-hydroxyindole acetaldehyde by MAO. This aldehyde is then rapidly converted to the excretory product 5-hydroxyindoleacetic acid by aldehyde dehydrogenase.

Role in physiology and pathophysiology

The selective localization of 5-HT in platelets and its vasoconstrictor properties suggest a role in blood clotting. Its role in gastrointestinal function (for example, peristalsis) is undetermined. A tumour of enterochromaffin or related cells (carcinoid) may develop in the gastrointestinal or respiratory tracts which secretes excessive quantities of 5-HT (in addition to polypeptides and prosta-glandins). 5-HT is probably important in the CNS (page 127). 5-HT may be involved in inflammatory responses or allergic and anaphylactic reactions but the evidence for this in man is not as strong as for histamine.

Actions of 5-hydroxytryptamine

5-HT has complex cardiovascular actions. In general it acts directly to constrict arteries and to give an increased peripheral resistance.

5-HT stimulates intestinal, bronchial and uterine smooth muscle, the adrenal medulla and ganglia of the autonomic nervous system. It is a potent stimulant of sensory nerve endings and gives pain when applied to an exposed blister base.

Two types of 5-HT receptor have been differentiated: those located on smooth muscle are labelled D receptors, while those located on nervous tissue (and the adrenal medulla) are labelled M receptors.

Pharmacological and therapeutic exploitation

There are no selective antagonists at M receptors available for clinical use.

Antagonists at D 5-HT receptors

Phenoxybenzamine and Phentolamine are potent antagonists at α-adrenoceptors (page 50) in addition to blocking responses to 5-HT.

Lysergic acid diethylamide (LSD) is a partial agonist at D 5-HT receptors.. The agonist activity may be relevant to its hallucinogenic properties (page 153).

Methysergide is an effective prophylactic in migraine (page 294). Its mechanism of action may involve inhibition of 5-HT-evoked local inflammatory response, although a selective vasoconstrictor effect on the dilated extracranial blood vessels plus a generalized increase in sensitivity of peripheral blood vessels to a variety of naturally occurring vasoactive compounds may also contribute. *Methysergide* also controls the increased intestinal motility but not the flushing (may be due to kinins, page 115, or prostaglandins) associated with carcinoid tumour. *Methysergide* is active orally. Side-effects are frequent (nausea, vomiting, diarrhoea, insomnia, nervousness, euphoria) and occasionally serious (peripheral vascular insufficiency, inflammatory fibroses).

Cyproheptadine is important only in so far as it shows pronounced and equal potency at both H_1 histamine and D 5-HT receptors. This is an obvious advantage in the treatment of various allergies, where both histamine and 5-HT might be involved. Cyproheptadine is given orally and side-effects are minor and similar to those of antagonists at H_1 histamine receptors (page 109).

PROSTAGLANDINS

Occurrence, biosynthesis and metabolism

The term prostaglandin (PG) is the generic name for a family of closely related cyclic, oxygenated, 20-carbon unsaturated fatty acids. The hypothetical basic 20-carbon skeleton of the prostaglandins has been given the name 'prostanoic acid'. On the basis of their structures the prostaglandins have been separated into six groups: A, B, C, D, E and F. All have in common a double bond at the 13, 14 position and an OH-group at C_{15}. In naming them the number of unsaturated carbon bonds is denoted by a subscript numeral and the subscript α or β denotes the orientation of an OH-group in position 9 below or above the molecular plane (*Figure 2.8*).

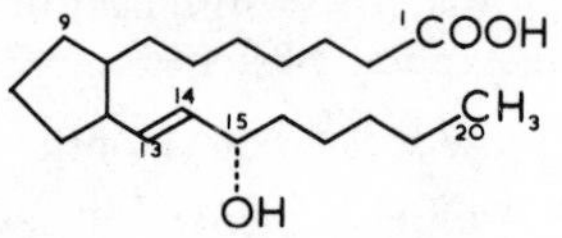

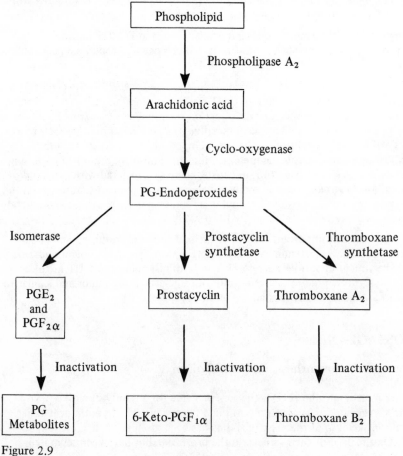

Figure 2.8

The prostaglandins are synthesized and released by virtually every tissue in the body. Since there is no evidence for storage of prostaglandins (except in the seminal fluid) the rate of release reflects that of biosynthesis. A wide variety of stimuli is capable of releasing prostaglandins.

It is believed that the substrates for prostaglandin biosynthesis are generated by the action of phospholipase A_2 on the phospholipid fraction of the cell membrane (*Figure 2.9*).

Figure 2.9

Released prostaglandin precursor (principally arachidonic acid) is acted on by an enzyme (cyclo-oxygenase) resulting in the formation of the prostaglandin endoperoxides. Non-steroidal anti-inflammatory agents such as *Aspirin* and *Indomethacin* act by inhibiting cyclo-oxygenase (page 118).

The endoperoxides are then converted to one or other of the prostaglandins. PGE_2 and $PGF_{2\alpha}$ are very rapidly metabolized in the kidneys, lungs and liver. A number of non-prostaglandin derivatives are also formed from the endoperoxides and these include thromboxane A_2 (synthesized predominantly by platelets) and prostacyclin (synthesized predominantly by heart, blood vessels and stomach). These are then broken down to the inactive metabolites thromboxane B_2 and 6-keto-$PGF_{1\alpha}$ respectively.

Role in physiology and pathophysiology

The prostaglandins are believed to be involved in many physiological processes, the most interesting being their possible involvement in reproductive physiology. In the male they have been implicated in erection, ejaculation, sperm motility and steroidogenesis, and in the female in uterine and Fallopian tube contractility, luteolysis (except human), ovulation, menstruation and labour (at term). There is good evidence that prostaglandins play a role in gastric secretion, maintenance of spontaneous smooth muscle tone and the control by −ve feedback of trans-mitter release at sympathetic nerve endings.

The prostaglandins have been implicated in many pathological processes, in particular the acute inflammatory response (page 117), fever (page 155) and various female reproductive disorders (dysmenorrhoea, anovulation, toxaemia of pregnancy, habitual abortion and premature labour). Their exact role in male infertility is undetermined.

Generation of prostacyclin by vessel walls could be the biochemical mechanism underlying their unique ability to resist platelet adhesion. A balance between formation of anti-aggregatory vasodilator substances (for example, prostacyclin) and pro-aggregatory vasoconstrictor substances (for example, thromboxane A_2) could contribute to the maintenance of the integrity of vascular endothelium and, when disturbed lead to formation of intra-arterial thrombi in certain pathophysiological conditions.

Actions of prostaglandins

Prostaglandins have many and varied pharmacological actions. *Table 2.16* summarizes the effects of the E and F prostaglandins.

Pharmacological and therapeutic exploitation

Clinical application is based on either mimicking physiological effects by exo-genous prostaglandins or, in pathological situations, preventing their synthesis.

The luteolytic and uterine smooth muscle stimulating properties of PGE_2 and $PGF_{2\alpha}$ form the basis of their use clinically. Both are currently marketed for use

Table 2.16

	Prostaglandin, for example, E_2	Prostaglandin, for example, $F_{2\alpha}$
BP	Decreases	Increases
Blood vessels	Dilates	Constricts
Capillary permeability	Increases	Little effect
Gastric secretion	Decreases	Little effect
Intestinal smooth muscle	Contracts*	Contracts
Bronchiolar smooth muscle	Relaxes	Contracts
Uterine smooth muscle	Contracts*	Contracts
Sensory fibres	Sensitizes*	?

* Generalization, the responses produced are often complex.

mainly in induction of labour and second trimester pregnancy termination. Side-effects are frequent but mild, and include nausea, vomiting, diarrhoea, flushing, shivering, headache and dizziness and when given iv, local tissue irritation and erythema. The use of more selective prostaglandin analogues, and in particular local application to the uterus, may help to overcome these side-effects. Another agent useful for the induction of labour (but not abortion) is *Oxytocin.* Combinations of prostaglandins and *Oxytocin* have been used successfully for induction of labour and abortion with a reduction in the incidence of side-effects due to the prostaglandin (a result of the lower dose now required).

One of the main objectives in prostaglandin research is to develop a selective luteolytic agent, sometimes referred to as the 'once-a-month' contraceptive tablet.

Inhibitors of prostaglandin synthesis are important clinically. *Aspirin* and similar drugs owe their anti-inflammatory properties and most probably their analgesic and antipyretic actions to inhibition of cyclo-oxygenase. These compounds are useful in relieving nausea, vomiting, diarrhoea, headache and uterine cramps, all symptoms of dysmenorrhoea thought to be due to hyperproduction of prostaglandins.

The clinical potential of drugs influencing thromboxane and prostacyclin metabolism is likely to be in atherosclerotic conditions associated with tendencies to thrombosis, in which platelet adhesion and aggregation are increased. Prostacyclin could be the prototype for the development of drugs which could more effectively combat the thrombi that lead to heart attack and stroke.

THE KININS

Occurrence, biosynthesis and metabolism

The kinins are bradykinin (a nonapeptide), kallidin (lysyl bradykinin, a decapeptide) and related vasodilator peptides. Bradykinin and kallidin are formed from the same circulating α_2 globulins (kininogens) by the action of specific proteolytic enzymes (kallikreins). Kallikreins are found in many organs and in urine, saliva, lymph, pancreatic secretions, blood, sweat and tears. Plasma kallikrein exists in the form of an inactive precursor (prekallikrein) but when plasma equilibrium is disturbed (change in pH, temperature or contact with water-insoluble materials), various activators (including Factor XII, the Hageman factor of blood clotting) convert it to its active form, with subsequent formation of kinins.

Kinins are rapidly destroyed in blood ($t_{1/2} < 1$ minute) by kininases (carboxypeptidases) which remove one or two amino acids from both bradykinin and kallidin to yield inactive peptides.

Role in physiology and pathophysiology

Kinins have been implicated in many physiological functions including functional and reactive hyperaemia, regulation of tissue blood flow, BP control and neonatal circulatory changes. They may be involved in various pathological states such as shock, allergy, inflammation, pancreatitis and the methysergide-resistant flushing and bronchoconstriction seen with carcinoid tumour.

Actions of kinins

The actions of bradykinin are typical of the vasodilator kinins.

On the cardiovascular system it has a potent relaxant effect on vascular smooth muscle (contrast angiotensin) causing a fall in systemic BP and a potent action in increasing capillary permeability (equipotent with PGE_1).

Bradykinin contracts the smooth muscle of the intestine, bronchioles and uterus and stimulates the adrenal medulla, sympathetic ganglia and sensory nerve endings (giving pain when applied to an exposed blister base).

No selective antagonist of bradykinin is available.

Pharmacological and therapeutic exploitation

Clinical studies suggest that kallikrein may be useful as an adjunct in the treatment of male infertility and in the treatment of diabetes (page 97).

The pharmacology of inflammation

Inflammation is an active defensive response of the body to injury of any kind. The inflammatory stimuli include infection with bacteria, viruses, rickettsiae, fungi or protozoa, infestation with helminths, chemical or physical trauma or antigen-antibody interaction. In acute inflammation, a succession of changes take place over a short period (minutes to days) which ends either by return of tissue to normal or by conversion to chronic inflammation. Chronic inflammation may last months or years and is characterized by periods of regression and repair which may be punctuated by further acute inflammatory changes.

THE INFLAMMATORY RESPONSE

General characteristics

An inflammatory stimulus to the skin results in the area becoming warm and red (increased blood flow), swollen (leakage of serum into the interstitial space due to increased protein permeability of microcirculatory vessel walls), and painful (stimulation of sensory pain fibres). Compare this situation with Lewis's triple response (page 107).

Emigration of leucocytes and phagocytosis

In the early stages of inflammation polymorphs aggregate along the inner margins of vessel (mainly venule) walls (margination), then pass through into tissues (emigration). At an inflamed site, polymorphs come within the chemotactic (= chemical attractive) orbit of living or dead bacteria (or tissues or plasma factors such as kinins or prostaglandins). Polymorphs move up the concentration gradient of the chemotactic stimulus and if not killed in the process, ingest the invading organisms or tissue debris (phagocytosis).

Repair and regeneration

When an inflammatory lesion subsides, vasodilatation diminishes and oedema disappears due to exuded fluid being reabsorbed into the lymphatics. Macrophages (monocytes and histiocytes) ingest dead polymorphs, bacteria and tissue debris.

When loss or destruction of tissues has occurred, new capillaries and fibroblasts grow into previously inflamed tissues. Collagen is laid down (fibrosis) and tissue becomes less vascular (granulation). Epithelium gradually extends over granulation tissue. Blood vessels, nerves and lymphatics grow into the repair tissue, more collagen is formed and fibres already laid down by fibroblasts shorten, drawing the edges of the wound together and forming a scar (cicatrix).

Chemical mediators

The following criteria should be satisfied by a putative endogenous chemical mediator of inflammation.

(1) It should be demonstrably present during the inflammatory reaction. The following have been demonstrated:

Release of histamine and 5-HT from mast cells and platelets.
Release of K^+ from all damaged cells.

116

Release of H^+ from hypoxic cells.
Formation of bradykinin and kallidin from kininogen.
Formation of prostaglandins from arachidonic acid.
Breakdown of lysosomes and activation of numerous enzymes including fibrinolysin, hyaluronidase and collagenase.

(2) It should produce effects which mimic one or more features of inflammation. The relevant effects of some putative chemical mediators are given in *Table 2.17.*

Table 2.17

Putative mediator	Oedema	Increased blood flow	Pain	Cell damage
Histamine	+	+	+	
5-HT	+	+	+	
Kinins	+	+	+	
Prostaglandins	+	+	+	
K^+			+	+
H^+			+	+

(3) Selective antagonists inhibiting one or more of its effects should inhibit similar components of the inflammatory reaction. Of the putative mediators, only specific antagonists for histamine and 5-HT are available. Antagonists at H_1 histamine receptors and those at D 5-HT receptors inhibit the inflammatory response but only during the first 30—60 minutes when these compounds are detectable in the exudate.

(4) Depletion of tissues of the postulated mediator, or inhibition of its means of production and release, should suppress appropriate components of the inflammatory reaction. Aspirin-like drugs inhibit cyclo-oxygenase *in vitro* and suppress the secondary phase of inflammation associated with prostaglandin presence in the exudate.

Thus, many of the features of inflammation can be explained by a combination of histamine with one or more of the other compounds observed to be present. Histamine (and 5-HT) are thought to be significant only during first 30—60 minutes of response. Prostaglandins and kinins are strong candidates for mediating the inflammatory response beyond 60 minutes.

ANTI-INFLAMMATORY DRUGS

These are compounds with the capacity to suppress the development of the local heat, redness and swelling associated with inflammation. Until recently, active drugs were discovered empirically by screening many hundreds of compounds in relatively crude animal tests. A few were found to be effective and marketed; the mechanisms of their actions were left to be worked out at some future date.

The analgesic — antipyretic group

This group includes *Aspirin* (acetylsalicylic acid) and other salicylates, *Indomethacin, Phenylbutazone,* mefenamic acid and ibuprofen. All are organic acids with affinity for plasma albumin binding sites. All relieve pain, reduce swelling and increase mobility in diseases such as acute rheumatic fever, osteo-arthritis and rheumatoid arthritis (page 317). They do not alter the course of the underlying disease.

Their anti-inflammatory action is due to suppression of prostaglandin formation by inhibiting cyclo-oxygenase. The order of potency to inhibit prostaglandin synthesis is: *Indomethacin* > *Phenylbutazone* > *Aspirin* > *Paracetamol* [acetaminophen].

Note that inhibition of cyclo-oxygenase may also explain the analgesic and anti-pyretic activity of the anti-inflammatory acids (page 155). The analgesic action of *Aspirin* involves both peripheral and central components. By preventing prostaglandin release in inflammation *Aspirin* will prevent the sensitization of the pain receptors to mechanical stimulation or to chemical mediators. This would also explain why *Aspirin* is less effective as an analgesic in uninflamed tissues.

Relative potencies as anti-inflammatory, analgesic or antipyretic agents may depend on susceptibility of different tissue cyclo-oxygenases to inhibition by these, drugs. Thus, in clinical concentrations *Aspirin* and *Indomethacin* inhibit cyclo-oxygenase in peripheral tissues and brain and each displays anti-inflammatory activity (a peripheral action) and antipyretic activity (a central action). *Paracetamol* inhibits only brain cyclo-oxygenase and whilst anti-pyretic has no anti-inflammatory activity.

Major toxic effects of aspirin and other salicylates are uncommon but minor toxic effects largely of gastrointestinal type are very common. Epigastric discomfort is common as is minor bleeding due to gastric erosion. With large doses excessive gastric bleeding is sometimes seen and in addition there may be ringing in the ears, dizziness, deafness, drowsiness and confusion. This syndrome is called salicylism and is similar to the pattern of toxicity produced by *Quinine*. Salicylates may also produce allergic disorders and may precipitate asthma in susceptible individuals. They may also produce renal damage manifest as increased urinary excretion of epithelial cells and leucocytes. The major toxic effects of large doses of salicylates are due to disturbances of respiration and acid-base balance. Respiration is stimulated and air hunger may develop. The overbreathing leads to a fall of the arterial PCO_2 and a respiratory alkalosis. Dehydration from vomiting, sweating and overbreathing is severe. Compensation occurs by bicarbonate loss in the urine so that plasma bicarbonate falls. In addition, lactic acid and ketoacids accumulate in the blood due to interference with normal carbohydrate and fat metabolism. *Aspirin* inhibits the formation of prothrombin, an effect which may result in haemorrhage and is reversible by injection of vitamin K. The excretion of uric acid is increased (a uricosuric effect) by inhibition of tubular reabsorption.

Paracetamol has no marked toxic effects on the gastrointestinal tract. It is there-fore a suitable alternative for patients sensitive to *Aspirin* who need an antipyretic or mild analgesic. However, *Paracetamol* may cause liver or kidney damage in high dosage.

118

Phenylbutazone (and *oxyphenbutazone*) is much more effective in rheumatoid arthritis and gout than salicylates but is a poorly tolerated drug with a wide range of toxic effects, notably gastrointestinal disorders, including peptic ulceration, hypersensitivity reactions and bone marrow disorders including fatal aplastic anaemia (page 315). It is usually reserved for cases that are unresponsive to other drugs and then used in short courses to reduce the risks.

Indomethacin has similar effects to *Phenylbutazone* and similar indications. It also produces severe gastrointestinal side-effects and vertigo but does not produce bone marrow depression.

Adrenocortical steroids and their synthetic analogues

This group includes *Hydrocortisone, Prednisolone, Prednisone, Dexamethasone, Betamethasone* and *Beclomethasone*. All supress initial and secondary characteristics of the inflammatory response including emigration of polymorphs, phagocytosis and the process of repair and regeneration. They are used to suppress inflammation in a wide variety of disease processes including systemic lupus erythematosus (autoimmune inflammation of skin and many other tissues); asthma (page 290), cranial arteritis, polyarteritis nodosa and some cases of rheumatoid arthritis (though chronic use is to be avoided, page 317). Their actions are palliative and the underlying cause of the lesion remains. Long term therapy holds many hazards (page 100).

Their mechanism of action is unknown but they do not inhibit cyclo-oxygenase. They may interfere with prostaglandin synthesis by decreasing the availability of substrate, stabilize lysosomal membranes thus preventing the liberation of lysosomal enzymes, one of which is phospholipase A_2, or induce the formation of an endogenous phospholipase A_2 inhibitor.

Penicillamine

This is useful for the removal (by chelation) of toxic metals (especially copper) from the body and in cystinuria (abnormal renal loss of cystine). It is a reserve drug for severe rheumatoid arthritis that has not responded to other treatments. Toxic effects are common and may be serious, such as renal tubular damage and thrombocytopenia.

Organic gold compounds

Sodium *Aurothiomalate* [gold sodium thiomalate] has long-lasting anti-inflammatory effects and is administered im at weekly intervals. These compounds are chiefly employed against the early stages of rheumatoid arthritis. Their mode of action is unknown but they are known to increase cross-linkages in collagen and inhibit lysosomal enzyme activity in inflammatory exudates. Toxic effects are frequent and include various skin reactions and, less commonly, thrombocytopenia, aplastic anaemia and hepatic and renal damage.

Chloroquine

This antimalarial (page 189) which may be indicated in those patients whose rheumatoid arthritis does not respond to the antipyretic analgesic drugs. The anti-inflammatory effect of *Chloroquine* may be brought about by inhibition of phospholipase A_2.

Despite this wide range of drugs the ideal anti-inflammatory and antirheumatic agent has yet to be discovered. The toxicity of these compounds in effective doses often leaves *Aspirin* as the mainstay of patient management.

Anticoagulant compounds

These are used: (1) to prevent the clotting of blood in extravascular situations, for example, blood samples, heart-lung machines, artificial kidneys; (2) in an attempt to prevent the formation of intravascular clots (thrombi).

Compounds also exist which may be used in an attempt to breakdown pre-existing intravascular clots.

The essential features of normal blood clotting are: (1) in response to certain triggers an inactive precursor prothrombin, normally present in the plasma, is converted to the enzyme thrombin; (2) this catalyses the conversion of the soluble protein fibrinogen to the insoluble polymer fibrin.

There are a number of theories dealing with the activation of prothrombin (cascade theory, thromboplastins, auto-prothrombins) and it is clear that Ca^{2+} and several 'factors' are involved. An initial stage involves contact with a foreign surface or tissue damage and the aggregation of platelets. It has been shown that thromboxanes encourage aggregation whilst prostacyclin inhibits aggregation (page 113).

THROMBUS FORMATION

Thrombi occur most commonly in the deep veins of the calf following surgery and bed rest when blood flow is sluggish and there may be changes in the blood, namely, elevated platelet count, increased stickiness of platelets and raised concentration of fibrinogen. Thrombus formation starts with the aggregation of platelets at the endothelium and filaments of fibrin are formed. Passing red cells become entangled and a solid mass (thrombus) is formed. Arterial thrombus formation shows some differences and typically occurs in a fast flowing circulation.

DRUG INTERFERENCE WITH COAGULATION OR THROMBUS FORMATION

There are a number of means by which compounds can affect coagulation.

Removal of calcium ions

In practice this method is restricted to *in vitro* application. Removal of Ca^{2+} inhibits several stages of the process. Ionized calcium can be removed by precipitation (as the insoluble fluoride, sulphate, oxalate) or by chelation (with sodium edetate). Blood for transfusion is often prevented from clotting by the use of citrate. A soluble complex is formed. Citrate has the advantage that it is metabolized in the Krebs' cycle.

Decreased platelet adhesiveness

Aggregation of platelets and their adhesion to the vessel wall is essential for clotting and thrombus formation. Dipyridamole, a smooth muscle relaxant originally developed to treat angina, exerts an anti-aggregating effect, possibly by potentiating endogenous prostacyclin. Prostacyclin prevents platelets clumping by increasing their cAMP concentration. It is suggested that Dipyridamole inhibits phosphodiesterase in the platelets.

Heparin

This occurs naturally in the body in granules of basophils and tissue mast cells, significant amounts can be extracted from connective tissue, liver and lungs. Heparin is a strongly acidic mucopolysaccharide, built up of sulphated glucosamine and glucuronic acid, with a high net −ve charge. The acidic groups are essential for activity and probably combine with basic groups in various clotting factors. The major action of *Heparin* is probably to prevent the formation of thrombin but the action of thrombin may also be reduced. The anticoagulant action requires the presence of heparin co-factor. This is a plasma α-globulin and may be identical with plasma antithrombin. The anticoagulant effects of *Heparin* are exerted both *in vivo* and *in vitro*. Despite the presence of heparin in the body and its anticoagulant activity there is no evidence that it plays any role in the physiological control of blood clotting.

Heparin is not absorbed orally and is therefore given by im or sc injection or continuous iv drip. It is metabolized in the liver by an enzyme known as heparinase. *Heparin* may be used *in vivo*, in extracorporeal circulations and to preserve blood samples.

The main danger associated with the use of *Heparin* is haemorrhage, especially if there are unsuspected lesions such as peptic ulcer. Transient alopecia may occur several months after use. Hypersensitivity and anaphylactic reactions are rare occurrences.

Antagonists to *Heparin*

Such a compound may be required in major haemorrhage resulting from heparin use (for minor bleeding cessation of administration is usually sufficient). *Protamine* sulphate is a simple, low MW protein which is strongly basic and combines with heparin forming a stable salt with no anticoagulant properties. It is given by slow iv injection, usually 1−1.5 times the dose of *Heparin* but the dose required declines with the time after *Heparin* administration. Because *Protamine* has some anticoagulant properties (inhibits thrombin/fibrinogen interaction), care must be taken not to exceed the amount required to neutralize *Heparin*.

The injection of *Protamine* may cause bradycardia, dyspnoea, flushing and a feeling of warmth but usually is not antigenic.

Oral anticoagulants

There are two groups of compounds each with essentially the same mechanisms and drawbacks. They are the coumarins, for example, *Warfarin* and nicoumalone [acenocoumarol] , and the indanediones, for examples, Phenindione. These compounds act by competing with vitamin K which is essential for the formation of prothrombin and Factors VII, IX and X. There is a delay in the onset of action as these factors must first be depleted. The action is exerted only *in vivo* and is affected by the vitamin K intake and the fat content of the diet (affects absorption of vitamin K).

Warfarin is completely absorbed after oral administration, is almost totally protein bound in the plasma and is metabolized in the liver. Its peak anticoagulant effect is exerted from 36 to 72 hours. The duration of this effect after withdrawing the drug is 4—5 days. Side-effects other than haemorrhage or interaction with other drugs (*see below* and page 265) rarely occur. Gastrointestinal upsets and cutaneous lesions have been reported.

The less widely used Phenindione is also completely absorbed after oral administration, is protein bound in the plasma and metabolized in the liver. Its peak effect is exerted from 24 to 48 hours and its duration is 1—4 days. Side-effects are more numerous and common including hypersensitivity reactions, renal damage, hepatitis and agranulocytosis. A product of the metabolism colours the urine red-orange which may alarm the patient.

Barbiturates and *Dichloralphenazone* may all reduce the anti-coagulant effects by inducing the metabolizing enzymes (page 265).

Aspirin causes a reduction in prothrombin concentration in the blood and may add to the effects of the oral anticoagulants. Gastric haemorrhage commonly produced by *Aspirin* may also cause problems in the presence of oral anticoagulants.

Phenylbutazone may increase the anticoagulant effects of coumarins by the inhibition of metabolism and displacement from protein binding.

Antagonists to the oral anticoagulants

Minor haemorrhages and excessively reduced prothrombin concentration respond to withdrawal of the drug. Some situations may need more rapid action, whole blood (containing the missing factors) or vitamin K (*Phytomenadione* [phytonadione]) may be given.

DISSOLUTION OF THROMBUS

In the normal clotting process *in vivo* the clot is finally broken down to fibrin degradation products by the action of fibrinolysin (plasmin); this is formed from an inactive precursor fibrinolysinogen (plasminogen) by an activator released in the clotting process. Activators of this mechanism may be used in an attempt to break down pre-existing thrombi. *Streptokinase* (from haemolytic Strepto-cocci) and urokinase (from urine) are both able to activate fibrinolysinogen. This procedure is most successful in dissolving fresh clots.

One danger associated with such attempts to dissolve clots is that fibrinogen and other factors may be used up in maintaining the clot with the resultant risk of haemorrhage. Should this occur inhibitors of fibrinolysin, *Aminocaproic* acid or *Tranexamic* acid may be used. Another danger associated with attempts at dissolution is the loosening of the clot from its site of attachment and subsequent movement through the circulation as an embolus.

3
Drug action on the central nervous system

INTRODUCTION

The brain has a multitude of functions and each of them involves an altered brain chemistry. Every thought, decision, perception and mood change is chemically (in its widest sense) mediated. In their simplest form the principles of drug action are the same as those described for the peripheral nervous system. Drugs affect these functions either by non-specifically modifying neuronal function (page 156) or by interfering with neurochemical transmission.

(1) Transmitters can be excitatory or inhibitory.
(2) Drugs act by mimicking or antagonizing neurotransmitters.
(3) Mimics may act directly (receptor agonists) or indirectly (releasing agents, uptake inhibitors, enzyme inhibitors).
(4) Antagonists may act directly (competitive and non-competitive receptor antagonists) or indirectly (preventing release, depleting transmitter stores).

In the CNS the situation is infinitely more complex for several reasons, including the following:

(1) The relative inaccessibility of some brain areas which hampers investigations.
(2) The number of neurones in the brain.
(3) Each neurone is in synaptic contact with thousands of other neurones.
(4) In addition to the two major transmitters of the periphery there are at least twenty other transmitters in the brain and, as in the periphery, each may be excitatory or inhibitory dependent on location.
(5) It is certain that transmitters can interact with several different receptors (as in the periphery) and likely that receptors exist in the brain which have no peripheral equivalent.
(6) Drug interaction with presynaptic receptors which then modulates the release of transmitters is a more frequent explanation of drug action in the brain than in the periphery.

To illustrate this, consider transmission between two brain areas X and Y (*Figure 3.1*).

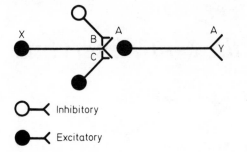

Inhibitory

Excitatory

Figure 3.1

Presynaptic excitatory and inhibitory neurones are shown. Three sites at which chemical transmission occurs are shown involving three different transmitters (A, B and C).

Assuming absolute selectivity of drug action and tonic activity in all pathways, the overall phenomenon of excitation at Y can be caused by mimics of transmitters A and C, or antagonists of B. Conversely, the phenomenon of inhibition at Y will be caused by a mimic of B, or by antagonists of A and C.

Accepting that the example is a massive over-simplification, and that most drugs interfere with more than one transmitter (for example, *Chlorpromazine*, page 140), some idea of the complexity emerges. Nevertheless, because there is a range of chemical transmitters in the brain which may be associated with certain brain areas (and therefore brain functions), and because some drugs have some selectivity of action, some degree of selective alteration of CNS activity is possible. Good examples are found in the pharmacology of Strychnine (page 128), *Levodopa* (page 131) and *Morphine* (page 143).

Chemical transmission in the CNS

AIMS

- To show how information on chemical transmission is gathered.
- To identify substances which are thought to be involved in chemical transmission processes and their status.
- To demonstrate the links between chemical transmission and nervous and mental diseases, thus putting drug action in the CNS on a rational basis.

INTRODUCTION

Proof of a chemical transmission process in the CNS is difficult to obtain; however, by analogy with the peripheral nervous system, chemical transmission in the CNS would be expected. Therefore, to understand drug action in the CNS it is necessary to identify the chemical transmitter with which the drug interacts.

CRITERIA FOR IDENTIFICATION OF A TRANSMITTER

(1) It must be present at the synapse.
(2) It should be stored in the presynaptic terminal.
(3) Processes for its synthesis should be present in the presynaptic neurone.
(4) It should be released on nerve stimulation.
(5) Postsynaptic application of the putative transmitter should mimic presynaptic stimulation.
(6) Processes for its inactivation should be present at the synapse.

Many techniques are required to determine whether these criteria are satisfied, including the following:

(1) Microelectrodes for recording from, or applying stimuli to, cells.
(2) Micropipettes either for application of putative transmitters or for removal of extracellular fluid for analysis.
(3) Biochemical and isotopic techniques for detection of transmitters or their precursors and metabolites.
(4) Histochemical fluorescence techniques for a more precise localization of putative amine transmitters.
(5) Immunological techniques for the localization of enzymes involved in transmitter synthesis and breakdown, or for identification of putative peptide transmitters.
(6) Lesion-making and neuroanatomy.

SUBSTANCES ACTING AS NEUROTRANSMITTERS

A large number of substances have been suggested to be chemical transmitters in the CNS, even though in many cases only a few of the above criteria have been satisfied, and in some cases the only evidence available is that the substance appears to be present in nerve terminals.

The substances most commonly quoted as having a neurotransmitter role include:

Amines

Most or all of the criteria have been fulfilled for ACh, NA, dopamine and 5-HT. Adrenaline-containing terminals have been inferred from immunofluorescence studies demonstrating the presence of the enzyme phenylethanolamine-N-methyl transferase. Histamine has also been considered for a neurotransmitter role on the basis of its regional localization, its disappearance after nerve tract lesions and its relatively high turnover rate.

Aminoacids

Glycine is believed to be the transmitter of the Renshaw cell and γ-aminobutyric acid (GABA) is also thought to be a neurotransmitter in various parts of the CNS, its presence in nerve terminals being inferred from the presence of its synthesizing enzyme glutamic acid decarboxylase. Glutamic acid and taurine are also contenders for a neurotransmitter role.

Peptides

The evidence for the peptides relies heavily on a combination of histological and immunofluorescence techniques. Candidate neurotransmitters include substance P, enkephalin, β-endorphin, angiotensin II, somatostatin and vasoactive intestinal polypeptide (VIP).

FUNCTIONAL SIGNIFICANCE OF NEUROTRANSMISSION

Examples will be given to illustrate the importance of understanding neurotransmission in the CNS when considering either drug action or disease processes.

The α-motoneurone—Renshaw cell circuit

A collateral of the α-motoneurone synapses with the Renshaw cell within the ventral horn of the spinal cord as demonstrated in *Figure 3.2.*

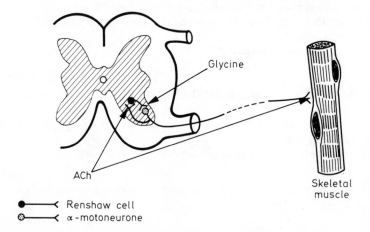

Figure 3.2 *The α-motoneurone-Renshaw cell circuit*

The collateral releases ACh which depolarizes the Renshaw cell (via nicotinic receptors). The induced Renshaw cell activity liberates glycine (an inhibitory transmitter) which causes hyperpolarization of the α-motoneurone cell body. Thus, this forms a —ve feedback loop, limiting activity in the α-motoneurone. Tetanus toxin prevents the release of glycine from the Renshaw cell, which explains the uncontrolled spasm of skeletal muscle seen after tetanus infection. Strychnine blocks the access of glycine to its receptors on the α-motoneurone, which explains why spasm of skeletal muscle is a feature of Strychnine poisoning.

The ascending monoamine tracts

Three ascending monoamine tracts have been identified in mammalian brain. Their cell bodies are located in specific areas of the midbrain and their axons transmit impulses to many brain areas (*Figures 3.3* and *3.4*).

128

The ascending nigrostriatal dopaminergic tract (*Figure 3.3*) plays an important role in the maintenance of gait and posture. Underactivity of this tract leads to a condition known as Parkinson's disease after the physician James Parkinson who first described it in 1817 (page 131).

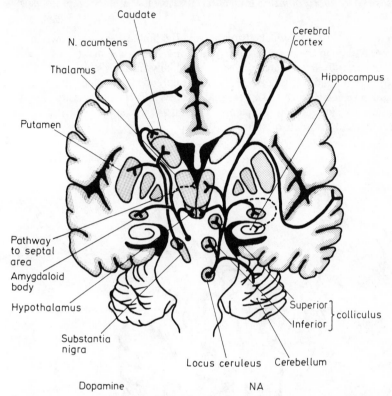

Figure 3.3 *Ascending dopaminergic and noradrenergic tracts; dopaminergic tracts only shown on left half of diagram, noradrenergic on right.*

The ascending NA and dopamine tracts to the limbic system are shown in *Figure 3.3.* The limbic system is a complex neuronal loop which connects the hippocampus, fornix bundle, mamillary body, thalamus, cingulate gyrus, septum and amygdala. The limbic system plays an important role in the regulation of mood. Thus, disorders of mood and behaviour are likely to have as their basis altered function of neurotransmitters in the limbic system. Many drugs which affect mood and behaviour can be shown to interact with either NA or dopamine. Empirically this has led to the monoamine theory of nervous and mental disease, which suggests that clinical depression is related to a functional monoamine deficiency, whilst mania and other behavioural excitations are related to a functional monoamine excess. At present it is not possible to define a separate role for any one of the monoamines in any one mental disorder. However, the theory receives support when the effects of drugs on the CNS are compared with their known mechanism of action. Thus, drugs which cause excitement are known to increase functional monoamine activity (*Cocaine* inhibits uptake of monoamines into nerve terminals, page 54, and therefore delays inactivation; Amphetamine releases stored monoamines from nerve terminals, page 48). Antidepressant drugs like *Imipramine* are also inhibitors of monoamine uptake. On the other hand, some drugs which cause sedation are known to decrease functional monoamine activity (*Reserpine* depletes neuronal stores, page 41), *Chlorpromazine* is an antagonist at monoamine receptors, page 140).

The ascending 5-HT tracts which also innervate the limbic areas are shown in *Figure 3.4.* Although the possible role of 5-HT in nervous and mental disorders has not been as fully investigated, it seems very likely that the monoamine theory of nervous and mental disease should be extended to include this amine also. There is some evidence to suggest that changes in 5-HT systems are closely linked to changes in sensitivity to painful stimuli, altered sexual behaviour, sleep patterns and disorders of appetite.

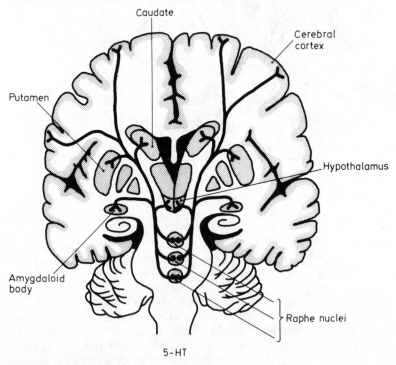

Figure 3.4 *Ascending 5 HT tracts*

It seems reasonable to suggest that many of the other transmitters listed on page 127 will also be implicated in disease processes within the CNS, but as yet sufficient evidence has not been collected to allow definitive statements to be made.

In the following sections the therapeutic significance of the interaction of drugs with these neurotransmitter systems will be discussed.

PARKINSON'S DISEASE

This disease provides a good example of a nervous disease which can be attributed to a defect in a central neurotransmitter system. It is also of interest because it demonstrates how investigations of chemical transmission processes in the CNS ultimately led to the development of a rational therapy for the disease.

Parkinson's disease is characterized by tremor and rigidity in skeletal muscle and akinesia (lit lack of movement — hypokinesia would be a more accurate description). When the disease is first recognized the symptoms and signs may be mild but the disease progresses and may ultimately lead to total incapacitation.

Before 1960 empirical medical treatment involved the use of anticholinergic drugs. These drugs were more effective against tremor than against rigidity and a high proportion of cases showed little or no improvement. Originally, *belladonna* (containing *Atropine*) was used but this was superseded by synthetic atropine derivatives such as *Benzhexol* and *Procyclidine.* Other drugs were developed from the antihistamines (*Benztropine, Orphenadrine*) but their efficacy in Parkinson's disease seems to correlate better with their antimuscarinic potency.

In 1960 a new therapy was introduced based on the dopaminergic nature of the nigrostriatal tracts in animals and the lack of dopamine in the striatum of brains taken from parkinsonian patients at autopsy. It was postulated that in Parkinson's disease there was a functional deficiency in neurotransmitter dopamine and that correction of that deficiency should lead to an improvement in the condition. Dopamine administration was of no use because it does not pass the blood brain barrier and has a very short $t_{1/2}$. Therefore, the precursor aminoacid *Levodopa* (L-DOPA) was used. This crosses the blood brain barrier and can be converted to dopamine within the brain by the enzyme aromatic L-aminoacid decarboxylase. *Levodopa* is now the drug of choice in the medical treatment of Parkinson's disease.

Three of the undesirable actions of *Levodopa* may also be explained in terms of overactivity in dopaminergic systems.

(1)   Vomiting — the chemosensitive trigger zone (CTZ) of the medullary vomiting centre (situated in the area postrema on the floor of the 4th ventricle close to the CO_2 sensing elements).

(2)   Involuntary muscle movements.

(3)   Some of the gastrointestinal disturbances which occur during *Levodopa* therapy may be peripheral in origin and related to the high doses required.

Some reduction in dosage may be obtained by combining *Levodopa* with an inhibitor of aromatic L-aminoacid decarboxylase which does not pass the blood brain barrier (for example, *carbidopa* and *benserazide*). In this case little of the *Levodopa* is metabolized in the periphery so that more is available for con- version to dopamine after penetrating the brain. Consequently lower oral doses are required.

Recently, dopaminergic drugs have been introduced which are not dopamine precursors but act as if they were agonists at dopamine receptors. Two such drugs are *Amantadine* and *bromocriptine*. Neither appears to be as effective as

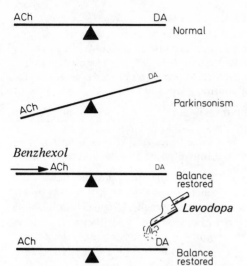

Figure 3.5 *The functional balance between ACh and dopamine (DA) in the striatum, the imbalance in Parkinsonism and its restoration by either antagonists at cholinoceptors or agonists at DA receptors*

Levodopa. In most cases of Parkinson's disease selected for medical treatment, **Levodopa** and an anticholinergic agent used together produce better results than either alone. This has led to the postulate that in the striatum there is a functional balance between ACh and dopamine neurotransmitters and that any change causing a decrease in the activity of dopamine relative to ACh (*Figure 3.5*) will produce the parkinsonian condition. The balance may be restored either by reducing functional ACh (for example, by atropine-like drugs) or by increasing dopamine (*Levodopa*).

Classification of mental disorders

Mental disorders involve disablement, considerable suffering and about 50 per cent of the hospital beds in the UK.

Until such time as the neurochemical classification of mental disease is possible, one based on the behaviour of patients must suffice. Such a psychiatric classification is as follows:

Psychosis

A major mental disorder characterized by derangement, loss of contact with reality and often delusions, illusions and hallucinations.

Organic (brain is abnormal at post-mortem examination)

Disturbance of consciousness, intellectual function and memory, ranging from clouding of consciousness, through delirium to dementia. Cause is brain damage

132

by injury, infection (for example, rabies), drug poisoning (for example, Ethanol, Pb) or old age.

Functional (brain is apparently normal at post-mortem examination)

Schizophrenia embodies a group of disorders characterized by retreat from reality, bizarre or regressive behaviour, auditory hallucinations and, commonly, delusions of grandeur or persecution (paranoia).

Manic-depressive psychosis is characterized by sustained phases of either excitement (hypomania, mania) or, more commonly, endogenous depression.

Neurosis

A relatively minor mental disorder due to unresolved conflicts causing exaggerations of normal mood or behaviour.

(1)   Anxiety neurosis. Unnecessary, easily provoked or persistent anxiety.
(2)   Neurotic (reactive) depression. Depression as a response to stress or problems (for example, bereavement, cf endogenous depression).
(3)   Hysteria. The use of symptoms to serve a personal purpose without awareness of motives for so doing (cf malingering).
(4)   Obsessional neurosis. Repeated and involuntary intrusion into the mind of thoughts or impulses.

The problem with such a classification is that symptoms characteristic of a particular disease may also be apparent in other disorders. In this way anxiety and depression are common to many psychiatric conditions.

It is assumed that functional mental disorders are associated with biochemical imbalances, though in no disorder is the imbalance currently understood. It is likely that the biochemical imbalances of schizophrenia and of depression will soon be established.

Drugs alleviate mental disorders by restoring the biochemical equilibrium, thus enabling the patient to surmount the effects; they rarely remove the cause.

Screening for new drugs

Animal studies with psychotropic and other centrally acting drugs have two aims: (1) to discover new drugs likely to be of help in treating disorders; (2) to learn more about mechanisms of drug action in an attempt to understand the biochemical correlates of mental disorders.

The tests may be either biochemical or behavioural.

Biochemical tests may give an idea of the mechanism of action and may provide a clue to the basis of the disorder, but they are complicated by the fact that drugs possess a variety of properties.

Behavioural tests in animals are empirical in nature and at best can only provide a rough guide to the type of drug under investigation. However, once the drug type has been established, the same test may give a reliable indication of relative potency in a series of related compounds. The different members of one drug group do have a common pattern of activity in a battery of screening tests, so such batteries can be used to predict membership of existing drug groups. Note, however, that almost all major advances in treatment were discovered accidentally, when a drug's 'side-effect' turned out to be more valuable than the originally planned therapeutic action.

It is not possible to produce accurate models of human mental illness in animals. However, by manipulation of the animal's environment it is possible to produce behavioural changes on which the effects of drugs can be studied. Such tests can be used in an attempt to predict therapeutic potential or to detect unwanted behavioural effects of drugs.

Behavioural tests rely on observing the effects of drugs on both basic and more complex animal behaviour. Basic functions of animal behaviour are motor activity, coordination (ability to stay on a rotating rod), exploratory and curiosity drives (simple maze, exploration of holes in a board).

More complex functions are learning, memory and emotionality which require tests including complex mazes with in-built reward (for example, food) or punishment (a mild noxious stimulus, for example, electric shock), systems for inducing anxiety (large brightly illuminated arena), conditioned behaviour in which the animals learn to respond to a standard stimulus such as a ringing bell either to obtain a reward or to avoid a punishment.

Note particularly that many measurements must be indirect, for example, anxiety can only be measured as an inhibition of some complex task. A detailed discussion of the use of these various behavioural tests is outside the scope of this book. However, summaries of the effects of three drugs (one each from the important psychotropic groups) are included on page 135, 140 and 163 to illustrate how the tests may be used to differentiate between them.

Antidepressants

DEPRESSIVE ILLNESS

The differences between endogenous and reactive depression, the complex clinical picture and lack of uniformity in classification, combine to make accurate assessment of drug treatment difficult. Following diagnosis, treatment may involve psychotherapy, family therapy, electroconvulsive therapy or drugs either alone or in combination.

Antidepressants may be divided into two groups as follows:

TRICYCLIC ANTIDEPRESSANTS

These have a chemical structure consisting of three fused rings (*Figure 3.6*). More recent developments include bicyclic and quadricyclic drugs.

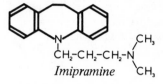

Figure 3.6 *A tricyclic antidepressant, imipramine*

Imipramine and amitriptyline

Imipramine and *Amitriptyline* have similar pharmacological profiles and will be considered together.

Mechanism of action

Both drugs inhibit the active uptake process which is responsible for the inactivation of neuronally released NA (page 53) and this property may be relevant to antidepressant action. However, these compounds have other pharmacological properties (for example, antagonist at muscarinic cholinoceptors, page 33) and can also inhibit uptake of other monoamines (for example, 5-HT). It is not possible at present to define the property most important for antidepressant activity.

CNS effects

An antidepressant drug might be expected to have a stimulating or mood-elevating effect in normal subjects but this is not so in the case of tricyclic antidepressants. One dose of 100 mg of *Imipramine* orally causes sleepiness, lightheadedness and sensations usually described as unpleasant in normal subjects. Repeating the dose increases the effect. In contrast, repeated dosage in a depressed patient results in mood elevation. The antidepressant response is not immediate but develops over 2—3 weeks of treatment. Depressed patients suffer from a characteristic early waking insomnia relieved by antidepressant drugs. Antidepressants diminish paradoxical sleep (page 157) and are not useful hypnotics in normal subjects.

At first sight *Imipramine* has a paradoxical effect in the experimental animal — it does not have excitatory effects. In fact it reduces locomotor activity (contrast with CNS stimulants like Amphetamine) and it increases barbiturate hypnosis. *Imipramine* also reduces exploratory activity in simple mazes and suppresses conditioned avoidance responses. Thus, these tests would not separate *Imipramine* from any group of drugs with sedative properties and therefore more specialized models have been developed which indirectly measure potentiation of endogenous monoamines. Unfortunately these tests (for example, prevention of *Reserpine* sedation) are relatively non-specific and give many false positives.

Peripheral effects

The tricyclic antidepressants have marked antimuscarinic actions and the most important consequences as far as the patient is concerned are: blurring of vision and precipitation of glaucoma in susceptible subjects, dry mouth, constipation and urinary retention. Tachycardia may also occur in part due to the anti-cholinergic effects and in part due to potentiation of NA.

Cardiovascular effects

A number of deaths have occurred during antidepressant therapy related to their cardiovascular actions. There is an increased incidence of cardiac arrythmias in patients taking tricyclic antidepressants and it has also been claimed that this group may precipitate congestive heart failure. Orthostatic hypotension also occurs with doses in the therapeutic range. This effect subsides with continued therapy. Two recently introduced antidepressants, viloxazine, a bicyclic drug, and mianserin, a quadricyclic drug, are less likely to cause cardiovascular problems.

Other side-effects

The most frequent problems are related to the cardiovascular and antimuscarinic actions. Other side-effects include tremor, headache.

Therapeutic uses

Apart from their antidepressant actions the tricyclic antidepressants (particularly *Amitriptyline*) have also been useful in treating nocturnal enuresis (bed wetting) in children. However, there have recently been warnings against the use of the tricyclic anti-depressants in very young patients and non-drug measures are preferred.

MONOAMINE OXIDASE INHIBITORS

It is by no means certain that the antidepressant actions of these compounds rely on their ability to inhibit MAO. Two MAO inhibitors will be discussed — *Phenelzine* and Tranylcypromine though they are not now widely prescribed (page 298).

Mechanism of action

These drugs inhibit MAO enzymes, including those enzymes in liver, sympathetic nerves and the monoamine neurones in the brain. When neuronal MAO is inhibited the intracellular monoamine concentration rises until the concentration achieved causes product inhibition of the synthetic pathway. Several amine oxidase enzymes exist and *Phenelzine* and Tranylcypromine are capable of inhibiting these various types which explains why they potentiate many drugs from a variety of pharmacological groups.

CNS effects

A single dose of *Phenelzine* produces little if any change in animal behaviour. After an injection of Tranylcypromine there is evidence of CNS stimulation with increased locomotor activity and an increased response to stimuli (for example, an exaggerated response to handling). These effects are similar to those of Amphetamine (page 151) and are probably due to the amphetamine-like structure of Tranylcypromine. A test commonly employed to predict antidepressant activity is the effect of a drug in a reserpinized animal. *Reserpine* causes sedation, reduced locomotor activity and hypothermia. The ability of drugs to either prevent or offset these effects is taken as an indication of therapeutic potential. There is a difference in the response to *Phenelzine* and Tranylcypromine in this model. Both drugs will prevent or delay the response to a subsequent dose of *Reserpine.* However, whereas Tranylcypromine will offset established *Reserpine* effects *Phenelzine* will not. This difference can be explained in the following way.

Reserpine acts on intraneuronal monoamine storage vesicles to cause accumulation of monoamines in the cytoplasm (*Figure 3.7a*), where mitochondrial MAO converts the amines to their inactive acid metabolites (page 52). The loss of central monoamines is manifest in sedation, loss of locomotor activity and hypothermia. Prior injection of an MAO inhibitor (*Figure 3.7b*) prevents the inactivation of the cytoplasmic monoamines so that the effects of *Reserpine* are prevented. However, if *Reserpine* is given first then the inactivation of the amines has already taken place and inhibition of MAO is ineffective in preventing the depletion. *Phenelzine,* therefore, will not offset an established *Reserpine* syndrome (*Figure 3.7c*). However, after reserpinization there is still a small residual pool of cytoplasmic monoamines and by its amphetamine-like properties Tranylcypromine can cause release from this pool and thus offset the effects of *Reserpine.*

MAO inhibitors elevate the mood of depressed patients and, like the tricyclic group, these effects do not appear immediately, requiring several weeks of treatment. Although MAO inhibitors suppress paradoxical sleep, they alleviate the sleep problem associated with depression.

Cardiovascular effects

MAO inhibitors cause postural hypotension. The mechanism is unclear but is probably peripheral and involves a decreased release of NA.

Side-effects

Acute overdosage may cause excitement, hallucinations, pyrexia and convulsions. Chronic toxicity includes: hepatotoxicity which does not seem to be simply related to dose or duration of treatment; excessive CNS stimulation which manifests itself as hypomania, tremor, insomnia and in some instances convulsions; orthostatic hypotension.

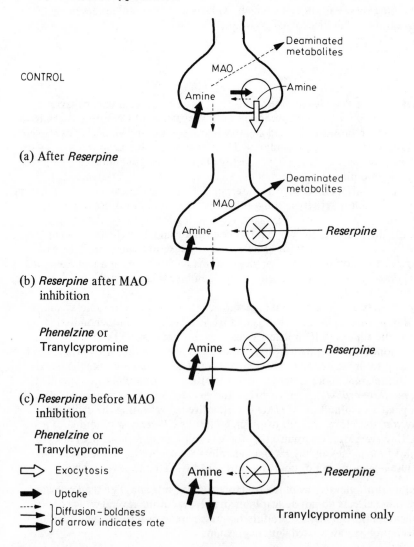

CONTROL

(a) After *Reserpine*

(b) *Reserpine* after MAO inhibition

    Phenelzine or Tranylcypromine

(c) *Reserpine* before MAO inhibition

    Phenelzine or Tranylcypromine

⇨ Exocytosis

➡ Uptake

⇢ } Diffusion–boldness of arrow indicates rate

Tranylcypromine only

Figure 3.7

An important problem is the change produced in the response to exogenous substances present in food or administered as drugs (pages 53 and 298). The potentiation of tyramine in foodstuffs is the best publicized effect where, because of the inhibition of gut and liver MAO, dietary tyramine is not

138

inactivated and achieves a high concentration in plasma. Tyramine is an indirectly acting sympathomimetic (page 48) and in high concentrations can provoke a hypertensive crisis.

Therapeutic uses

The primary use of *Phenelzine* and Tranylcypromine is in the treatment of depression. They have also been useful in narcolepsy and occasionally in hypertension.

Neuroleptics

Neuroleptic (mood regulating) drugs are useful in the treatment of psychoses and may be referred to as major tranquillizers or ataractic (lit not disturbed) drugs.

RESERPINE

Reserpine has a depressant action on the brain producing tranquillization. Psychotic patients receiving *Reserpine* become more relaxed, sociable and cooperative. They show indifference to environmental events and a tendency to sleep, but are easily aroused. The tranquillizing effect of *Reserpine* has been exploited clinically but is now seldom used because of unwanted effects.

Mechanism of action

Depletion of monoamines (page 41) in the brain is thought to be the basis for the neuroleptic action of *Reserpine.*

Unwanted effects

Lethargy, nightmares, mental confusion, vertigo, severe depression and suicidal tendencies can result from depletion of central monoamines. *Reserpine* depletes peripheral stores of monoamines allowing parasympathomimetic activity to dominate, for example, diarrhoea.

The decline in usage of *Reserpine* as a neuroleptic agent was accelerated by the introduction of drugs more closely approximating to an ideal neuroleptic, which abolish pyschoses without clouding consciousness. These drugs belong to several different chemical groups.

PHENOTHIAZINES

Phenothiazine has a tricyclic structure (*Figure 3.8*) and is the nucleus of numerous derivatives with neuroleptic activity, for example, *Chlorpromazine*.

THIOXANTHENES

Substitution of the N in position 10 of phenothiazine (*Figure 3.8*) by C produces thioxanthene. Some derivatives of thioxanthene have neuroleptic activity similar to that of *Chlorpromazine*, for example, flupenthixol.

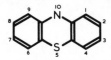

Figure 3.8 *The phenothiazine nucleus*

BUTYROPHENONES

Butyrophenones are tricyclic compounds but are unrelated chemically to either phenothiazine or thioxanthene. Some butyrophenones have neuroleptic activity similar to that of *Chlorpromazine*, for example, *Haloperidol.*

NEUROLEPTIC ACTIVITY

Phenothiazines, thioxanthenes and butyrophenones produce qualitatively similar effects on mood and behaviour, differing only in potency. Butyrophenones are generally most potent, *Haloperidol* is about 200 times more active than *Chlorpromazine*.

These drugs exert a relatively selective depressant effect on conditioned responses. In man, they reduce defensive hostility, attention and emotional responses. Intellectual activities are not altered appreciably. The most obvious effect of *Chlorpromazine* is a dose-related depression of behaviour. With low doses there is a taming effect in aggressive animals. As the dose is increased there is reduced locomotor activity and at high doses the animals become immobile and catatonic. In the catatonic state the animal has increased muscle tone and will maintain an abnormal posture imposed on it by the experimenter. Induction of catatonia distinguishes *Chlorpromazine* from the non-specific depressants (page 156) and the anxiolytics (page 163). It is also possible to demonstrate inhibition of conditioned behaviour (for example, escape behaviour in response to a bell) with doses too low to modify an unconditioned response (such as escape behaviour in response to mild noxious stimuli). This again is in contrast to the effects of non-specific depressants with which both conditioned and unconditioned responses are similary affected.

These neuroleptics are the drugs of choice in the treatment of both functional and organic psychoses, notably the schizophrenias. Neuroleptics are also effective antagonists of the centrally acting sympathomimetics and the hallucinosis produced by mescaline, LSD and similar compounds.

MECHANISM OF NEUROLEPTIC ACTION

The similar effects of chemically different neuroleptics on behaviour and mood is ascribed to their common ability to block dopamine receptors in the limbic

140

system, a part of the brain controlling emotion, behaviour and mood. This property suggests that psychoses are manifestations of excess dopaminergic activity in the limbic system. Such an abnormality has not yet been substantiated independently.

OTHER EFFECTS DUE TO DOPAMINE ANTAGONISM

Blockade of dopamine receptors in the brain by neuroleptics is not restricted to the limbic system.

Antagonism of dopamine in the caudate and putamen causes rigidity and tremor of skeletal muscle (page 131, *Figure 3.9*). These extrapyramidal motor effects are most prominent with butyrophenones, for example, *Haloperidol* and phenothiazines with a piperazine group at position 10 in the nucleus (*Figure 3.8*), for example, *Fluphenazine, Prochlorperazine, Trifluoperazine*.

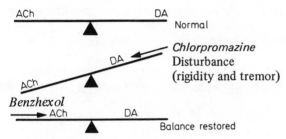

Figure 3.9 *Functional balance between ACh and dopamine (DA) in the striatum, its disturbance by neuroleptics (for example,* chlorpromazine*) and its correction by antagonists at muscarinic cholinoceptors (for example benzhexol); c.f. Figure 3.5*

Centrally acting anticholinergic agents such as *Benzhexol* which relieve Parkinson's disease (page 131) reduce neuroleptic-induced motor effects. Tranquillization with a piperidine-substituted phenothiazine, for example, thioridazine, may be preferable therapy because this type has a low incidence of extrapyramidal motor disturbances. This is attributable to the ratio of anticholinergic : antidopaminergic activity being greater in piperidine phenothiazines than in other neuroleptics.

Nausea and vomiting induced by **Apomorphine**, an agonist at dopamine receptors, acting on the CTZ in the brain stem medulla is prevented by *Chlorpromazine*. *Chlorpromazine* is effective against vomiting caused by other drugs acting directly on the CTZ, for example, *Morphine* and vomiting occurring post-operatively (page 301). *Chlorpromazine* is less effective against vomiting produced by vestibular stimulation, as in motion sickness, than phenothiazines with greater anticholinergic activity.

Neuroleptics antagonize dopamine-mediated inhibition of prolactin release from the anterior pituitary gland and may cause an excess flow of milk (galactorrhoea, page 75).

Blockade of dopamine receptors in the hypothalamus may be responsible for the fall in body temperature caused by *Chlorpromazine* and similar drugs.

EFFECTS NOT DUE TO DOPAMINE ANTAGONISM

Neuroleptic drugs can block central and peripheral receptors other than those for dopamine. Receptors that may be affected include those for ACh (muscarinic), catecholamines (α-adrenoceptors) and histamine (H_1). Blockade of non-dopamine receptors is most marked with phenothiazines and least with butyrophenones.

Clinically useful effects

Numerous effects can result from neuroleptic blockade of non-dopamine receptors, some of these are clinically useful, including the following:

(1)   The anticholinergic activity in alleviating motion sickness (*Prochlorperazine, Promethazine*).
(2)   The antihistamine activity in alleviating allergic reactions (*Promethazine, Trimeprazine*).
(3)   The sedative activity in suppressing restlessness caused by mental disturbances or alleviating itching (pruritus) associated with jaundice (*Promethazine, Trimeprazine*).
(4)   The potentiating effect on the action of other central depressants particularly narcotic analgesics (*Chlorpromazine*).

Unwanted effects

Some effects resulting from blockade of non-dopamine receptors are unwanted, for example, on the cardiovascular system (orthostatic hypotension), the gastro-intestinal tract (constipation) and the eye (blurring of vision).

Sensitization reactions to phenothiazines occur as blood dyscrasias, cholestatic jaundice and skin rashes.

CHOICE OF NEUROLEPTIC

There is no convincing evidence that combinations of neuroleptics are more beneficial than one drug alone. The choice of drug depends on the acceptability of a particular unwanted effect in individual patients. The differing abilities of neuroleptics to induce extrapyramidal motor effects (page 141) and autonomic disturbances (*see above*) have been noted. Outpatient treatment of psychotic or agitated patients who may not take their tablets regularly is facilitated by the use of long-acting preparations, for example, *Fluphenazine decanoate* despite the common occurrence of extrapyramidal motor effects with piperazine-substituted phenothiazines.

Narcotic analgesics and their antagonists

All are structurally related to *Morphine*, the most important of the alkaloids extracted from the latex of the opium poppy (*Papaver somniferum*). They are termed narcotic analgesics because in addition to relieving pain they also cause narcosis – a state of stupor and insensibility. They are also called opiates (derived from opium) or opioids (acting like opium).

They produce their effects by interacting with receptors for the peptide neuro-transmitters, enkephalins and endorphins.

ENKEPHALINS AND ENDORPHINS

The term enkephalin refers to two similar pentapeptides differing in one terminal aminoacid. The term endorphin usually refers to larger fragments of the anterior pituitary hormone β-lipotropin but sometimes to any endogenous peptide possessing *Morphine*-like activity.

Enkephalins

The aminoacid sequences of the two enkephalins are:
     Tyr-Gly-Gly-Phe-Met   =   met-enkephalin
     Tyr-Gly-Gly-Phe-Leu   =   leu-enkephalin

Highest concentrations are found in the striatum and limbic system, moderate concentrations are found in the brain stem (pons and medulla) and low concentrations in the cerebellum and cortex. They have been identified in the periphery (for example, gastrointestinal tract).

They have been identified as neuronal in origin and they fulfil most of the criteria for neurotransmitter function. Since they were only identified in 1975, knowledge of their pharmacological actions and physiological role is sparse. Some speculation appears on page 144.

Endorphins

β-Lipotropin is a pituitary hormone consisting of 91 aminoacids. It is a fragment of the ACTH-endorphin prohormone (MW 31,000). Sequence 61–65 of β-lipotropin corresponds to metenkephalin, aminoacid 61 being the tyrosine residue. Fragments commencing at residue 61 possess *morphine*-like activity, the most important being:

α-endorphin	sequence 61–76
β-endorphin (C-fragment)	sequence 61–91
γ-endorphin	sequence 61–77
C′ fragment	sequence 61–87

Though the endorphins are primarily pituitary in origin, some have been identified in neurones of the thalamus and hypothalamus. They have not been identified in the periphery. It is anticipated that other peptides possessing opioid activity await identification, notably a precursor of leu-enkephalin.

Pharmacological action and physiological role

Structural correlations

Figure 3.10 compares the structures of *Morphine* and the enkephalins. The terminal tyrosine of enkephalin corresponds to the phenol group of *Morphine*, the amino groups are held in the same spatial plane.

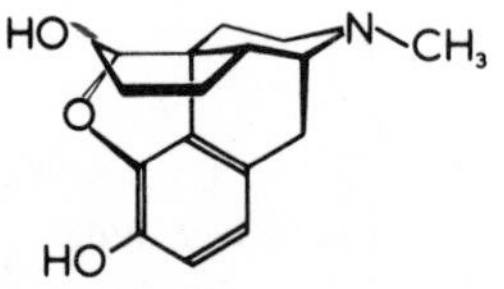

Morphine

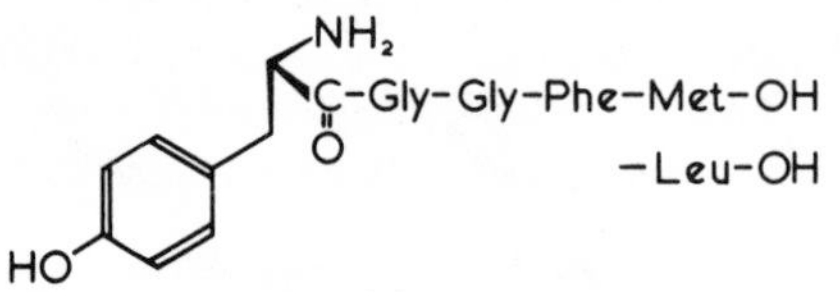

Enkephalins

Figure 3.10

Peripheral models

Instrumental in the discovery of these peptide transmitters and current research into their physiological role has been the existence of at least two peripheral neuroeffector junctions at which opiates and endorphins inhibit transmitter release. These are the guinea-pig ileum and mouse vas deferens (transmitters being ACh and NA respectively). These two sites have been extensively used as models of central mechanism of action since potency ratios between agonists are the same as those for analgesic activity in man, as are agonist/antagonist ratios. It is known that in the CNS the opioids/transmitters also act presynaptically by inhibition of transmitter release (though not necessarily of ACh or NA).

Pharmacological actions

These are similar to those of *Morphine*. They possess analgesic and respiratory depressant activities, have similar effects on single brain neurones to *Morphine* and in most instances *Naloxone* is an effective antagonist.

Tolerance develops to them and there is cross-tolerance with narcotic agonists. Their durations of actions vary from the enkephalins (a few minutes), through the derivatives of β-lipotropin (similar to *Morphine*), to synthetic peptides rendered resistant to peptidases (several hours).

Physiological role   This is unclear; no satisfactory explanation currently exists as to why — if they possess a physiological role — the injection of their antagonist (*Naloxone*) should do little. There is also the paradox of their addictive nature.

144

Current interest is centred on the following:

(1) *Naloxone*'s actions in the absence of exogenous opiates. The most promising areas are *Naloxone*'s ability to antagonize analgesia produced by electrical stimulation of certain brain areas, acupuncture, stress, pain or placebo. All imply an involvement of enkephalins or endorphins.

(2) Endorphins and mental disorders. Both *Naloxone* and some derivatives of β-lipotropin (particularly the non-opioid des-Tyr-γ-endorphin) have been shown to be effective in some types of schizophrenia. A role of endorphins in hypothalamic control of appetite has also been postulated.

(3) Interactions with other pituitary hormones. Many interactions are likely; that with prolactin is most extensively studied.

OPIOID RECEPTORS

Most work has measured specific binding sites and these may not be synonymous with receptors that have pharmacological let alone physiological function. The highest density of binding sites is in components of the limbic system (page 129) and hypothalamus, then in descending order, basal ganglia, spinal cord and lower medulla. This distribution is not quite the same as that of the enkephalins. More than one type of opioid receptor exists. That for the classical addictive analgesics has been designated μ (*Morphine*), that for the non-addictive analgesics κ (keto-cyclazocine).

THE NARCOTIC ANALGESICS

Derivatives of *Morphine* can possess two types of activity: (1) they can act as agonists causing the well-known effects of analgesia, respiratory depression, cough suppression, vomiting and constipation; (2) they can act as selective inhibitors of the effects exerted by the opioid agonists.

Some derivatives (for example, *Morphine*) are termed 'pure' agonists, whilst others are pure antagonists (*Naloxone*). All other derivatives fall between these two extremes and the spectrum of activity is summarized in *Figure 3.11*.

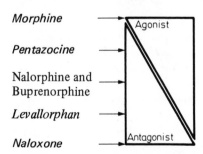

Figure 3.11 *Relative opioid activities*

Note *Pentazocine* and buprenorphine which possess both agonist and antagonist activities. These are the partial agonists sometimes referred to as 'narcotic antagonist analgesics'.

Agonist actions are both central and peripheral.

Central agonist actions

The narcotic analgesics have selective depressant and excitatory actions on centres throughout the CNS. The depressant actions include analgesia, sedation, anaesthesia, respiratory depression and cough suppression. Excitatory actions (which may be due to depression of inhibition or to direct stimulation) are hallucinations, convulsions, ADH release, miosis and vomiting. The narcotic analgesics also cause euphoria.

Whether the net effect is excitation or depression depends on the drug and the species. *Pethidine* is more likely to cause convulsions than is *Morphine* whilst *Methadone* will cause less sedation than *Morphine* in man. *Morphine* is sedative in man but convulsant in cats.

In man the overall effect of any opioid is usually depressant.

Individual actions

Analgesia

Analgesia is produced both by effect on the pain pathways (pain threshold) and on the reaction to the stimulus (pain tolerance). The latter is associated with the drug's euphoriant action. A patient will state that the pain is still perceived but that it does not matter so much.

The narcotics are more effective against dull constant pain, though sharp stinging pain can be reduced. This suggests some selectivity of action on one of the two major pain pathways.

Their analgesic action is enhanced by salicylates (summation) and neuroleptic drugs (unknown mechanism) but reduced by barbiturates. The individual drugs differ in the following ways:

Ratio of excitation to depression Excitatory manifestations (*see above*) are more likely to follow administration of *Pethidine, Codeine* derivatives, or some partial agonists.

Maximum analgesic activity Diamorphine (heroin) has the greatest analgesic activity, then in descending order *Morphine* (and *Methadone*, dipipanone, dextromoramide, levorphanol, phenazocine), *Pethidine, Dihydrocodeine, Codeine* and dextropropoxyphene [propoxyphene].

Oral versus parenteral efficacy This is a function of lipid solubility. Note that *Morphine* (*Figure 3.12*) has two hydroxyl groups and is relatively insoluble in lipid and therefore shows poor oral efficacy, whilst *Pethidine* is less polar and is effective orally.

Duration of action Diamorphine and fentanyl are short acting, most others act for longer than these.

Incidence of undesirable side-effects at satisfactory analgesic doses Sedation may or may not be clinically undesirable. Vomiting is always undesirable in an analgesic. *Codeine* is capable of causing the same degree of analgesia as 10 mg *Morphine* (im) but this would be accompanied by excessive vomiting.

146

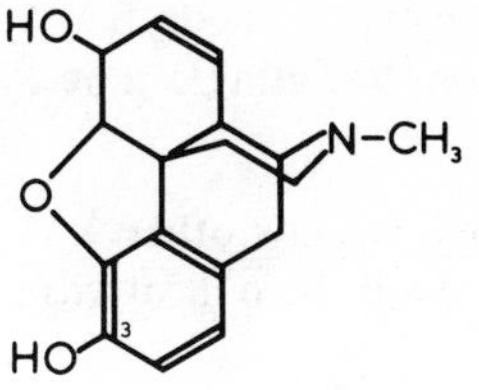

Morphine

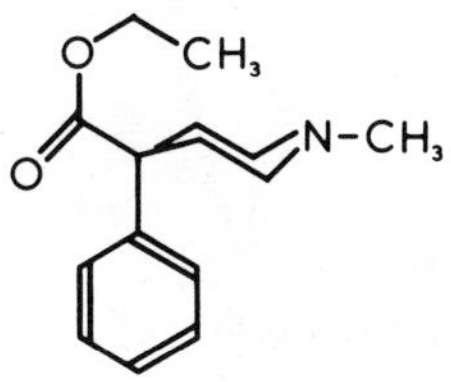

Pethidine

Figure 3.12

Respiratory depression

Analgesia caused by any opioid will be accompanied by depression of respiratory rate (changes in tidal volume may be variable). There is an increase in the threshold of the medullary centres to the excitatory effects of CO_2. Arterial PCO_2 rises. The resultant periodic breathing is characteristic of narcotic poisoning.

Whilst respiratory depression is the cause of death in *Morphine* poisoning, man can tolerate the consequences of severe respiratory depression when caused by an opioid since it can occur without cardiovascular depression. This contrasts with that caused by some non-specific depressants (barbiturates) when vasomotor depression and hypotension accompany hypoventilation.

Cough suppression

The derivatives of *Morphine* are the only clinically useful drugs which depress the cough centre (situated in the medulla near the respiratory centres). Some derivatives of *Morphine* possess greater antitussive activity relative to analgesic activity. Quantitative separation is seen in derivatives with bulky substituents at position 3 (*Figure 3.12*), hence, *Codeine* and Pholcodine which are effective antitussives at sub-analgesic doses. Qualitative separation has also been achieved. Only those stereoisomers equivalent to D-*Morphine* possess narcotic-like activity (generally these are l-rotatory, though there are some exceptions). Dextromethorphan possesses no analgesic or respiratory depressant activity yet retains antitussive activity. It is equipotent with *Codeine.*

Emetic action

All the derivatives of *Morphine* can cause vomiting. The mechanism is by stimulation of the CTZ. Vomiting can be especially troublesome if the patient is ambulatory. Subsequently, opioids can depress the vomiting centre. Thus, if vomiting is going to occur it will happen soon after injection. Vomiting can be controlled with neuroleptic drugs.

Selectivity of emetic action is seen with Apomorphine which has few other Morphine-like actions. Apomorphine is known to be a mimic of the neurotransmitter dopamine (page 141).

Miotic action

All the derivatives stimulate the oculomotor centre and cause pupillary constriction (parasympathetic innervation). They may complicate the use of pupil size as an index of depth of anaesthesia (page 160), though it is a useful sign of opiate poisoning. Tolerance to this excitatory action occurs slowly; thus, miosis is still present in addicts.

Peripheral agonist actions

Gastrointestinal effects

Morphine causes an increase in tone of the stomach, duodenum, small intestine and colon leading to decreased intestinal propulsion. Sphincters throughout the tract are particularly sensitive. This is the mechanism of opiates' constipative action. Hence the use of Kaolin and Morphine for diarrhoea of assorted causes. A selective opiate constipative agent is Diphenoxylate. This drug lacks analgesic and respiratory depressant actions at constipative doses but dependence has been described after excessive self-medication. Poisoning is treated as for Morphine poisoning (page 267). A proprietary preparation also contains a subtherapeutic dose of Atropine to minimize self-medication.

Histamine release

Morphine in common with other basic drugs (Tubocurarine, Atropine) can displace histamine from its binding site. This is of clinical importance if the patient has a history of allergic conditions. The consequences are irritation at the site of injection, bronchospasm (which may be fatal in an asthmatic) and peripheral vasodilatation leading to postural hypotension.

Tolerance

Tolerance is a decreasing response to continued drug use, which is generally surmountable by increasing drug dose.

Tolerance develops to some actions of *Morphine* with remarkable speed and to a considerable extent. An addict may tolerate 500 times the clinical dose of *Morphine.* Generally, tolerance develops quickest to the depressant actions, there being little tolerance to the miotic, emetic and convulsant actions. Whilst tolerance may be apparent after single injections of opiates in man and certainly after about six consecutive injections (as in postoperative pain), this may be of little clinical significance (*see below*). The mechanism of tolerance is unknown but is not due to increased biotransformation.

Physical dependence

Physical dependence is defined on page 252. It cannot occur unless the subject has developed tolerance. The withdrawal symptoms are generally opposite to the original effects of agonists (for example, diarrhoea, hyperventilation, mydriasis) though vomiting will occur.

The symptoms will develop at the time of the next regular dose and reach peak severity in 36–72 hours. The symptoms will last for about a week.

If opiates are used to relieve acute pain (for example, six injections), withdrawal symptoms, though detectable, may pass unnoticed if the patient is not anticipating any reaction.

The treatment of dependence is theoretically simple and effective. Hospitalization is essential. The addictive drug (commonly *Diamorphine*) is withdrawn and a derivative which has a longer duration of action and which causes less euphoria substituted (commonly *Methadone*). The dose given is just sufficient to prevent withdrawal symptoms. Over a period of weeks (dependent on severity) the dose of the substitute is reduced gradually during which time whatever biochemical imbalance was responsible for the syndrome returns to normal (page 252). Intense psychiatric supervision is necessary. Following this the patient is clinically cured. The difficult part is the rehabilitation which must follow.

It should be stressed that the risk of inducing severe dependence in a patient during treatment for acute pain (the 'therapeutic addict') is remote. Treatment of dependence is more relevant to illicitly obtained drugs and in these instances there are complicating factors — pathological, psychological and sociological.

THE NARCOTIC ANTAGONISTS

The narcotic antagonists should be considered from two viewpoints (*Figure 3.11*): (1) their use in the treatment of agonist overdose; and (2) the use of partial agonists as analgesics.

Use as antagonists (for example, *Naloxone*)

Naloxone will antagonize the pure agonists more effectively than the partial agonists. The characteristics of the antagonism in all cases are competitive. Its major use is to offset postoperative respiratory depression notably in the neonate. *Naloxone* has a short duration of action (30 minutes). The partial agonists (especially Nalorphine) can also be used, though they are ineffective as antagonists of other partial agonists (*Pentazocine*) and will aggravate non-narcotic-induced respiratory depression.

All derivatives possessing antagonist activity will precipitate the withdrawal syndrome in narcotic addicts. The symptoms thus precipitated will appear in seconds and last for 24 hours (cf the withdrawal syndrome precipitated by abstinence).

Use of partial agonists as analgesics (for example, *Pentazocine*)

The partial agonists share with the pure agonists analgesic, respiratory depressant, cough suppressant, constipative and emetic activities. They differ in that they normally cause dysphoria, they can cause hallucinations (which are normally of a persecutory nature) and they do not cause dependence of the pure agonist type.

Two derivatives are currently available: (1) *Pentazocine* has analgesic potency similar to *Pethidine*, causes dysphoria though hallucinations are uncommon and is a weak antagonist, thus no therapeutic use as such. A very rare form of dependence has been described — it is different from that to pure agonists (even weak agonists like *Codeine*). Withdrawal symptoms are abdominal pain, sweating, lacrimation and rhinorrhoea, and can be tolerated without medication. (2) Buprenorphine differs from *Pentazocine* in that it has a higher maximum analgesic action and a long duration of action. It is strongly sedative and causes neither euphoria nor dysphoria. Psychotic effects have not been reported. Vomiting (especially in the ambulatory patient) may be more frequent than that characteristic of the group. Currently the drug is only available for parenteral use. *Naloxone* is not an effective antagonist when injected after buprenorphine though it can prevent its action when given before. *Doxapram* (page 152) is an effective antidote to buprenorphine overdosage.

Stimulants and hallucinogens

Though one transmitter may be excitatory at one site and inhibitory at another, it is possible to generalize that some transmitters are more likely to be excitatory and others inhibitory. In this way glycine and GABA are generally inhibitory.

Stimulants either enhance excitation or reduce inhibition. Following drug-induced excitation there is commonly a phase of depression.

ACh → ↑ saliva

STIMULANTS

a **Centrally acting sympathomimetics** (for example, Amphetamine)

Amphetamine causes stimulation throughout the CNS, particularly of the reticular formation. This, in combination with other actions (*see below*) results in prolonged alertness, postponement of fatigue, motor stimulation, suppression of appetite (anorexia), confusion and anxiety. Hallucinations are rare.

It retains potent peripheral sympathomimetic activity (page 48).

Its central mechanisms of action include release of NA and dopamine (it causes a behaviour pattern characteristic of all agonists at dopamine receptors), release of 5-HT, inhibition of monoamine uptake and inhibition of MAO.

Whilst the D- and L-isomers have equal potency in the periphery, dexamphetamine [dextroamphetamine] is four times more potent as a central stimulant.

Acute poisoning is characterized by delirium and autonomic symptoms. Treatment involves acidification of urine to promote excretion (page 247) and *Chlorpromazine* (neuroleptic and α-blocking actions are of benefit). Death is due to cardiovascular collapse.

Chronic toxicity: displays tolerance and severe psychic dependence and a psychosis almost identical to paranoid schizophrenia.

Common clinical use was as an appetite suppressant, though it is no longer used since newer derivatives cause less central and cardiovascular stimulation and have a low dependence liability. Current use is restricted to the rare condition of narcolepsy.

Table 3.1

Structural change	Consequence	Drug
N-substitution	More selective central stimulation	Methylamphetamine
Side-chain rendered less flexible	Decreased central and autonomic stimulation; retention of MAO inhibitory activity	Tranylcypromine
Bulky substitution on ring	Decreased central and autonomic stimulation; retention of anorectic activity	*Fenfluramine*
Ring methoxylation	More selective hallucinogen	Mescaline

Structural manipulation of the molecule affords more selective derivatives (*see Figures 1.28* and *1.29* for structural characteristics of directly and indirectly acting sympathomimetics).

Table 3.1 summarizes the consequences of modification of the Amphetamine molecule.

b Convulsants

Drugs can cause convulsions by many different mechanisms at sites between the spinal cord and cerebral cortex.

Strychnine

Poisoning is treated with short-acting neuromuscular blocking agents and sedatives (mechanism of action is described on page 128).

Bicuculline and picrotoxin

These are antagonists of the inhibitory transmitter GABA.

Nikethamide

Mechanism of action of *Nikethamide* is not known. Since the respiratory stimulant dose is lower than the convulsant dose, it was once used in the treatment of barbiturate poisoning. However, the dose necessary to stimulate respiration in a comatose subject is a convulsant dose. Since the abandonment of such drugs, the prognosis for barbiturate poisoning has significantly improved.

Doxapram

Unlike *Nikethamide*, the ratio between respiratory stimulant and convulsant doses is satisfactory and the drug is used as a respiratory stimulant when no more specific drug/facility is available. Its relative selectivity of action may be related to peripheral stimulation of chemoceptors.

Whilst the above drugs have negligible clinical use, several are valuable in neurophysiological and pharmacological research.

c Methylxanthines

The three related alkaloids Caffeine, Theophylline and theobromine have useful central and peripheral actions. They stimulate the central nervous system, skeletal and cardiac muscle; relax smooth muscle and cause diuresis.

For central stimulation their order of potency is Caffeine $\gg$ Theophylline $>$ theobromine. For cardiac stimulation, smooth muscle relaxation and diuresis the order is Theophylline $>$ theobromine $>$ Caffeine.

At oral doses of 200 mg, Caffeine postpones fatigue with no adverse effects. A cup of strong tea or coffee contains about 150 mg Caffeine. The lethal dose in man is unknown.

The presumed mechanism of action is to inhibit phosphodiesterase causing an accumulation of cAMP. The sequence of events is illustrated in *Figure 3.13.*

152

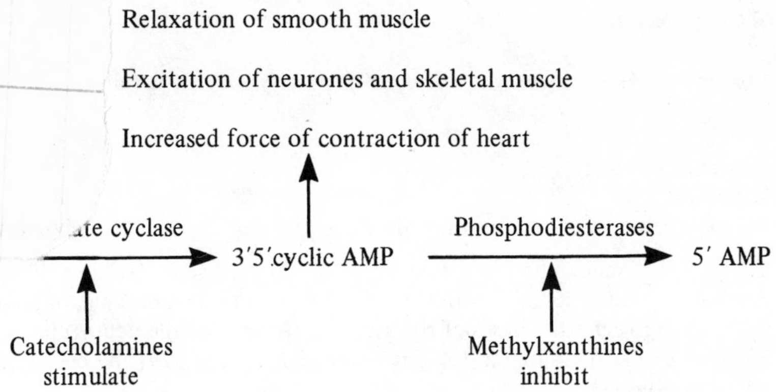

Relaxation of smooth muscle

Excitation of neurones and skeletal muscle

Increased force of contraction of heart

.te cyclase   3′5′cyclic AMP   Phosphodiesterases   5′ AMP

Catecholamines
stimulate

Methylxanthines
inhibit

Figure 3.13

Aminophylline and *Choline theophyllinate* [oxtriphylline] are the commonest theophylline complexes, useful primarily in asthma.

HALLUCINOGENS

A hallucination is a sense perception not based on objective reality. Though normally thought of as visual, drugs can alter all the senses (tactile, auditory, taste, pain, etc.).

Many drugs cause hallucinations by various mechanisms. In few cases are the mechanisms of action understood. Note that in the following list not all hallucinogens can be classified as 'stimulants':

(1)   Centrally acting sympathomimetics (page 151). Whilst Amphetamine can occasionally cause hallucinations following parenteral administration, its methoxylated derivatives (mescaline, dimethoxy-methylamphetamine) are potent hallucinogens. They cause vivid visual hallucinations, though the mechanism is unknown.

(2)   LSD. Vivid visual hallucinations. Mechanism presumed to be related to the drug's ability to interact with central neutotransmitter 5-HT.

(3)   *Cocaine.* Euphoria, indifference to pain, tactile hallucinations. Mechanism presumed to be related to inhibition of neurotransmitter uptake (page 54).

(4)   Narcotic antagonist analgesics (*Pentazocine*). Dysphoria, visual hallucinations commonly persecutory. Mechanism presumed to be interference with endorphins and enkephalins.

(5)   Nitrous oxide (N_2O). Analgesia lowering of sensory threshold, notably auditory distortion. Mechanism unknown though may also involve endorphins and enkephalins.

(6)   Cannabis, main active constituent Δ^9-tetrahydrocannabinol (THC). Lowering of sensory threshold, euphoria, time distortion.

Hallucinogens have no therapeutic use as such.

Acute toxicity

Bizarre behaviour under drug influence; toxicity specific for drug group.

Chronic toxicity

Psychoses may occur at any time after drug taking.

The fact that schizophrenic patients commonly experience hallucinations provides both a rationale for the choice of drugs in schizophrenia (antagonists of hallucinogens) and the bases of the assorted theories of the neurotransmitter imbalance of schizophrenia (the dopamine, 5-HT, page 129, and endorphin, page 145, hypotheses).

Antipyretic analgesics

This group of drugs usually combine antipyretic, analgesic and anti-inflammatory actions. Their anti-inflammatory properties and peripheral toxicity are presented on page 117). Therefore, in this section only two drugs, *Aspirin* and *Paracetamol*, will be covered in any detail.

ANTIPYRESIS

Body temperature is controlled from a hypothalamic integrating centre ('thermostat') which detects changes in deep body (core) and environmental (cutaneous) thermoceptors and then adjusts the functioning of peripheral effector systems (*Figure 3.14*).

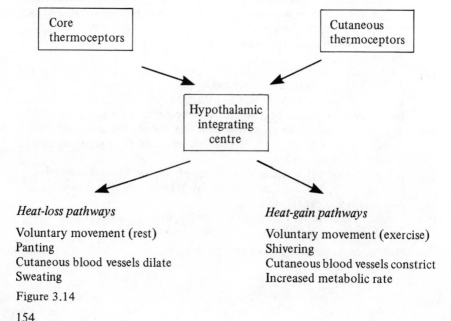

Heat-loss pathways

Voluntary movement (rest)
Panting
Cutaneous blood vessels dilate
Sweating

Heat-gain pathways

Voluntary movement (exercise)
Shivering
Cutaneous blood vessels constrict
Increased metabolic rate

Figure 3.14

In fever (for example, as a result of infection or after injection of pyrogenic substances) the hypothalamic thermostat behaves as if it had been reset at a higher temperature. Thus, effectors raise the core temperature so that it is higher than normal (febrile state). There is some doubt about the mechanisms by which pyrogenic substances induce a febrile state but some evidence suggests that prostaglandins are involved. Prostaglandins have been detected in the cerebrospinal fluid (CSF) of febrile animals and hypothalamic injection of prostaglandin E_1 causes fever.

ANALGESIA

The role of the various central neurotransmitters in the response to pain is as yet poorly understood. Recent work suggests that the enkephalins may be involved (page 143) and may be the endogenous equivalent of the opioids. No such statement can be made for the antipyretic analgesics but other substances including the prostaglandins and substance P have been implicated.

When the pain involves a peripheral inflammatory response, there is an obvious role for a drug with an anti-inflammatory action. However, it seems likely that there is also a central component, since *Paracetamol* can relieve pain even though it is not anti-inflammatory, whereas *Phenylbutazone* is not antipyretic, is a more potent anti-inflammatory agent than *Aspirin* and yet a weaker analgesic.

Aspirin

Antipyretic action

Aspirin acts as though to reset a central thermostat to its pre-febrile level so that the abnormally high temperature is detected and heat loss effectors (for example, sweating) are brought into play. *Aspirin* will not reduce core temperature when the thermostat is operating normally or when the body temperature is otherwise elevated (for example, during excessive physical exercise).

Aspirin will inhibit a febrile response and at the same time prevent the appearance of prostaglandins in the CSF. Thus, it has been argued that by inhibiting cyclo-oxygenase *Aspirin* prevents the production of the prostaglandin mediators of fever.

Analgesic action

Aspirin analgesia has a peripheral component, particularly when inflammation is the origin of pain. In addition, a central component seems likely and *Aspirin* is useful for the relief of many types of mild pain.

Other CNS actions

In high doses *Aspirin* first causes stimulation (notably of respiration with resultant acid-base disturbance) and then depression of the CNS. Confusion,

155

dizziness, tinnitus and high-tone deafness can occur and as the dose is increased delirium, psychosis, stupor and coma may ensue. Nausea and vomiting may occur and though there is a peripheral component (gastric irritation) a central effect is also involved since iv *Aspirin* can cause vomiting which is abolished by ablation of the medullary CTZ.

Paracetamol

Antipyretic and analgesic actions

Paracetamol is approximately equipotent with *Aspirin* as an antipyretic and analgesic but differs from *Aspirin* in that it lacks anti-inflammatory action. This is because *Paracetamol* inhibits central more than peripheral cyclo-oxygenase.

Other CNS actions

In some individuals relaxation, drowsiness and euphoria have been reported following ingestion of *Paracetamol*, but this may be related to relief from pain rather than a direct action on the CNS. After very high doses CNS stimulation, excitement and delirium may occur followed by sedation and stupor. Other toxic effects are mainly peripheral in origin with delayed liver damage being the most serious consequence of acute overdosage and renal damage being possible after chronic abuse.

Many proprietary mixtures which include *Aspirin* or *Paracetamol* are available, as are preparations in which *Aspirin* is presented in a soluble form. The application of such preparations is discussed on pages 292 and 317.

The state of consciousness and the non-specific depressants

The majority of central depressants cause non-specific depression of all central neuronal activity (that is, whilst consciousness is lost, other brain functions are also depressed). This contrasts with some other central depressants which have selective effects on certain brain areas or neurotransmitters (for example, neuroleptic drugs, narcotic analgesics, anti-emetics, cough suppressants).

THE PHYSIOLOGICAL BASIS OF CONSCIOUSNESS

The reticular formation contains areas responsible for the sleep-wake cycle (reticular activating system). The sleep and wake centres have inherent rhythmicity and are mutually inhibitory. The wake centre is dominant. Their

Table 3.2   *Non-specific depressants*

Organic solvents
    Clinically useful   General anaesthetics ether, chloroform, Halothane
    Socially used   Ethanol
    Clinically useless   Acetone, petrol, etc.
Iv Anaesthetics   Thiopentone*, Althesin^R
Sedatives and hypnotics   *Chloral Hydrate, Diazepam,* some barbiturates
Some anticonvulsants†   *Phenobarbitone*
Some anxiolytics   *Chlordiazepoxide*

† The classification of anticonvulsants (page 167) and anxiolytics (page 163) in a list of non-specific depressants is later qualified.

regular control of the cycle is influenced by many factors which can: (1) maintain wakefulness, for example, unusual sensory stimuli (noise, light, pain), excessive limbic activity (anxiety), volitional desire to stay awake and various unsatisfied urges; (2) encourage sleep, for example, absence of the above.

SLEEP AND INSOMNIA

The depth of sleep can be measured by EEG recordings (*Figure 3.15* illustrates typical records).

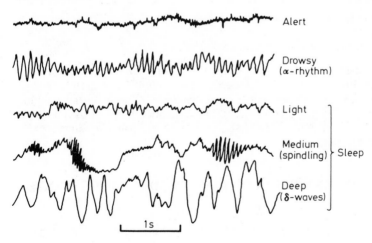

Figure 3.15 *EEG patterns*

Note the fast electrical activity of 'alertness'; α-rhythm (typical of drowsiness, eyes closed); the bursts of activity during sleep (spindling) and the δ-waves (high voltage, low frequency).

There is an additional stage of sleep called paradoxical sleep. This is characterized by rapid eye movements (REM), an increase in electrical activity, difficulty in arousing the subject and dreaming.

157

The course of a night's sleep is summarized in *Figure 3.16.*

Note that deep sleep occurs early and the incidence and duration of paradoxical sleep increases as the course of sleep progresses. Paradoxical sleep is thought to be a psychological necessity and its reduction (by drugs) undesirable.

Anxiety is the most common cause of insomnia, followed by ingestion of caffeine-containing drinks and then pain.

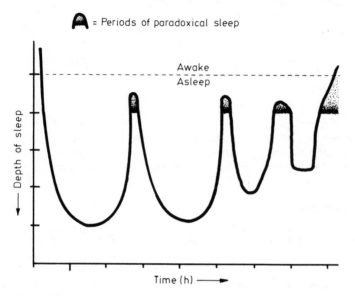

Figure 3.16

There is no drug that causes natural sleep. The majority of drugs used to treat insomnia are either non-specific depressants (for example, barbiturates) or relatively selective anxiolytics which reduce the cause of insomnia and encourage natural sleep (for example, *Nitrazepam*). The distinction between the two mechanisms is not absolute (page 163). Insomnia due to pain can sometimes be treated with analgesics.

MECHANISMS OF ACTION OF NON-SPECIFIC DEPRESSANTS

If the chemical structures of drugs taken from *Figures 3.17* and *3.18* are compared, it is apparent that there is no structural similarity, yet they act by the same mechanism.

Hence the term 'structurally non-specific depressants'. It is believed that they act by occupying a biophase to prevent its normal physiological function. It follows that for structurally non-specific drugs the same biological effect will be produced at the same relative saturation of the biophase (Ferguson's principle, page 66).

The nature of the biophase is lipid. There is a good correlation between potency as anaesthetics and lipid solubility expressed as oil/gas partition coefficient (*Figure 3.17*).

158

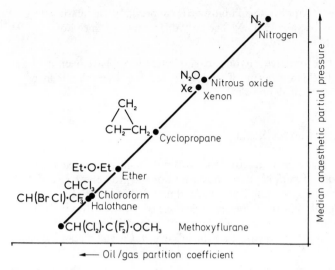

Figure 3.17

The location of this biophase is likely to be: (1) lipid portions of pre-synaptic and post-synaptic neuronal membranes. The result of drug occupation of (that is, solution in) this lipid will distort membrane structure and prevent ionic movements (membrane stabilization); (2) lipid portions of enzymes, notably of energy-producing systems.

ANAESTHESIA

Anaesthesia refers to a reversible drug-induced absence of all feeling and sensation.

Anaesthetics depress all parts of the brain in a predictable order. A progressive depression descends through the CNS, the cortex (loss of inhibition leading to excitation), the midbrain (sedation leading to anaesthesia), the spinal cord (loss of reflexes) and finally medulla (respiratory and vasomotor depression leading to death).

The sequence of events is illustrated by Ethanol (a weak general anaesthetic):

(1) Tranquillization (removal of anxiety).
(2) Excitation (loquaciousness, recklessness).
(3) Dysarthria (slurring of speech).
(4) Ataxia (staggering).
(5) Sedation.
(6) Hypnosis.
(7) Anaesthesia.
(8) Medullary depression.
(9) Coma.
(10) Death.

159

This sequence of events applies to all non-specific depressants (inhalational and iv anaesthetics, sedatives, anxiolytics). The only differences are speed of induction and margin of safety.

The terms 'anxiolytic', 'sedative', 'hypnotic' and 'anaesthetic' have been used but it is more accurate to think in terms of anxiolytic, sedative, hypnotic or anaesthetic doses of non-specific depressants.

Stages and planes of anaesthesia

These were defined many years ago for ether without premedication and were based on observations of peripheral manifestations of the progressive depression of the CNS, notably change in pupil size, skeletal muscle tone, respiratory pattern, eye movements and the presence or absence of various reflexes (corneal, laryngeal, pharyngeal). With the replacement of ether by other anaesthetics and the use of pre-anaesthetic medication the original stages and planes are less relevant to modern anaesthesia.

The most useful index of surgical anaesthesia is the absence (or near absence) of sympathetic responses to pain (BP, heart rate, pupil size). Pupil size (constricted) and respiratory pattern (diaphragmatic assuming the patient is breathing spontaneously) are also confirmatory indices.

The depth of anaesthesia may also be assessed from EEG records. There is an increase in electrical activity equivalent to the stage of excitation, a distortion of rhythm equivalent to surgical anaesthesia and electrical silence indicating death.

The general anaesthetics

Since the mechanism of action is occupation of a lipid phase in the brain, a most important consideration is their ability to reach that phase. This governs speed of anaesthetic induction (page 241). Since any lipid-soluble compound (organic solvent) is potentially an anaesthetic, the only difference between clinically useful and useless agents is whether anaesthesia is or is not accompanied by undesirable effects; for example, petrol is a general anaesthetic but causes bronchial irritation, liver and kidney damage.

Inhalational anaesthetics

Though a homogeneous group the clinically useful anaesthetics differ in the following:

Physical properties

N_2O and cyclopropane are gases at normal temperature and pressure. Some agents are highly inflammable (ether), others explosive (cyclopropane). Halothane has ideal physical properties (it is inert).

Speed of induction

N_2O is the fastest (the least soluble in blood, page 240), ether the slowest. Halothane is intermediate.

Potency

The volatile anaesthetics are more potent than the gases (for example, anaesthetic concentrations are: N_2O — 100 per cent; cyclopropane — 30 per cent; Halothane — 2 per cent; methoxyflurane — 1 per cent.

Analgesic activity

N_2O is a potent analgesic at sub-anaesthetic concentrations (20 per cent) and is useful as an analgesic (for example, in labour). Halothane has no analgesic activity.

Muscle relaxation

Major surgery requires neuromuscular blocking agents, though ether causes some peripheral neuromuscular blockade (*Table 1.3*).

Production of cardiac arrhythmias

Cyclopropane and any anaesthetic containing a halogen can sensitize the myocardium to the actions of catecholamines causing arrhythmias.

Hypotension and respiratory depression

Medullary depression will occur, though if respiration is maintained artificially medullary depression is usually unimportant.

Liver damage

Liver damage is the most common toxic action of organic solvents.

Summary

The most commonly used inhalational anaesthetic is a mixture of N_2O (50–70 per cent) and Halothane (1 per cent).

The formulae of some inhalational anaesthetics are included in *Figure 3.17.*

Intravenous anaesthetics

The advantages of iv anaesthesia are: rapid (few seconds) and pleasant induction, simple equipment, little postoperative vomiting, short duration, no respiratory irritation. The disadvantages are: inability to control depth of anaesthesia easily, severe respiratory and vasomotor depression and no analgesia at sub-anaesthetic doses.

Thiopentone and methohexitone are barbiturate derivatives (page 165). They are widely used. Specified disadvantages are necrosis on extravascular injection and fatal exacerbation of acute intermittent porphyria. This disease is an absolute contraindication of all barbiturates. Recovery from Thiopentone is due to drug redistribution (page 237).

Althesin^R is a mixture of two steroids — alphaxalone and alphadolone. Neither is sufficiently water soluble but in combination they have a mutual solubilizing effect. Very rapid onset and recovery — free of the specific disadvantages of barbiturates. Recovery is due to rapid biotransformation (cf Thiopentone). The formulae of some iv anaesthetics are included in *Figure 3.18*.

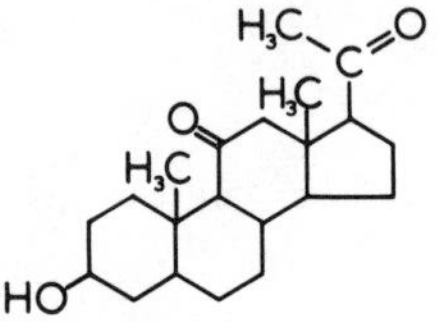

Alphaxalone

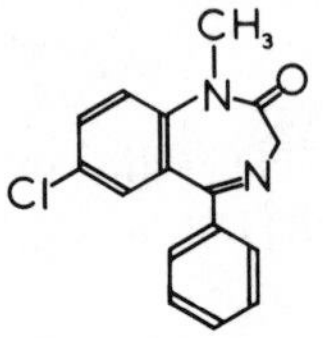

a Benzodiazepine
(*Diazepam*)

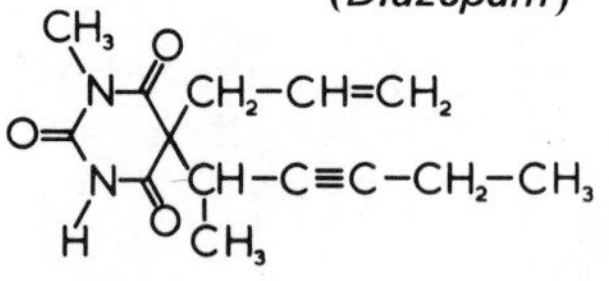

a Barbiturate
(Methohexitone)

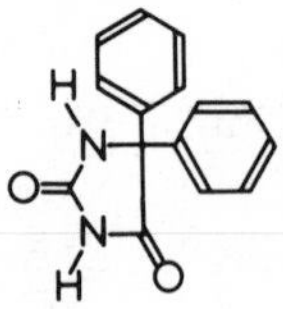

Phenytoin

Figure 3.18

Diazepam (*see below*) and lorazepam are not really classified as anaesthetics but are used extensively by the iv route to cause deep sedation.

PRE-ANAESTHETIC AND POSTANAESTHETIC MEDICATION

Drugs commonly used before, during and after anaesthesia include: muscarinic blocking agents (*Atropine*) to reduce secretions; anxiolytics (*Diazepam*) to allay anxiety and cause amnesia; neuroleptic drugs (droperidol), to allay anxiety and minimize risk of vomiting; neuromuscular blocking agents (Suxamethonium, Tubocurarine) to cause skeletal muscle relaxation; narcotic analgesics (*Morphine, Pentazocine*) and antagonists of some of the above (*Neostigmine, Naloxone*).

NEUROLEPTANALGESIA

This is the technique of preparing a patient for major surgery using a combination of a potent short-acting narcotic analgesic (for example, fentanyl) with a neuroleptic agent (droperidol). Whilst the patient remains conscious and can (up to a point) follow instructions, such is his 'indifference' to his circumstances that surgery can be performed.

ANXIOLYTICS, SEDATIVES AND HYPNOTICS

The difficulties of the classification of central depressants into the above three categories has already been noted (page 160). Derivatives of benzodiazepine supply the vast majority of anxiolytics which, dependent on dose, are clinically useful as sedatives and hypnotics.

Benzodiazepines (*Diazepam*)

The structure of *Diazepam* is included in *Figure 3.18*. Whilst *Diazepam* causes the same progressive depression of the central nervous system as that listed on page 159, it has a wider margin of safety than the barbiturates (page 165). *Figure 3.19* illustrates this difference.

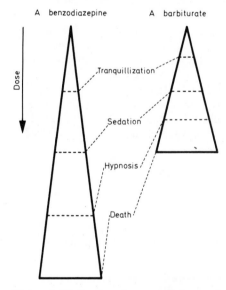

Figure 3.19 *Progressive central depression*

Diazepam has a relatively selective depressant action on components of the limbic system thereby reducing anxiety at doses which have little effect on the reticular activating system (that is, little sedative effect). It also has a relaxant effect on skeletal muscle (mediated centrally) of value in the treatment of anxiety in which skeletal muscle tone is increased.

It causes amnesia (characteristic of all non-specific depressants) and whilst this is undesirable in patients taking the drug long term, it can be valuable in pre-anaesthetic medication (for example, in dentistry).

It possesses anticonvulsant activity (page 304), has a long $t_{1/2}$ and the drug can accumulate.

As is characteristic of the drug group *Diazepam* has neither antidepressant nor neuroleptic properties.

Unwanted effects are common to similar drugs: lapses in attention (use of machinery, driving), drowsiness and sedation. Its actions summate with similar drugs (*Table 3.2*). Psychic and physical dependence can develop (page 252).

In experimental animals the behavioural profile of *Diazepam* is superficially similar to that of *Chlorpromazine.* It has a taming effect in experimental animals, it reduces locomotor activity and suppresses conditioned avoidance responses. However, the sedation is not accompanied by catatonia. Indeed, there is a reduction in muscle tone.

Other derivatives are available (for example, *Chlordiazepoxide, Nitrazepam,* lorazepam).

The clinical differences between these (and the many other benzodiazepines) are negligible. The custom of using some (for example, *Chlordiazepoxide*) for day-time tranquillization and others (such as *Nitrazepam*) for night-time sedation probably reflects either marketing policy or the relative doses in available preparations (page 296).

In the original classification of non-specific depressants (*Table 3.2*), the inclusion of the benzodiazepines was qualified. Recent work has suggested that these drugs enhance the activity of the inhibitory transmitter GABA by interacting with a receptor associated with, though distinct from, the GABA receptor. An endogenous ligand for this receptor (related to β-carboline) has recently been proposed. Whilst further research will clarify this interesting speculation of the biochemical basis of anxiety, the continuous injection of *Diazepam* into a subject will produce the same progressive depression of the CNS as that caused by other non-specific depressants (*Figure 3.19*).

The alcohols (Ethanol)

The alcohols are non-specific depressants — Ethanol being the derivative with fewest side-effects. It is widely used in self-medication, for social purposes and as an anxiolytic.

Excessive consumption leads to dependence (page 252), psychosis and liver damage.

The drug is oxidized in the liver by the route shown in *Figure 3.20*. Note the toxic acetaldehyde in the pathway but as the aldehyde dehydrogenase step is normally rapid it does not accumulate.

Some drugs (*Metronidazole,* page 185; *Monosulfiram,* page 183; *Chlorprop-amide*, page 95) are inhibitors of aldehyde dehydrogenase, and Ethanol consumption is contraindicated during therapy with them. Disulfiram is an inhibitor of aldehyde dehydrogenase and is useful in the aversion treatment of alcohol addiction. During Disulfiram treatment, if the patient takes Ethanol, acetaldehyde accumulates and causes unpleasant effects including nausea and vomiting.

$$CH_3CH_2OH \xrightarrow[\text{dehydrogen-ase}]{\text{Alcohol}} CH_3CHO \xrightarrow[\text{dehydrogen-ase}]{\text{Aldehyde}} CH_3COOH \longrightarrow CO_2 + H_2O$$

Ethanol   Acetaldehyde   Acetic acid

$$CH_3OH \dashrightarrow H \cdot CHO \dashrightarrow H \cdot COOH \dashrightarrow$$

Methanol   Formaldehyde   Formic acid

Figure 3.20

The central pharmacology of methanol is identical to that of Ethanol. It is also biotransformed via the same pathway (*Figure 3.20*) but the enzymes are less capable of handling formaldehyde and formic acid. These accumulate and cause blindness (chronic toxicity) or severe acidosis (acute toxicity).

Poisoning by a third commercially available alcohol, ethylene glycol (antifreeze), is characterized by CNS depression (coma, respiratory depression) and severe nephrotoxicity.

Chloral and its derivatives

The pharmacological properties of chloral and its derivatives are due to their biotransformation to trichloroethanol.

They are used at sedative and hypnotic doses, are relatively safe and are useful as sedatives in children.

Chloral hydrate is a non-specific depressant, though it has too narrow a margin of safety to be used as an anaesthetic. Gastric irritation often occurs and the drug should always be taken in dilute form and never on an empty stomach. Allergic reactions (urticaria, erythema) sometimes occur.

Dichloralphenazone and *Triclofos* are more palatable complexes of *Chloral hydrate* and gastric irritation rarely occurs.

Patterns of dependence on chloral derivatives are similar to alcohol dependence. Poisoning is treated in the same way as barbiturate poisoning.

The barbiturates

Chemically related to barbituric acid (itself without depressant activity). Structural modification (*Figure 3.18*) leads to depressants which differ only in onset and duration of activity.

The only justifiable clinical uses of barbiturates are: (1) the specific use of *Phenobarbitone* as an anti-epileptic drug (page 304); (2) the use of Thiopentone and methohexitone as iv anaesthetics (page 162).

Although many barbiturate derivatives of intermediate duration of action have been used as sedatives and hypnotics in the past and are still commercially available (for example, pentobarbitone, amylobarbitone [amobarbital], butobarbitone) they are no longer recommended for this use because they have too narrow a margin of safety.

Barbiturate poisoning and its treatment

Barbiturates are directly responsible for about 50 per cent of all drug deaths. The number of prescriptions for and the number of deaths directly attributed to the barbiturates and the benzodiazepine anxiolytics in 1974 in England and Wales are shown in *Table 3.3*.

Table 3.3

	No. of prescriptions	*No. of deaths*
Barbiturates	8,500,000	1,600
Non-barbiturate hypnotics	9,500,000	120
Anxiolytics	22,000,000	50

The characteristics of barbiturate poisoning (typical of all non-specific depressants) are: coma; hypothermia; shallow, regular and infrequent breathing; hypotension, imperceptible pulse. Death is usually due to inhalation of vomit.

The treatment of poisoning is artificial ventilation, forced diuresis and intensive care. The practice of using non-specific CNS stimulants (*Nikethamide,* Amphetamine) has virtually been abandoned.

Note that the term 'non-barbiturate', though often used, may be pharmacologically misleading. Thus, methaqualone, which is not chemically related to barbituric acid is pharmacologically identical.

TOLERANCE AND DEPENDENCE

The definitions of tolerance and dependence are given elsewhere (pages 149 and 252).

Tolerance is due to two components, as follows:

(1)   Induction of liver microsomal enzymes which accelerate drug biotransformation — most of the depressants are biotransformed to an appreciable extent even if this is not the mechanism of recovery (for example, Thiopentone, Halothane).

(2)   An unknown mechanism other than the above which is presumably at the level of the biophase in the CNS.

Cross-tolerance exists between all members of the group though cross-tolerance is most marked between members of the same chemical group (for example, barbiturates).

All the non-specific depressants are drugs of psychic and physical dependence and are the most common cause of addiction in the UK (there are about 300,000 Ethanol addicts). The severity of dependence is a function of the potency of the drugs (barbiturates the greatest, benzodiazepines the least); the incidence is a function of availability (Ethanol the greatest).

Symptoms of dependence are tolerance, adjustment of life style around periods of drug taking, anxiety, amnesia, sluggishness, nutritional deficiencies and ataxia.

Symptoms of withdrawal are craving, tremor, anxiety, EEG changes, hallucinations and, if severe, grand mal convulsions. Deaths have occurred during withdrawal.

Assuming regular drug taking, the time for dependence development is a function of potency (barbiturates a few months, Ethanol and benzodiazepines a few years).

Treatment involves hospitalization, gradual reduction in drug intake (and where applicable switching to a less potent drug) and intensive psychiatric supervision.

ANTICONVULSANT DRUGS

Epileptic convulsions are due to the presence in the brain of an unstable neuronal membrane which can fire off spontaneously at high frequency.

The attack is self-potentiating by +ve feedback (post-tetanic potentiation).

By virtue of their membrane stabilizing action, many non-specific depressants are effective anticonvulsants. The mechanism is thought to be prevention of post-tetanic potentiation rather than stabilization of the ectopic focus.

In some cases there is poor separation between anticonvulsant and general depressant actions (for example, *Phenobarbitone* is sedative), though in others good separation is achieved (for example, *Phenytoin*).

The types of epilepsy and methods of treatment are described in detail elsewhere (page 301).

4
Antiparasitic chemotherapy

LEARNING OBJECTIVES

After studying this section you should know the following:

- The name of each of the principal current antiparasitic chemotherapeutic and chemoprophylactic agents.
- The mechanism of its cytotoxic action.
- The basis of its selectivity: (*a*) towards parasite rather than host cells; (*b*) towards some parasites rather than others.
- Something of its useful place in therapeutics.
- Something of its side-effects and disadvantages.

THE PLAN OF THIS SECTION (*Table 4.1*)

On pages 170–179 the biochemically selective drugs are classified according to their sites of primary cytotoxic action with cross-reference to their therapeutic use. On pages 179–183 the distributionally based selectivity of antiparasitic chemotherapeutic agents is covered with cross-reference to their therapeutic use. The remainder of the section places these same drugs, and others found empirically to be selective but by as yet unknown mechanisms, in a therapeutic context by classifying the parasitisms with cross-reference to their mechanisms of toxicity and selectivity.

DEFINITIONS

Antiparasitic chemotherapy is the treatment of symptomatic parasitism with chemicals of known constitution. Human parasitisms fall into the three following groups:

(1) Infestation of organs with metazoa (insects, arachnids, worms).
(2) Infection of tissues or cells with unicellular organisms (protozoa, bacteria, fungi, Mycoplasmas, Rickettsiae, Chlamydiae, viruses).

169

(3) Invasion of organs or tissues by aberrant human cells (malignant neoplasms).

Toxicity means injury or disturbance of function. The cytotoxic action may result in the death of cells (cytocidal effect) or prevention of their multiplication (cytostatic effect) without cell death. In the latter case the body's chemical (antibody) and cellular (phagocytic) defence mechanisms can usually clear the residual static infecting population. Most drugs can be cytocidal in high concentration and cytostatic in lower concentration: which is seen in practice depends on the body concentration attained with normal therapeutic doses.

The scale of measurement of cytotoxic action is really a continuous quantitative one (median cytotoxic concentration) but is often expressed verbally as sensitivity or resistance of a parasite to clinically attainable concentrations of a chemotherapeutic agent. If a parasite population acquires increased resistance (reduced sensitivity) to a chemotherapeutic agent it also shows cross-resistance to other agents having the same mechanism of cytotoxic action.

Selectivity means that one kind of cell is more affected than another. So selective toxicity means (qualitatively) that one kind of cell is injured while another is not or (quantitatively) that one kind of cell is more injured than another by the same dose or is injured at a lower dose than another. The injury may be reversible or irreversible, structural or functional, beneficial or detrimental to the recipient organism.

The scale of measurement of selective toxicity is the chemotherapeutic index = median toxic dose to host/median curative dose.

A prodrug is a chemical precursor of the active drug. It has no pharmacological action itself (so the effect resulting from its administration does not correlate in time or intensity with the body concentration of the prodrug) but is metabolized in the body to an active drug.

The basic assumption of human antiparasitic chemotherapy is that parasite cells differ from human cells. By chemical exploitation of these differences, toxicity to the parasite can be achieved without harm to the host. There are many ways of classifying these differences (and hence the origin of selectivity). We shall adopt a simple two-way classification into biochemical and distributional bases of selectivity.

Biochemical selectivity

The chemotherapeutic agent has a greater toxicity to parasite than to host cells, even when the sites of toxic action in both are exposed to the same concentration. This may be only a quantitative difference (for example, dihydrofolate reductase, page 174, or cytoplasmic membrane, page 178) or a qualitative one (for example, cell wall synthesis, page 171, or dihydrofolate synthetase, page 173).

SITE OF TOXIC ACTION

This may be such as to make the chemotherapeutic agent cytotoxic to all phases of the parasite's life cycle, including the adult resting phase; for example, cytoplasmic membrane (page 178), energy-yielding metabolism (page 178), muscle (page 178).

It may be such as to make the chemotherapeutic agent cytotoxic only to parasites in the rapid growth and multiplication phase of their life cycle; for example, cell wall synthesis, nucleic acid synthesis and replication (page 173), protein synthesis (page 176).

Table 4.1   *Classification of mechanisms of selectivity and mechanisms of toxicity to be discussed.*

	Page
Biochemical selectivity	170
Inhibition of cell wall synthesis	171
Inhibition of nucleic acid synthesis	173
Interference with supply of precursors	173
DHF	173
THF	174
Nucleotides and nucleosides	174
Direct interference with nucleic acid synthesis	175
Alkylating agents	175
Nitrogen mustards	175
Busulphan	175
Inhibition of RNA-polymerase	176
Inhibition of protein synthesis	176
t-RNA binding to ribosomes	177
Peptide bond formation	177
Translocation	177
Increased permeability of the cytoplasmic membrane	178
Energy yielding metabolism	178
Muscle function	178
Distributional selectivity	179
Accumulation by the parasite	179
Distribution into the parasite's environment	180
Administration to the parasite's environment	181
Gut	181
Skin	182
Eye	183

INHIBITION OF CELL WALL SYNTHESIS

Bacterial and fungal, unlike mammalian, cells provide themselves with an exoskeletal cell wall. Drugs which interfere with the synthesis of cell wall material therefore show a qualitative biochemically selective action.

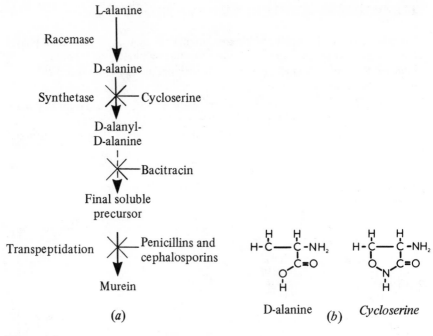

Figure 4.1

Cycloserine, Bacitracin, penicillins and cephalosporins inhibit the formation of the insoluble mucopeptide murein, which is a major constituent of the cell wall of Gram +ve bacteria and Gram −ve cocci (*Figure 4.1a*). It is, in part, formed of D-alanine. *Cycloserine* is a rigid structural analogue of D-alanine (*Figure 4.1b*). It competes for those enzymes in murein synthesis which produce and utilize D-alanine(alanine racemase and D-alanyl-D-alanine synthetase). It is concentrated by bacterial cells and so is more effective *in vivo* than on the isolated enzymes. Although it has a broad antibacterial spectrum, it is reserved for use in tuberculosis where it has second-line status due to CNS toxicity.

Bacitracin, a polypeptide antibiotic, is bactericidal to the same spectrum of organisms as are the penicillins. As well as inhibiting murein synthesis, which it does at a stage intermediate between *Cycloserine* and the penicillins, it also disorganizes the cytoplasmic membrane (page 178).

Penicillins (example, *Benzylpenicillin* [penicillin G], page 196) and cephalosporins (for example, *Cephaloridine,* page 198) are structural analogues of D-alanyl-D-alanine which inhibit the transpeptidation or cross-linking reaction which creates the insoluble murein polymer from its soluble immediate precursors. They have similar spectra of antibacterial activity, basically all Gram +ve bacteria and Gram −ve cocci are sensitive. They are the most selective chemotherapeutic agents available. Resistant bacteria secrete a β-lactamase enzyme (penicillinase or cephalosporase) which hydrolyses and inactivates the drug. Individual members of this group have significant differences in properties and use.

INHIBITION OF NUCLEIC ACID SYNTHESIS

Interference with supply of precursors

Pteridine enzyme precursors are essential for purine and pyrimidine synthesis. Because cells have stores of preformed intermediates there is a long lag between an attack on an early stage of this replicative metabolism pathway and the resulting inhibition of growth and multiplication.

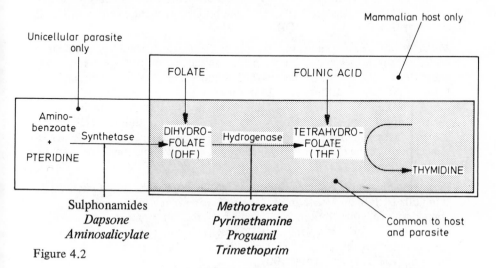

Figure 4.2

Many bacteria, unlike mammalian cells, cannot absorb folate and so utilize aminobenzoate to synthesize dihydrofolate (DHF) (*Figure 4.2*).

Drugs which interfere with the synthesis of DHF from aminobenzoate

Sulphonamides, sulphones and sodium *Aminosalicylate* necessarily show qualitative biochemical selectivity.

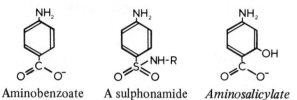

Aminobenzoate   A sulphonamide   *Aminosalicylate*

Figure 4.3

All are structural analogues of aminobenzoate (*Figure 4.3*) and compete with it for DHF synthetase; the enzyme makes a functionless DHF analogue from sulphonamides.

Sulphonamides (for example, *Sulphamethizole*) have a patchy spectrum of bacteriostatic activity and may cause renal toxicity unrelated to their effect on aminobenzoate metabolism (page 195). Sulphones (for example, *Dapsone*) are selective for leprosy bacteria. *Aminosalicylate* is selective for tuberculosis bacteria (page 201).

Drugs which interfere with the synthesis of tetrahydrofolate (THF) from DHF

Methotrexate, Pyrimethamine, Proguanil and Trimethorprim can only show a quantitive biochemical selectivity. They inhibit DHF reductase (*Figure 4.2*); all are structural analogues of DHF.

Methotrexate is a large and complex close analogue which cannot penetrate into bacteria and protozoa. It does enter mammalian cells but only shows quantitative selectivity for those with the highest THF turnover (most rapid cell division). It has a much higher affinity than DHF for DHF hydrogenase so it is virtually an irreversible inhibitor (folic acid will not overcome its effects but folinic acid [leucovorin], by supplying THF directly, will). It can cure choriocarcinoma and is useful (with other drugs) in acute leukaemias (page 203). The host toxicity is typical of drugs the selectivity of which is only for cell populations with rapid multiplication (page 205).

Pyrimethamine has a simpler structure which allows penetration into parasites. It inhibits DHF hydrogenase from malaria parasites much more than the homologous enzymes from mammalian or bacterial sources (that is, it shows quantitative biochemical selectivity). It is useless in the treatment of clinical malaria but a valuable prophylactic agent for non-immune persons in an area where malaria is endemic (page 190).

Proguanil is a prodrug; the drug formed from it in the body has properties very like those of **Pyrimethamine.**

Trimethoprim is another simple DHF analogue which is able to penetrate parasite cells. It inhibits DHF hydrogenase from bacterial sources (and malaria parasites) much more than the homologous enzyme from mammalian sources (that is, it shows quantitative biochemical selectivity). There is a long lag before inhibition of growth and multiplication is effected. It is combined with a sulphonamide (sulphamethoxazole) as *Co-trimoxazole* to achieve very efficient synergism by sequential blockade of the THF synthetic pathway (*Figure 4.2*).

Drugs which interfere with the supply of nucleoside and nucleotide precursors of DNA

Some structural analogues of purines and pyrimidines are incorporated into the cell's metabolic pathways with the synthesis of functionless intermediates which suppress nucleic acid synthesis.

Purine analogues

Mercaptopurine inhibits many steps in the synthesis and interconversion of

174

purine ribonucleotides. Selectivity is limited to the most rapidly dividing cells. It is useful in the treatment of acute leukaemias (with other agents, page 203). *Azathioprine* is a prodrug from which *Mercaptopurine* is released in the body.

Pyrimidine analogues

Fluorouracil: the false nucleotide produced blocks deoxyribonucleotide (thymidylate) synthesis.

Cytarabine: its derivatives compete with cytidine derivatives and cause profound inhibition of DNA synthesis. Both show selectivity limited to rapidly multiplying cell populations and are useful in the palliative treatment of malignant neoplasms.

Idoxuridine: its derivatives are incorporated into DNA. It shows some anti-neoplastic activity but selectivity affects the replication of certain DNA viruses (page 203).

Drugs which directly interfere with nucleic acid synthesis

Alkylating agents

Nitrogen mustards (*Mustine* [mechlorethamine], *Cyclophosphamide, Melphalan, Chlorambucil*). All effective antineoplastic drugs in this class possess two alkylating groups (cf Phenoxybenzamine, page 50). The highly reactive cyclic cations formed spontaneously in watery solution (*Figure 4.4*) bind to side

Figure 4.4

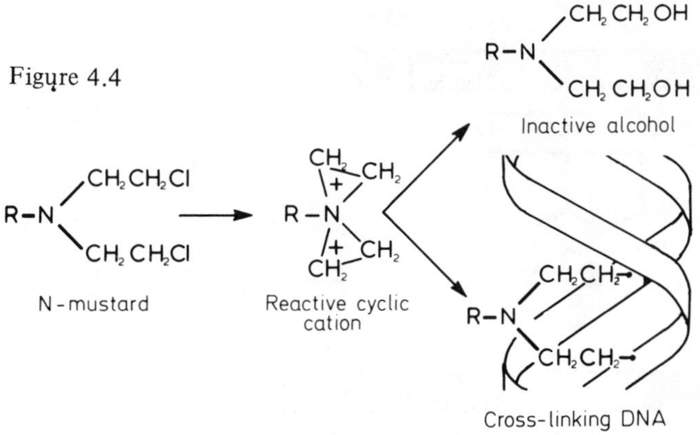

N-mustard → Reactive cyclic cation → Inactive alcohol / Cross-linking DNA

chains of large molecules, especially the guanine codon of DNA. This causes functional damage to the DNA perhaps mainly by cross-linking it to other macromolecules. Any unbound cyclic cation is spontaneously hydrolysed to an inactive alcohol. This happens too fast with *Mustine.* The other examples are chemical derivatives in which the production and inactivation of the cyclic cation proceed more slowly. As a group they show selectivity limited to rapidly multiplying cell populations and the expected host toxicity (page 206).

Cyclophosphamide is a prodrug metabolically activated by ring cleavage in the liver.

Busulphan does not ionize; it alkylates —SH in cysteine and is the treatment of choice in chronic myelogenous leukaemia.

INHIBITION OF RNA-POLYMERASE

Rifampicin combines with and inhibits the RNA-polymerase in bacteria but not that in mammalian cells. It is bactericidal to Gram +ve bacteria and *M. tuberculosis* and has low host toxicity. Gram —ve bacteria have a low permeability to *Rifampicin.* It is reserved for use in tuberculosis (page 201).

INHIBITION OF PROTEIN SYNTHESIS

To help in the understanding of this section you should revise the stages of protein synthesis on ribosomes. Most mammalian protein turnover is slow

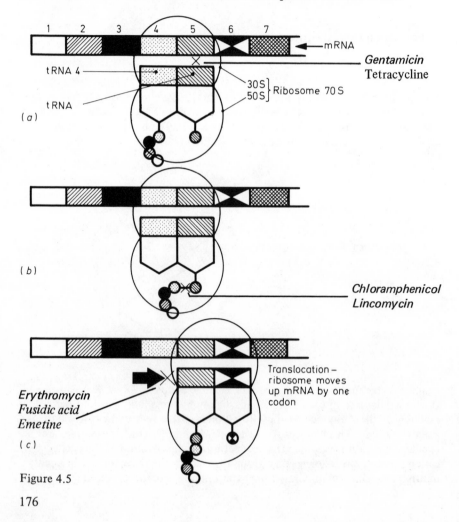

Figure 4.5

176

(fibrinogen apart) compared with that associated with cellular multiplication. Quantitative biochemical selectivity for bacterial rather than mammalian protein synthesis is possible because bacteria contain only 70S (a measure of their density) ribosomes whereas most mammalian ribosomes are 80S.

Drugs which inhibit tRNA binding to ribosomes

Amino sugar antibiotics (*Streptomycin, Gentamicin, Kanamycin, Neomycin*) bind irreversibly to the acceptor part of the 30S subunit (*Figure 4.5a*) and distort it so that aminoacyl-tRNA cannot bind to its acceptor site. Bacteria resistant to these antibiotics have ribosomes which do not bind them. Amino sugar antibiotics are highly polar water-soluble bases not absorbed from the gut. All show ototoxicity (damage to the hair cells of the inner ear) resulting in impaired balance and hearing. They have a fairly broad spectrum which includes *M. tuberculosis.* Resistance develops readily so another drug should be given at the same time.

Streptomycin is mainly useful in tuberculosis (page 201).

Gentamicin and *Kanamycin* are useful in treating life-threatening infections by Gram —ve bacilli, their spectrum includes Pseudomonas (Ps.), they show renal toxicity.

Neomycin is too toxic for systemic use. It may be given orally to reduce the bacterial flora of gut (page 181).

Peptide bond formation

Chloramphenicol is a dipeptide. One molecule binds to each 50S subunit (*Figure 4.5b*) and blocks peptidyl transferase activity. It has a broad spectrum but is reserved for typhoid fever and *H. influenzae* meningitis. A dose-related reversible anaemia is a common toxic effect but 1 patient in 40,000 is hypersensitive and suffers total irreversible bone marrow depression (page 315).

Lincomycin and *Clindamycin* are also dipeptides which bind reversibly to the 50S subunit and block peptidyl transferase. They are active on all isolated bacterial ribosomes but *in vivo* mainly affect Gram +ve bacteria including Bacteroides (page 200).

Translocation

Erythromycin: one molecule binds to the donor site of each 50S subunit (*Figure 4.5c*) and blocks translocation. Resistant bacteria lose this binding ability. It has a narrow spectrum, similar to *Benzylpenicillin* and a patient who requires this but is allergic to it provides the clearest indication for the use of *Erythromycin* (page 198).

Fusidic acid is chemically unrelated to but has properties very like *Erythromycin;* it is expensive.

Emetine affects the ribosomes of eukaryotic (nucleated) cells (the 60S subunit of 80S ribosomes). It has been observed that the resulting inhibition of transloca-tion and protein synthesis is maintained in Entamoeba but is only transient in the mammalian host, which explains the selectivity. It is reserve therapy for amoebiasis (page 187).

The foregoing mechanisms operate on actively growing and multiplying parasites only, while the following mechanisms also operate on non-multiplying parasites.

INCREASED PERMEABILITY OF THE CYTOPLASMIC MEMBRANE

Damage to the cell membrane allows leakage of vital intracellular solutes. This mechanism ensures a wide spectrum of susceptible parasites and a cytocidal effect on non-growing cells but limits selectivity.

Polyene antibiotics (*Nystatin* and *Amphotericin*)

These bind to sterols in the cell membrane (abundant in fungal, intermediate in mammalian, none in bacterial or viral membranes) and damage it, increasing its permeability. They show useful selectivity for certain fungi (not those of ring-worm) but also substantial host toxicity.

Nystatin is too toxic for systemic use; it is useful locally so that its biochemical selectivity is reinforced by distributional selectivity (page 182).

Amphotericin [amphotericin] shows slightly less host toxicity and so may be parenterally administered for systemic fungal infections (page 191).

Polypeptide antibiotics (*Colistin* and *Polymyxin* [B])

These bind to and injure the cytoplasmic membrane causing death of Gram −ve bacilli. They are not absorbed from the gut. Sometimes they are given parenterally for a life-threatening Pseudomonas infection.

Miscellaneous

Streptomycin (page 177) and Bacitracin (page 172) also damage cell membranes. This aspect of their action contributes to their bactericidal effect but also to their host toxicity.

ENERGY YIELDING METABOLISM

Most aerobic organisms derive their energy by similar mechanisms, so that inter-ference with this process has not been a fruitful source of selectively toxic drugs.

Anaerobes differ significantly from the human host so selective interference with their anaerobic pathways is possible. *Metronidazole* and *Nimorazole* interfere with the function of ferredoxin — a Fe-S-protein acting as an electron transfer agent in plants, anaerobic bacteria and protozoa. They are lethal to anaerobic protozoa (Trichomonas, Entamoeba) and bacteria (Bacteroides, *Clostridium (Cl.) difficile* and *Borrelia vincenti*) with little host toxicity (page 165).

MUSCLE

Worms need their motility to stay in their intestinal environment; paralysis therefore leads to their expulsion. *Piperazine* is a functional ACh antagonist at worm neuromuscular junctions with little effect at those of mammals (frog muscle has intermediate sensitivity). It is well absorbed from the gut and effective in roundworm (Ascaris) and threadworm (Enterobius) infestations (page 185). Host toxicity is negligible.

Distributional selectivity

Even though a drug may be equally toxic at its biochemical sites of action in host and parasite cells, it may still be useful as a chemotherapeutic agent if the sites of action in the parasitizing cells can be exposed to a higher concentration than those in the host cells. There are three ways in which this can come about.

SELECTIVE ACCUMULATION BY THE PARASITE

Tetracyclines (for example, *Tetracycline*)

These drugs affect a wide range of parasites: those affected — many bacteria (but not Pseudomonas or Proteus), Mycoplasmas, Rickettsiae and Chlamydiae (large viruses) — accumulate tetracyclines to a high intracellular concentration by a carrier-mediated transport process requiring ATP. *Tetracycline*-resistant cells — fungi, mammalian cells and resistant bacteria — do not do this.

After selective absorption tetracyclines bind reversibly to the acceptor part of the smaller subunit of the ribosome and prevent the binding of amino-acyl-tRNA and therefore protein synthesis (cf. page 177). Unlike amino sugar antibiotics, tetracyclines do this in both 70S and 80S isolated ribosomes.

They are broad spectrum antibiotics with low host toxicity (page 199).

4-Aminoquinolines (*Chloroquine* and *Quinine*)

These are concentrated in all nucleated cells but very concentrated by malaria parasites in erythrocytes. *Chloroquine* resistance in malaria is associated with a loss of this concentrating mechanism.

After selective concentration these basic drugs with flat ring systems intercalate into DNA between layers of base pairs of the double helix. This disturbs the structure and function of the starter DNA employed by DNA polymerase. They inhibit DNA synthesis at the same high concentration in isolated systems from all cells.

These are the drugs of choice for patients clinically ill with malaria, they clear the blood though they do not clear the liver of malaria parasites (page 190). In amoebic liver abscess (page 188) the amoebae selectively accumulate the *Chloroquine* by engulfing nuclear material. They show little toxicity in anti-parasitic doses; large doses have an anti-inflammatory action utilized in rheumatoid arthritis (page 317) and show retinal toxicity.

Malathion

This is a prodrug activated to the organophosphorus anticholinesterase malaoxon selectively by insects, which also inactivate malaoxon slower than mammals. Thus, it is the malaoxon rather than the prodrug which is selectively 'accumulated' by the parasite. It is useful in treating louse infestations (page 184).

Miscellaneous

Cycloserine (page 172),
Griseofulvin (*see below*).

SELECTIVELY DISTRIBUTED INTO A LIMITED COMPARTMENT WHICH FORMS THE PARASITES' ENVIRONMENT

Skin

Griseofulvin is very poorly absorbed from the gut but that which is absorbed is selectively concentrated in the keratin precursor cells of skin. As these differentiate it is strongly bound to keratin. The mechanism of its toxicity is unknown but it is fungistatic to ringworm fungi which parasitize keratin — skin, nails, hair. The keratin formed during treatment resists invasion by fungal hyphae but treatment must be continued until static fungus and infected keratin have been shed. It is reserved for hair and nail infections with dermatophytes (page 190).

Thyroid gland

Sodium iodide (^{131}I) is rapidly and efficiently trapped by thyroid parenchymal cells, incorporated into thyroid hormone and deposited in the colloid of the follicles. β-Irradiation has only a short range so it is destructive only to nearby thyroid parenchymal cells. ^{131}I is disappointing as treatment for thyroid carcinoma because the malignant cells often show less than normal I^--pump activity. It is more useful in diagnosis and treatment of hyperthyroidism.

Bone marrow

[32]Phosphate is concentrated in bone and rapidly dividing cells so bone marrow receives most of its β-irradiation (average range 2 mm). It is the treatment of choice for polycythaemia vera (excessive erythrocyte production) but increases the incidence of leukaemia.

Urinary tract – urinary antiseptics (page 200)

Nitrofurantoin is rapidly and completely absorbed from the gut; with healthy kidneys glomerular filtration prevents an antibacterial blood concentration being attained; renal tubular abstraction of water from the nascent urine results in a bactericidal concentration in the urine.

The mechanism of bacterial toxicity is unknown. It has a broad spectrum (but Proteus and Pseudomonas are resistant). Sensitive bacteria rarely become resistant. Renal failure results in an ineffective urine concentration and a toxic blood concentration.

Nalidixic acid is disposed like *Nitrofurantoin.* It shows some biochemical selectivity – it inhibits DNA synthesis in Gram –ve bacilli – reinforced in use by distributional selectivity. Resistance develops readily. Use and limitations are as for *Nitrofurantoin.*

Liver

Chloroquine in amoebic liver abscess (pages 180 and 187).

SELECTIVELY ADMINISTERED TO A LIMITED COMPARTMENT WHICH FORMS THE PARASITES' ENVIRONMENT

Lumen of gut

All of these drugs, when swallowed, are poorly absorbed from the gut and there-fore are selectively toxic to parasites within the gut lumen.

The amino sugar antibiotic *Neomycin* is toxic to bacteria (page 177) but when given systemically is toxic to the host too. Gut absorption is negligible because it is highly polar (page 231). It is used in bowel preparation for intestinal surgery to reduce the bacterial content of any spills and of wall seams with the intention of reducing postoperative infective complications (efficacy unproven). Along with dietary protein restriction it does reduce the bacterial ammonia and amine production which is responsible for the encephalopathy (disturbance of conscious-ness, coma) of liver failure (*Figure 4.6*).

Nystatin is not absorbed because it is insoluble in water. It is useful orally for Candidiasis (page 190) of the gut.

Dichlorophen and *Niclosamide* are water-insoluble unabsorbed drugs which kill

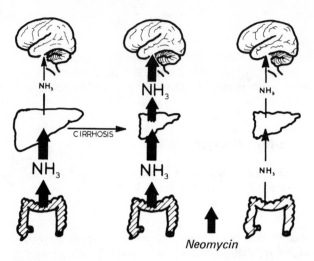

Figure 4.6

intestinal metazoa, probably by damaging their cell membranes. They are useful for tapeworm infestations (page 185).

Viprinium embonate [pyrvinium pamoate] is a water-soluble unabsorbed drug which kills intestinal metazoa, probably by interference with glucose uptake. It is useful for threadworm infestations (page 185).

Bephenium is not absorbed because it is a quaternary ammonium agonist at nicotinic receptors causing depolarising neuromuscular blockade (like Suxamethonium, page 21) and spastic paralysis of worms (page 186).

Skin

Antibacterial antibiotics

So little of a drug applied to the unbroken skin is absorbed into the systemic circulation that the more systemically toxic antibiotics can safely be used on the skin. The advantages of such a reliance on distributional selectivity — pathogens are less likely to be resistant and it avoids the need for penicillins, sulphonamides, *Streptomycin* or *Chloramphenicol* to be applied to the skin (all have a strong tendency to induce skin allergy, page 321).

Gentamicin, Neomycin, Chlortetracycline and sodium *Fusidate* are toxic by inhibition of protein synthesis (page 177).

Bacitracin is toxic by inhibition of cell wall synthesis (page 172) and also by damage to cytoplasmic membranes. The latter mechanism probably determines the renal toxicity of the drug which limits its biochemical selectivity and systemic usefulness.

Antifungal drugs

Nystatin is useful for mucocutaneous Candidiasis (page 191).

182

Insecticides

Gamma benzene hexachloride makes the cytoplasmic membranes of insect neurones leaky and so causes convulsive death of the insect. Selectivity is great, but entirely distributional; it is useful against skin and hair dwelling mites and lice. Spread on the skin as powder or emulsion, very little is absorbed by the host but much penetrates the chitinous exoskeleton of ectoparasites. The dose per unit body mass received by parasite and host is vastly different, partly because of different permeability and partly because of different mass to surface area ratios.

Antiseptics

Chlorhexidine, Cetrimide, Benzalkonium act at all cell membranes and rely for their selectivity on poor penetration of the unbroken skin.

Hexachlorophane [hexachlorophene] is a chlorinated phenol bactericidal to Gram +ve bacteria. Regularly applied to the skin it gradually accumulates; the number of organisms in the surface layers is gradually but substantially reduced. Misuse, for example, whole body immersion of babies in strong solutions allows sufficient to be absorbed through the skin to give CNS toxicity, even death.

Eye

Similar considerations apply as to the choice of antibiotics for skin use (page 182).

Gentamicin, Neomycin, Chlortetracycline and *Chloramphenicol* are toxic by inhibition of protein synthesis (page 177).

Polymyxin is toxic by damage to cytoplasmic membranes (page 178).

Sulphacetamide shows biochemical selectivity based on competition with amino-benzoate for DHF synthetase (page 173) reinforced by distributional selectivity. It has pharmacological properties exactly like *Sulphadimidine* (page 195) but physical properties which allow ocular use, that is, it is very soluble and a 30 per cent solution has a pH of 7.4.

Idoxuridine shows some biochemical selectivity based on metabolic acceptance as a pyrimidine, and incorporation into a functionless DNA (page 175) reinforced by distributional selectivity.

DRUG RESISTANCE IN PARASITES

Origin

Usually spontaneous mutation; frequency 1 per $10^6 - 10^7$ cell divisions.

Selection

Mutants have no advantage, and may be at a disadvantage, compared with the wild type in a drug-free environment but they survive and multiply, selected by the administration of a drug to which the wild type is sensitive but the mutant strain is resistant. A single mutation may confer a high degree of resistance (one step) or just a small increment of resistance to which others can be added (multi-step) with selection to a high degree of resistance by prolonged or repeated inadequate drug dosage.

Spread

Spread is by cross-infection or by transfer of genetic material by:

(1)   Transduction — by a bacteriophage (for example, *Staphylococcus* [*Staph.*] *aureus*).
(2)   Conjugation (for example, Shigellae and *E. coli*).

Mechanisms

(1)   Inactivation of the drug. (*a*) β-Lactamase inactivation of penicillins and cephalosporins. *Staph. aureus* is most often discussed but this occurs in other species too, including Gram −ve bacteria but not in Streptococci (Str.) The gene confers the ability to synthesize the β-lactamase enzyme, production of which is induced by contact with the antibiotic. (*b*) Acetylation of *Chloramphenicol.* (*c*) Acylation of amino sugar antibiotics.
(2)   Loss of permeability to, or uptake process for drug. (*a*) Bacterial resistance to tetracyclines (page 179). (*b*) Neoplastic cells resistance to antimetabolites. (*c*) Plasmodia resistant to *Chloroquine* (page 179).
(3)   Increased production of a metabolite which competes with the drug. Aminobenzoate production is increased in some sulphonamide-resistant cells: DHF in plasmodia resistant to *Pyrimethamine* (page 189).
(4)   Enhanced activity of alternative metabolic route by-passing the inhibited pathway. Neoplastic cells resistant to purine or pyrimidine analogues.
(5)   Increased production of drug-sensitive enzyme. (*a*) *Cycloserine* resistance — increased production of alanine racemase and D-alanyl-D-alanine synthetase. (*b*) *Methotrexate* resistance in neoplastic cells — increased production of DHF hydrogenase.
(6)   Modification of drug sensitive site. (*a*) Ribosome loses ability to bind, for example, *Streptomycin, Erythromycin.* (*b*) RNA polymerase loses ability to bind *Rifampicin.* (*c*) DHF synthetase decreases affinity for sulphonamides.

Chemotherapy of metazoal infestations

ECTOPARASITES

Scabies

Scabies is infestation with the mite *Sarcoptes scabiei.* The fertilized females burrow into the horny layer of the skin. This is symptomless at first but an allergic itching rash develops later. Transmission is by close bodily contact. Treatment involves completely covering the body surface, except the face, on two successive days with *gamma benzene hexachloride* (page 182), *Benzyl benzoate* or *Monosulfiram* (like Disulfiram, this shows a toxic interaction with Ethanol, page 165). The mites are all killed by this process but the rash takes about three weeks to clear. Renewal of symptoms is due to reinfestation.

Pediculosis

Pediculosis is infestation with the louse *Pediculus humanus*. Head, body or pubic hair areas may be affected. *Gamma benzene hexachloride*, *Monosulfiram* or *Malathion* (page 180) are effective insecticides.

ENDOPARASITES

Worms

Classification of parasitic worms:

(1) Flatworms; (*a*) tapeworms, (*b*) flukes (includes schistosomes)
(2) Roundworms; (*a*) Ascaris (often called 'roundworm'), (*b*) threadworms, (*c*) hookworms, (*d*) filariae.

Infestation with worms can occur in two basic sites:

(1) The worms live in the tissues of the host; (*a*) lymphatics, skin, connective tissue − filariae, (*b*) liver, bile ducts, lungs − flukes and some schistosomes, (*c*) blood vessels − schistosomes.
     The problems in the development of drugs effective against tissue-resident worms are the difficulty in creating a laboratory model of the infestation and the difficulties inherent in field trials (the need to count worms).

     Effective, if rather toxic, drugs have been developed empirically. Their mechanisms of toxicity and selectivity have been little studied and these parasitisms are not endemic in the UK (*Table 4.2*).

Table 4.2 *Metazoal infestations not endemic in the UK*

Worm:	Vector	Drug
Tissue infestation		
Schistosoma (Bilharzia)	Fresh water snail	*Niridazole*
Filaria	Biting flies	*Diethylcarbamazine*
Intestinal infestation		
Ancylostoma (hookworm)		*Bephenium*
Strongyloides		*Thiabendazole*

(2) The worms live in the lumen of the alimentary canal which has a low PO_2 and are therefore anaerobes; (*a*) tapeworms, (*b*) all roundworms except filariae.

185

Most worms in an infesting population are adult. Therefore, interference with nucleic acid or protein synthesis, which so successfully achieves selective toxicity in bacteria because they are rapidly growing and multiplying, is inappropriate.

Biochemical selectivity has been achieved with some drugs, for example, the worms depend on muscular activity to stay in the gut lumen; drugs (for example, *Piperazine*) biochemically selective for parasite muscle have been developed. However, distributional selectivity is the principal method employed because: (1) the worms are located in a limited compartment; (2) the factors limiting absorption of chemicals from this compartment into the systemic circulation are known; and (3) the worm's pellicle is highly permeable.

Beef tapeworm (*Taenia saginata*)

Successful treatment depends on the scolex (head) of the worm being made to relinquish its hold on the mucosa of the upper jejunum.

Dichlorophen or *Niclosamide* kill the tapeworm, probably by damaging its cytoplasmic membranes and making them leaky. These are water-insoluble compounds, not absorbed from gut (page 182). Since the worm is not passed whole but partially digested, the scolex may be unrecognizable. The criterion of cure is 12 weeks without recurrence of segments in the stool.

Roundworms

Threadworms (Enterobius) inhabit the colon and rectum. They are common in children, causing irritation and sleeplessness when the females emerge from the anus at night to lay eggs. Reinfestation is common so treat the entire household simultaneously.

Roundworms (Ascaris) inhabit the small intestine.

Piperazine is effective against both threadworms and Ascaris. It blocks the action of neurotransmitter ACh at the roundworm's neuromuscular junction by functional antagonism; flaccid paralysis of a worm allows its expulsion by peristalsis. Though well absorbed from the gut *Piperazine* has hardly any neuromuscular blocking activity in mammals (page 178) and very low toxicity to the host.

Bephenium is effective against Ascaris causing spastic paralysis of the worm by an agonist action at muscle ACh receptors. It is a quaternary ammonium compound so little is absorbed by the host (page 231).

Viprinium is effective against threadworms. It is a red dye which kills anaerobic worms probably by blocking their active uptake of glucose. It is prescribed as the insoluble embonate salt therefore not absorbed by the host (page 182).

Chemotherapy of protozoal infections

TRICHOMONAS

Trichomonas vaginalis is a flagellated protozoon causing a venereally transmitted vaginitis and, to a lesser extent, urethritis.

Metronidazole or *Nimorazole* orally is safe and effective. These are biochemically selective, acting on the ferredoxin important to anaerobes (page 178). Recurrence is usually due to reinfection; if repeated treat the sexual partner even if symptom-free. Show a Disulfiram-like interaction with Ethanol (page 165).

AMOEBIASIS

Entamoeba histolytica (Figure 4.7)

Transmission is by the anal-oral route. Cysts are swallowed and hatch in the small intestine to motile amoebae which multiply by binary fission. Low in the large intestine some encyst and are excreted in the faeces.

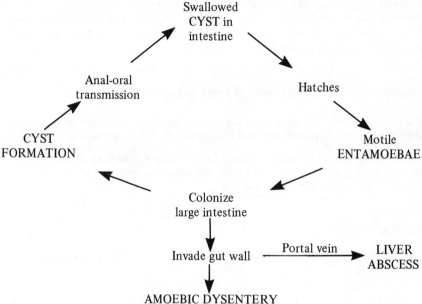

Figure 4.7

About 10 per cent of the world population harbour intestinal Entamoeba as a harmless commensal.

Symptoms — amoebic dysentery — occur when, for an unknown reason, the amoebae invade the wall of the large intestine, cause ulcers and phagocytose red blood cells.

Amoebae may gain access to the liver via the portal vein where they cause tissue necrosis and a bacteriologically 'sterile' abscess.

Classification of amoebicidal drugs

Drugs systemically active against both intestinal and liver parasites

These are useful in treating the acute attack with or without complications.

187

Metronidazole is now the drug of choice. It kills tissue-invading forms. It is biochemically selective (page 178).

Emetine is obsolescent. It is reserved for addition to *Metronidazole* therapy in the desperately ill patient. Given by sc injection it only kills tissue-invading forms. It is biochemically selective (page 177) but very toxic, causing nausea, diarrhoea and damage to the myocardium.

Drugs systemically active only against liver parasites

These are useful in treating amoebic liver abscess only. *Chloroquine:* after malarially parasitized erythrocytes, the liver is the organ which most concentrates *Chloroquine.* Though the concentration there achieved is inadequate to eliminate the malarial parasite (page 189) it is adequate to eliminate *Entamoeba histolytica* (presumably because they phagocytose liver nuclear material further concentrating the *Chloroquine*).

Drugs orally active only against luminal parasites

These are used after all symptoms and signs of infection have subsided, to clear the bowel lumen of Entamoeba and thus terminate the carrier state.

Diloxanide is directly amoebicidal but the mechanism is unknown; it is presumed to be biochemically selective since most *Diloxanide* is absorbed and excreted in the urine but causes little host toxicity.

MALARIA

Plasmodium falciparum, Plasmodium vivax and two other species (Figure 4.8)

In a human with the disease, every 24—72 hours, depending on which of the four pathogenic plasmodial species is causing the infection, red cells loaded with parasites rupture, releasing their contents. This has two consequences: (1) a febrile attack; and (2) infection of other red cells with one parasite each, which then multiply by binary fission to set up the next cycle. Occasionally, the single parasite in a blood cell fails to multiply but instead differentiates into a male or female gametocyte. It is these only which are infective to the anopheline mosquito — the primary (because fertilization and zygote formation occur in it) host — when it takes a blood meal. The infective particles resulting from development of the zygote enter man from the mosquito's salivary glands when it takes another blood meal. If he is not immune they first enter liver cells where they multiply by binary fission — the pre-erythrocytic stage — to burst forth after about 11 days to infect the blood. In all but *P. falciparum* malaria (for example, *P. vivax*) some also infect other liver cells where cyclical development continues for up to ten years as the exo-erythrocytic cycle.

Thus, in falciparum malaria the development of immunity or treatment with a drug which clears the blood (such as *Chloroquine*) can genuinely rid the body of

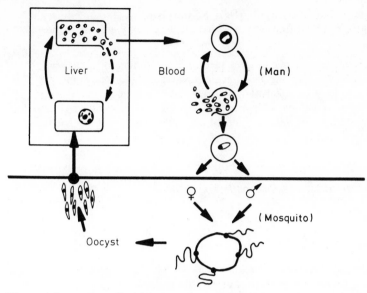

Figure 4.8 = *not in P. falciparum*

the parasites. In *P. vivax* and other malarias, however, only the symptoms are cured, not the disease, and relapse can occur.

Drugs for radical cure — *Primaquine*

This is rapidly absorbed from the gut. Neither the antimalarial effect nor the host toxicity is directly related to the blood concentration of *Primaquine*; it is a prodrug which gives rise in the body to an oxidizing agent — the active species.

Radical cure implies clearing the liver of parasites in the exo-erythrocytic cycle and is therefore not relevant to *P. falciparum* malaria. The only drug available, *Primaquine*, is toxic — do not attempt radical cure in a very ill patient; first clear the blood and get him fit to withstand the treatment.

The mechanism of toxicity is not clearly understood. *Primaquine* binds to DNA (but does not intercalate) and interferes with the phagocytic activity and mitochondrial function of the parasite. The mechanism of selectivity is presumably biochemical.

It is active against the pre-erythrocytic and exo-erythrocytic forms and gameto-cytes but not against the blood form of the parasite which causes the symptoms. Plasmodium does not seem to develop resistance to *Primaquine.*

Host toxicity is principally to the blood: methaemoglobinaemia and haemolysis occur because the active species is a strong oxidizing agent (similar toxicity is shown by other oxidizing drugs, for example, sulphonamides, sulphones and *Nitrofurantoin*). Oxidizing agents can damage haemoglobin and -SH containing enzymes. Erythrocytes possess a reducing mechanism which protects these susceptible targets from oxidation, so damage occurs only when the capacity of the reducing system is exceeded: it is the pentose phosphate cycle (6 molecules

189

of glucose-6-phosphate produces NADPH + 5 molecules of glucose-6-phosphate via pentoses) the essential first step of which is catalysed by glucose-6-phosphate dehydrogenase.

Deficiency of this enzyme occurs as an incompletely dominant sex linked abnormality and has a high incidence in areas where malaria is endemic. The abnormality may have been naturally selected there because it confers some natural immunity to malaria. If *Primaquine* is given to a patient with glucose-6-phosphate-dehydrogenase deficiency its blood toxicity is very much greater than normal.

Drugs for clinical cure — *Chloroquine, Quinine*

Clinical cure implies quickly clearing the blood of parasites. Since *P. falciparum* displays no exo-erythrocytic cycle, clinical cure provides radical cure; for the others (for example, *P. vivax*) it does not and relapse can occur.

The mechanism of toxicity is intercalation into DNA, suppression of DNA replication and therefore suppression of parasite multiplication (page 179). The mechanism of selectivity is distributional: these drugs are selectively concentrated by the erythrocytic parasite, therefore only in these is a concentration adequate to produce the toxic effect achieved. Resistance to *Chloroquine* has begun to emerge (not yet in tropical Africa), probably because it is now being used prophylactically. In this situation *Quinine* or sequential therapy with *Pyrimethamine* and *Sulfadoxine* is valuable.

Drugs for prophylaxis — *Pyrimethamine* and the prodrug *Proguanil*

These properly provide suppressive treatment rather than prophylaxis. They do not stop the contraction of malaria, or its establishment in the liver; they do stop the symptomatic cyclical infection of blood cells. They should be taken daily from one week before to one month after any visit to an endemic area. For mechanisms of toxicity and selectivity *see* page 174).

Resistance occurs readily and there is cross-resistance between *Pyrimethamine* and *Proguanil*. Its mechanism involves increased synthesis of DHF so resistant parasites are more sensitive to sulphonamides because they are more dependent on DHF synthetase.

Some protozoa not endemic in the UK are listed in *Table 4.3.*

Table 4.3 *Other protozoal diseases and their therapy*

Protozoon	Drug
Leishmania	*Sodium stibogluconate*
Giardia	*Metronidazole*
Toxoplasma	*Pyrimethamine* and a sulphonamide

Chemotherapy of fungal infections

KERATIN INFECTIONS (RINGWORM OR DERMATOPHYTOSES)

The fungal mycelia have special affinity for keratin, for example, athlete's foot (tinea pedis). Usually controlled by adequate hygiene.

Ringworm infection of skin

Benzoic acid and *Salicylic* acid ointment: *Benzoic* acid has fungistatic activity while *Salicylic* acid is keratolytic — fungus-laden layers are shed and access of the fungistatic drug to deeper layers is improved.

Tolnaftate (narrow spectrum — dermatophytes only) fungicidal. *Miconazole* (broad spectrum) fungicidal by impairing glutamine uptake through cytoplasmic membrane.
Ointment is useful in treatment and powder in prevention.

Ringworm infection of hair or nails

The mechanism of the fungistatic effect of *Griseofulvin* is unclear. The mechanism of its selectivity is distributional (page 180) — the very small fraction of each oral dose which is absorbed is taken up selectively by keratin precursor cells. Treatment must continue until all infected keratin has been shed (can be more than one year for toe nails). Growing dermatophytes also concentrate the drug.

MUCOCUTANEOUS INFECTION

The yeast Candida is a normal inhabitant of the mouth and gut. Opportunist overgrowth occurs when the normal flora is suppressed — broad spectrum antibiotics — or when the normal defences are suppressed — steroids, suppressed immune system (antineoplastic drugs), in debilitation, diabetes or pregnancy. This occurs commonly in the mouth and throat (thrush) and vagina. *Nystatin* (page 178) is fungicidal to many species of fungus by damaging their sterol-containing cell membranes. It is too toxic for systemic use so in practice its selectivity is distributional and it is only useful against mucocutaneous Candida. It is not absorbed from the gut so the oral route is useful for alimentary infection and local application (pessaries) for vaginitis. *Clotrimazole* is a broad spectrum fungicidal drug which impairs amino acid transport through cytoplasmic membrane.

DEEP TISSUE INFECTION

This tends to occur only in patients whose defences have been seriously impaired by steroids or cytotoxic drugs.

Amphotericin is a close relative of *Nystatin* but sufficiently less toxic to allow

191

its slow iv infusion: renal toxicity which is dose related and reversible with lower doses is nevertheless seen in 80 per cent of patients.

Flucytosine is selectively taken up by susceptible fungi: prodrug giving rise to *Fluorouracil*.

Clotrimazole systemically is being evaluated.

Chemotherapy of bacterial infections

PRINCIPLES OF TREATMENT

Before committing a patient to a course of antibiotic therapy ask — is it necessary?

Table 4.4   *Common pathogenic bacteria, infections and drugs of choice*

Genus species	Infection	Antibacterial agents 1st choice	2nd choice
Gram +ve cocci			
Staph. aureus	Pneumonia	Benzylpenicillin *	Erythromycin
	Wound	Cloxacillin	Gentamicin
Str. pyogenes	Throat	Penicillin V	Erythromycin
	Middle ear		
Str. pneumoniae	Pneumonia	Benzylpenicillin	Erythromycin
	Meningitis		
Gram +ve bacilli			
C. diphtheriae	Diphtheria	Antitoxin	Benzylpenicillin
Cl. perfringens	Gas gangrene	Benzylpenicillin	Metronidazole
Gram −ve cocci			
N. meningitidis	Meningitis	Benzylpenicillin	
N. gonorrhoeae	Gonorrhoea	Benzylpenicillin	Co-trimoxazole
Gram −ve bacilli			
H. influenzae	Bronchitis	Ampicillin	Co-trimoxazole
	Meningitis	Chloramphenicol	Ampicillin
E. coli	Urinary tract	Co-trimoxazole	Ampicillin
			Cephaloridine
			Gentamicin
Klebsiella	Urinary tract	Gentamicin	Cephaloridine
	Pneumonia		
Proteus	Urinary tract	Carbenicillin	Kanamycin
Ps. aeruginosa	Urinary tract	Carbenicillin	Gentamicin
	Septicaemia		
S. typhi	Typhoid	Chloramphenicol	Ampicillin
Others			
Tr. pallidum	Syphilis	Benzylpenicillin	Erythromycin
Bacteroides	Various	Metronidazole	Clindamycin
M. tuberculosis	Tuberculosis	Rifampicin	Streptomycin
		Isoniazid	
		Ethambutol	Pyrazinamide
Mycoplasma	Pneumonia	Tetracycline	Erythromycin

* Only for strains not producing β-lactamase

The basis of rational treatment is the bacteriological diagnosis. The clinical diagnosis from the patient's history and physical signs often allows a provisional bacteriological diagnosis (for example, exacerbation of chronic bronchitis — *Haemophilus (H.) influenzae*; lobar pneumonia — Pneumococcus: urinary tract infection — *Escherichia(E.) coli*) on which basis an antibiotic is chosen. A definitive bacteriological diagnosis requires isolation of the organism responsible. The time required depends on the test employed (for example, Gram stain — ½ hour; culture and identification of pathogens — 12—24 hours; sensitivities to antibacterial drugs — 48 hours). When the bacteriological diagnosis and sensitivities are known, the initially chosen therapy may require modification but not if the patient is improving, for example, falling temperature and resolving of inflammation. *Table 4.4* lists some common infecting organisms and appropriate antibacterial agents.

Routes of administration

The object of chemotherapy is to attain an antibacterial concentration in the infected tissues to assist host defences in eradicating infection. In general, the serum concentration should exceed the minimum inhibitory concentration *in vitro* (mic) by a factor of 5. *Table 4.5* is a reference table. *Table 4.6* summarizes prescribing information on some commonly used antibiotics.

Antibiotics are usually administered by mouth but inadequate doses and infrequent administration encourage the emergence of resistant organisms. In a

Table 4.5 *Sensitivity of important pathogenic bacteria to the principal antibiotics: usual minimum inhibitory concentration (µg/ml)*

Drug	BP	A	CL	CE	E	L	G	T
Staph. aureus[1]	0.03	0.06	0.12	0.12	0.12	0.5—2	0.06	0.12
Staph. aureus[2]	R	R	0.25	5	0.12	0.5—2	0.06	0.12
Str. pyogenes	0.01	0.03			0.03			
Str. pneumoniae	0.01	0.06						
Cl. perfringens	0.12	0.25					R	
N. gonorrhoea	0.01	0.04	0.5				1	
N. meningitidis	0.03	0.06	0.5			R	1	
H. influenzae	0.5—2	0.25	16	8	1—8		1	
E. coli[3]	R	8	R	3	R	R	0.5	1
Klebsiella	R	16—5	R	2—R	R	R	0.25	
Proteus	R	R	R	R	R	R	0.25	
Bacteroides	8—R	R	R		1—4	0.5	R	
Serum concentration (µg/ml)[4]	0.5	2.5	2.5	5	1.5	2.5	4	2.5

BP = *Benzylpenicillin*	A = *Ampicillin*	CL = *Cloxacillin*
CE = *Cephaloridine*	E = *Erythromycin*	L = *Lincomycin*
G = *Gentamicin*	T = *Tetracycline*	R = *resistant*

[1] *Benzylpenicillin*-sensitive.
[2] β-Lactamase-producing.
[3] Sensitivity varies considerably with species.
[4] Approximate mean concentration achieved with recommended dose.

severe infection the antibiotic should be given parenterally at a dose and dosage interval which provides subtoxic peak concentrations and antibacterial trough concentrations. Iv administration ensures that the necessary dose is received — to

Table 4.6   *Prescribing of some commonly used antibiotics*

Drug	*Serum $t_{1/2}$ (h)	Elimination	Usual dose	Route of admin.	Dosage interval (h)
Benzylpenicillin	0.5	ts	0.5 MU	im iv	6
Ampicillin	0.5	ts	250 mg	oral im	6
Cloxacillin	0.5	ts	500 mg	oral im/iv	6
Flucloxacillin	0.5	ts	250 mg	oral im/iv	6
Cephaloridine	1.5	gf	0.25–1 g	im iv	6
Cephalexin	0.5	gf m	250 mg	oral	6
Erythromicin	3	m	500 mg	oral iv	8
Lincomycin	5	gf m	500 mg	im	8
Gentamicin	2.5	gf	80–160 mg	im iv	8
Tetracycline	8.5	gf m	250 mg	oral	8
Co-trimoxazole	8	ts	S 400 mg T 80 mg	oral	12

gf = Glomerular filtration   m = Metabolism
ts = Tubular secretion   * Mean values for normal individuals
S = Sulphamethoxazole   T = Trimethoprim

avoid chemical neutralization avoid mixing one antibiotic solution with another or with iv infusion fluid.

Duration of therapy

This should be decided at the outset but may be amended in response to objective clinical observations, for example, temperature, pulse rate, resolution of signs. Prolonged therapy in the asymptomatic patient is occasionally necessary, for example, recurrent urinary tract infections, pulmonary tuberculosis.

Additional therapy

Chemotherapy may deal with the bacteria but other measures may be necessary to improve the patient's condition (for example, respiratory infection — physiotherapy; abscess — drainage; osteomyelitis — removal of sequestrum; wounds — debridement).

Prophylactic therapy

This is rarely indicated but *see* page 197.

Failure to respond

If the patient does not improve, consider the following:

- Failure of the patient to take the drug — commonly occurs in patients on prolonged therapy, the example, pulmonary tuberculosis.
- Inadequate dose — check mic (*Table 4.5*).
- Additional measures required, for example, drainage of pus.
- Incorrect route of administration, for example, a pleural abscess may require instillation of an antibiotic because of difficulty in penetrating the wall of the cavity and meningitis may require *Benzylpenicillin* intrathecally.
- Response modified because of co-existing disease (anaemia, malignancy) or other drug therapy (steroids, cytotoxic drugs).

Factors modifying the response

(1) Age: premature and newborn infants have immature livers and cannot detoxify certain drugs (for example, *Chloramphenicol*, sulphonamides). Poor renal excretion may result in drug accumulation (for example, *Gentamicin*). Renal function declines in old age and dose adjustment may be necessary.

(2) Pregnancy: the possibility of teratogenicity.

(3) Renal disease: causes accumulation, for example, amino sugar antibiotics. Tetracyclines are contraindicated.

Antibacterial drug combinations

There are certain rules governing the use of antibiotic combinations. Only three are possible:

(1) Bacteriostatic with bactericidal — this combination should never be used. Bactericidal drugs only kill growing bacteria. If growth is prevented by a bacteriostatic drug antagonism of the bactericidal drug may be important, for example, there is a higher mortality in pneumococcal meningitis when *Tetracycline* is given in addition to *Benzylpenicillin.*

(2) Bacteriostatic with bacteriostatic — these are simply additive with the exception of Trimethoprim and sulphamethoxazole (*Co-trimoxazole*) in which synergism converts two bacteriostatic drugs into one bactericidal combination.

(3) Bactericidal with bactericidal — this may be synergistic, for example, binding of penicillinase by *Cloxacillin* allows *Ampicillin* (penicillinase susceptible) to be used. Occasionally, they may be antagonistic, for example, *Gentamicin* and *Carbenicillin in vitro.*

The advantages of combination therapy are to: (1) reduce the emergence of resistant strains during long term therapy, as in tuberculosis; (2) increase the antibacterial spectrum, for example, in severely ill patients, patients with impaired host defences, multiple infecting organisms.

SULPHONAMIDES

For mechanisms of toxicity and selectivity *see* page 173.

This group contains hundreds of compounds but modern usage depends on the degree of absorption and protein binding of the different drugs. Most are absorbed by mouth and are variably bound to plasma albumin (competing with other acidic drugs, for example, oral anticoagulants, *Tolbutamide, Phenylbutazone*). Many undergo acetylation in the liver to a less soluble metabolite which together with the parent compound is eliminated by glomerular filtration and tubular secretion. The proportion eliminated is increased if the urine is alkaline.

Renal toxicity depends on crystalluria — limited solubility of the sulphonamide or its metabolite.

Sulphamethizole is highly soluble, even in acid urine where high concentrations are obtained. It is useful mainly for urinary tract infections; frequent doses are necessary.

Sulphadiazine shows low protein binding which facilitates diffusion into the tissues and CSF. Useful in bacterial meningitis when it is usually given iv.

Sulphamethoxazole was selected for combination with Trimethoprim as *Co-trimoxazole* because it possesses similar pharmacokinetic characteristics. The few toxic effects are attributable to the sulphonamide but folate metabolism can be disturbed in the elderly by the Trimethoprim.

Sulphacetamide is reserved for topical application to the eye due to its unique physical properties — high solubility, a 30 per cent solution has pH 7.4.

Sulphasalazine (a combination of sulphapyridine and a salicylic acid derivative) is used exclusively in the management of ulcerative colitis and Crohn's disease as a means of delivering the salicylate to the desired site of action in the colon where it is released by bacterial hydrolysis.

PENICILLINS

All penicillins have in common fused lactam and thiazolidine rings (*Figure 4.9*). Alteration of the side chain improves the performance of the drug in different situations but results in a reduction of potency against organisms normally sensitive to *Benzylpenicillin* (*Table 4.5*). The basic structure can be altered so

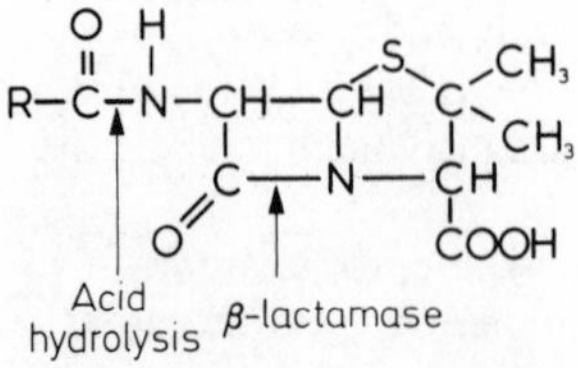

Figure 4.9

that it: (1) becomes resistant to hydrolysis by gastric acid but absorption from the gut remains incomplete although adequate for most clinical purposes; (2) is made resistant to penicillinase; (3) has a broader spectrum of antibacterial activity.

196

For mechanisms of toxicity and selectivity *see* page 172. *Benzylpenicillin* [penicillin G] is very potent (*Table 4.5*) and is the drug of choice in certain infections. It is inactivated (hydrolysed) by gastric acid so it must be administered parenterally. After im injection absorption is rapid and the drug is widely distributed throughout the body but does not readily pass the blood brain barrier. There is no significant metabolism. Elimination is by tubular secretion — 60—90 per cent of the administered dose is eliminated in one hour. Excretion can be delayed and serum levels increased by *Probenecid* which competes for the renal tubular active secretion mechanism for organic acids.

Spectrum of activity — bactericidal at very low mic against Gram +ve and −ve cocci and Gram +ve bacilli (*Table 4.4*): sensitivities vary. Penicillinase opens the β-lactam ring and renders the drug inactive.

Procaine penicillin [penicillin G procaine] combines equimolar amounts of *Benzylpenicillin* and procaine. Peak blood levels are reached in four hours and the drug is still detectable 24 hours later. It is used prophylactically in accident units following trauma.

Penicillin V (phenoxymethylpenicillin) is acid stable. Chemical variants are available in tablet or elixir form. It is very effective in the treatment and prophylaxis of streptococcal infections. Prophylaxis is generally ill-advised except in the following cases:

(1)   To prevent streptococcal infections in patients with rheumatic fever and glomerulonephritis.
(2)   In patients with heart valve disease undergoing dental treatment. Dental treatment produces bacteraemia which leads to infection of and further damage to congenitally or rheumatically damaged endocardium.

Cloxacillin is resistant to both penicillinase and gastric acid. Food interferes with its absorption but even in the fasting state this is incomplete and a higher serum concentration is obtained by the im route, which is preferred in the acutely ill patient.

Flucloxacillin has the same antibacterial spectrum as *Cloxacillin*, but absorption is more complete after oral administration. Higher serum concentration of free drug is also obtained because the proportion bound to plasma protein is less than that of *Cloxacillin*. Both drugs should be reserved for infections with penicillinase-producing staphylococci: they should never be prescribed for infections due to an organism sensitive to *Benzylpenicillin* or *Ampicillin* because they are much less potent.

Methicillin is highly resistant to staphylococcal penicillinase although less resistant to penicillinases produced by other bacteria. It is reserved for infections with penicillinase-producing staphylococci. It is hydrolysed by gastric acid and so must be given parenterally.

Ampicillin has a wider spectrum of activity than penicillin. It is acid stable and adequate serum concentrations are obtained after oral administration. It is, however, susceptible to penicillinase and like *Benzylpenicillin* it is rapidly eliminated by renal tubular secretion. Therapeutic concentrations are found in bile so it is useful for biliary tract infections (cholecystitis) and to eliminate the carrier state in typhoid fever. It may be given parenterally if required. Oral absorption is not complete and a recent derivative *Amoxycillin* achieves a peak blood concentration about twice that of *Ampicillin*, but comparative studies have shown no advantage for either drug. Food does not interfere with the absorption of *Amoxycillin.*

Carbenicillin is penicillinase-sensitive and acid labile (given iv). It is reserved for infections with Pseudomonas.

Host toxicity

None of the above compounds is toxic in the ordinary sense. Indeed, it is almost impossible to 'poison' a patient with penicillin (except by administering it into the CSF). The predilection of this group lies in the production of sensitivity reactions. This is most marked with *Ampicillin.* Reactions are of two kinds: (1) immediate, for example, shock, collapse and death; (2) delayed, for example, rash, urticaria, oedema, fever and serum sickness syndrome.

A rash with *Ampicillin* is more common at a dose of 2 than 1 g/day. It usually occurs when *Ampicillin* is prescribed irrationally for a viral infection, typically a sore throat; for example, infectious mononucleosis (*Penicillin V* is the treatment of choice for a streptococcal tonsillitis).

There is a gradation in reactions produced — the first reaction is usually mild. Always ask a patient if he is sensitive to penicillin before prescribing any of the above drugs. Treatment consists of *Adrenaline, Hydrocortisone*, antihistamines.

Other toxic reactions — nephritis and haemolytic anaemia — may occur, usually in patients on long-term therapy, for example, for subacute bacterial endocarditis.

CEPHALOSPORINS

The basic nucleus closely resembles that of penicillin (*Figure 4.9*) as do the mechanisms of toxicity and selectivity.

Cephaloridine is not absorbed from the gut as it is destroyed by endogenous bacteria. It is given im or iv and is eliminated by glomerular filtration at a rate which correlates well with the creatinine clearance. This explains why the drug accumulates when renal function is impaired.

Cephalothin must be given iv as im injection is irritant and painful. It is more extensively bound to plasma proteins than *Cephaloridine.* It is metabolized in the serum, liver and tissues and therefore accumulation occurs less readily. *Cephalexin,* may be given by mouth.

Host toxicity

Allergy, rashes, nephrotoxicity (especially if *Cephalothin* is combined with *Gentamicin*). They may be administered with caution to a patient sensitive to penicillin.

ERYTHROMYCIN

For mechanisms of toxicity and selectivity *see* page 177. Absorption of the base from the gut is delayed by food. The drug is widely distributed throughout the body with the exception of the CSF. Significant metabolism occurs and elimination is via the bile and urine. Low doses are bacteriostatic but high doses are bactericidal. The spectrum of activity is similar to *Benzylpenicillin* but it is active against penicillinase-producing staphylococci. Host toxicity is minimal and allergy rare. The estolate derivative should not be prescribed for more than 2 weeks because it may produce an intrahepatic obstructive jaundice.

AMINO SUGAR ANTIBIOTICS

For mechanisms of toxicity and selectivity *see* page 177. This group has several members with similar pharmacological characteristics. They are all soluble in water and strongly basic — absorption from the gut is therefore negligible. Distribution is predominantly extracellular; there is little penetration into tissues and no passage across the blood brain barrier. There is no significant metabolism and elimination is by glomerular filtration; no tubular secretion or reabsorption occurs. Excretion correlates well with the creatinine clearance.

Persistent high serum concentrations will produce high tone deafness by damaging the organ of Corti, as well as producing some vestibular damage and also result in renal tubular damage. This situation can be avoided by modifying the dose (*see* page 233).

Streptomycin is a second line in the treatment of tuberculosis. It is a potent cause of skin allergy and can cause foetal eighth nerve damage in pregnancy.

Gentamicin is the most useful member of the group. It has a wide spectrum of activity particularly against Gram —ve bacilli (including Pseudomonas) and also Staphylococcus.

Neomycin is the most toxic member of the group and is given by mouth for 'sterilization' of the gut either preoperatively or in the management of liver failure (page 181). It is also useful topically but note that some systemic absorption can occur with toxicity and sensitivity as a result (pages 182 and 212).

TETRACYCLINES

This group contains several members with a wide spectrum of bacteriostatic activity which includes most Gram +ve and Gram —ve cocci and bacilli as well as Mycoplasmas, Rickettsiae and Chlamydiae. For mechanisms of toxicity and selectivity *see* page 179. Absorption from the gut is incomplete but quite adequate. Two factors account for variability in absorption: (1) the hydrochloride derivatives are soluble in water giving an acid solution; in a neutral or alkaline medium (the intestine) they tend to precipitate out or do not dissolve; (2) they are chelating agents and will complex with divalent ions, for example, Ca^{2+}, Al^{2+}, Mg^{2+} (milk, antacid mixtures) and *Ferrous sulphate* significantly reducing bioavailability.

Disposition varies according to the degree of protein binding, biliary excretion and reabsorption (enterohepatic circulation) and tetracyclines are widely distributed throughout the body, including the CSF (concentration 10 per cent that of serum). They complex with calcium in growing long bones and the enamel of developing teeth and should never be prescribed in pregnancy or in children under the age of 7 years. Elimination occurs in both urine (glomerular filtration and tubular secretion) and faeces (biliary excretion).

Tetracycline — highest peak serum concentration.
Oxytetracycline — least well absorbed.
Chlortetracycline — most toxic.
Lymecycline.

Doxycycline — completely absorbed — need only be administered once daily and may be given if renal function is impaired and there is no alternative. It is expensive.

Host toxicity

Superinfection: because of their wide spectrum and incomplete absorption tetracyclines eliminate commensal organisms in the bowel, allowing the over-growth of organisms naturally resistant to them, for example, *Candida albicans*, resistant Staphylococcus, Pseudomonas. Renal tubular damage has occurred with outdated preparations but the anti-anabolic effect (inhibition of protein synthesis) of in-date tetracyclines can cause a raised blood urea concentration in normal patients and aggravate the uraemia and associated metabolic abnormalities in patients with chronic renal failure. Tetracyclines (with the exception of doxycycline) and their metabolites accumulate when renal function is impaired. Other side-effects include photosensitization and rashes.

CHLORAMPHENICOL

This is bacteriostatic and well absorbed when administered by mouth. Its wide distribution includes the CSF. It is metabolized and little unchanged drug is eliminated in the urine. Its conjugation mechanism in the liver is immature in the newborn, therefore it easily accumulates to toxic concentrations. It acts by inhibiting protein synthesis (page 177) and this is responsible for its major side-effect, that is, depression of the bone marrow. Therefore, monitor the full blood count (including platelets) every 48 hours in patients receiving the drug. In sensitive subjects unpredictable development of complete marrow aplasia may occur and is fatal in all cases. This has restricted its use to infections with *Salmonella (S.) typhi* and to meningitis due to *H. influenzae*.

LINCOMYCIN AND CLINDAMYCIN

These are absorbed after oral administration and are bactericidal for Gram +ve and —ve cocci and bacilli but are also active against Gram +ve and —ve anaerobes (including Bacteroides). They are widely distributed and penetrate bone particularly well. However, diarrhoea is a frequent side-effect and may be severe if pseudomembranous colitis develops — an enterotoxin produced by an anaerobe resistant to these antibiotics (*Cl. difficile*) is often responsible for the diarrhoea and colitis — an example of superinfection, treatable by *Metronidazole*. For mechanisms of toxicity and selectivity *see* page 177.

URINARY ANTISEPTICS

These exert antibacterial activity in the urine but have little or no systemic antibacterial effect (*see* page 181). Toxic effects may still occur despite this, especially if there is renal impairment. In this situation the drugs are useless since adequate urinary concentrations are not achieved.

Nitrofurantoin is active against Gram +ve and −ve organisms. It often causes nausea and vomiting and occasionally a peripheral neuropathy.

Nalidixic acid is mainly active against Gram −ve organisms.

TUBERCULOSIS

Eradication of *Mycobacterium (M.) tuberculosis* from patients is now almost always achieved provided the patient takes the right drugs for the prescribed course. Antituberculous drugs have two kinds of action, as follows:

(1) Sterilization of tuberculous lesions − *Rifampicin* and *Pyrazinamide* are most potent with *Isoniazid* moderately potent.
(2) Prevention of development of resistance to other sterilizing drugs − *Isoniazid* and *Rifampicin* have greatest activity in this regard with *Streptomycin* less effective and *Ethambutol* weaker still.

Current antituberculosis chemotherapy involves triple therapy with *Rifampicin*, *Isoniazid* and *Ethambutol* for three months (longer if *M. tuberculosis* can still be isolated from the sputum) with administration of the first two drugs being maintained for a further six months.

In countries outside Western Europe and North America *Rifampicin*, because of its great expense, is used more economically. Very low rates of relapse have been found using a thrice weekly regimen for eight months with *Streptomycin*, *Isoniazid, Pyrazinamide*, and *Rifampicin* (thrice weekly for four months).

Streptomycin used to be the first line of treatment in combination with *Isonazid* and sodium *Aminosalicylate*; the large dose needed of the last named was associated with unpleasant gastrointestinal upset.

The mechanism of the antituberculosis activity of *Isoniazid* is unclear. It is well absorbed and crosses the blood brain barrier (may elevate mood). It is acetylated in the liver at a rate which is genetically determined (page 257) and toxic effects are more likely in slow acetylators. Polyneuropathy is reversed by *pyridoxine*. Liver damage (hepatitis-like) can be very severe. *Rifampicin* has a wider spectrum of potent antibacterial activity (page 176) but is reserved for use in tuberculosis because resistance readily develops and allergic reactions are common if interrupted therapy is practised. Abnormal liver function tests are common but usually transient. Hepatic microsomal enzyme induction results in a reduction of the efficacy of the low dose oestrogen oral contraceptives.

Ethambutol is prescribed on a weight basis as high doses may damage visual acuity. About 90 per cent is excreted unchanged in the urine so dosage adjustment is necessary if renal function is impaired.

Pyrazinamide is much better than *Ethambutol* in short-course (eight month) therapy. It may cause hepatic dysfunction.

Chemotherapy of viral infections

Viruses are obligatory intracellular parasites because they have the genetic information for reproduction but no mechanism for carrying it out. The simplest consist of a single piece of nucleic acid containing just enough codons to reproduce itself. The large majority, including most human pathogens, also contain coding for a simple protein coating, to be worn when the virus particle is extracellular, which confers antigenicity and affinity for specific cells. A few large complex viruses (Chlamydiae) also contain lipoprotein and enzymes — these are susceptible to *Tetracycline* but diseases caused by them are uncommon.

The nucleic acid content of viruses allows their classification into: (1) DNA viruses, for example, herpes simplex, chickenpox (herpes zoster/varicella), small-pox (variola major) and vaccinia. (2) RNA viruses, for example, poliomyelitis and influenza.

THE VIRAL REPLICATION PROCESS

(1)   Virus particles exist free in the environment or host ECF.
(2)   Adsorption onto specific cell surfaces.
(3)   Penetration into susceptible cells.
(4)   Lysosymal digestion of the protein coat. The liberated nucleic acid by-passes or takes over genetic control of the infected cell.
(5)   Synthesis of early proteins (nucleic acid polymerases).
(6)   Synthesis of RNA or DNA (multiple replicates of virus nucleic acid).
(7)   Synthesis of proteins for coat.
(8)   Assembly of virus particles.
(9)   Release from the host cell with cell damage or death, induction of release of interferon and inflammation (gives localizing symptoms) and repair.

Thus, the peak of multiplication has usually passed when illness becomes clinically obvious and there is little that an antiviral drug can be expected to do therapeutically.

ANTIVIRAL THERAPY

Vaccines

The particles are most exposed when extracellular — Stage (1) above — but are then metabolically inert. Immunological attack directed against the protein coat works well. There are vaccines for prophylaxis of influenza, measles, poliomyelitis, rabies, rubella, smallpox and yellow fever. Passive immunity can be confered with Human Normal Immunoglobulin against hepatitis and measles.

Drugs

Amantadine seems to act at Stage (2) or (3). A beneficial effect in parkinsonism

202

(page 131) was discovered as a side-effect during tests of the antiviral action. It reduces the incidence of influenza A infections if administered continuously during epidemics; it may reduce the duration of illness if taken after the onset of symptoms. It is also effective in herpes zoster (shingles).

Idoxuridine acts at Stage (6), being incorporated into DNA synthesis to make a functionless product. Therefore, it is lethal to all cells actively synthesizing DNA (page 175) and very toxic if used systemically.

Mechanism of selectivity Cells infected with herpes simplex make DNA about 1000 times faster than normal cells; therefore, there is some biochemical selectivity which is reinforced in use by distributional selectivity — local application as eyedrops in herpes simplex of corneal epithelium (page 183). Skin — herpes simplex and zoster.

Vidiarabine is effective against DNA virus replication but very toxic (bone marrow depression) when used systemically; only justified in, for example, herpes simplex encephalitis.

Methisazone seems to act on Stage (7) or (8). When given to unvaccinated small-pox contacts it reduced the incidence and mortality of smallpox. Toxicity — vomiting.

The most promising experimental leads for the future are probably the inducers of interferon.

Chemotherapy of malignant neoplasms

In the past, due to poor therapeutic responses and a high incidence of undesirable side-effects, chemotherapy was considered only as a last resort, after the apparently more successful treatments — surgery and radiotherapy — had failed. Recent progress (particularly with intermittent combination chemotherapeutic schedules) holds considerable promise and chemotherapy is now the preferred form of treatment of the leukaemias, lymphomas, choriocarcinomas and certain other tumours.

The main problem in cancer chemotherapy is the lack of highly selective agents. With those currently used, many rapidly dividing normal cells (for example, bone marrow, gut epithelium, spermatogenic cells, lymphoid tissue, hair follicles, foetus) are also killed.

The limited success (enhanced tumour regression, longer remission periods, decreased side-effects) of intermittent combination therapy has been obtained by rather empirical clinical methods. Developments in knowledge of cell cycle kinetics (and pharmacokinetics) provide some understanding of the mechanisms involved.

CELL KINETICS AND DOSE STRATEGY

Cellular replication involves passage through a cell cycle (*Figure 4.10*).

In general, anticancer drugs may be described (Bruce's classification) as being either cell-cycle phase-dependent or phase-independent.

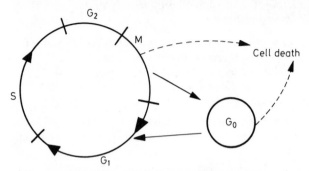

Figure 4.10 G_0 = *resting phase (non-proliferating cells).*
G_1 = *variable (usually long) period prior to DNA synthe-sis (cells grow in size). S = period (6−8 hours) of DNA synthesis. G_2 = period ($\cong$ 2 hours) prior to mitosis (tetraploid). M = mitosis*

Cell-cycle phase-dependent drugs act chiefly on cells in certain phases of the cell cycle (but not G_0). When a tissue culture is treated with drugs in this group the percentage of colony-forming cells surviving falls rapidly at first with increasing dose but reaches a plateau where further increase in dose produces no further increase in cell death (*Figure 4.11*, curve D): Colaspase and *Prednisolone* (G_1), *Methotrexate, Mercaptopurine, Cytarabine*, and procarbazine (S); and *Vinblastine* (M).

Cell-cycle phase-independent drugs act on cells in any phase of the cycle including a slight effect on the G_0 phase. Cell survival in tissue culture falls progressively with increasing dose (*Figure 4.11*, curve I). *Cyclophosphamide, Fluorouracil*, actinomycin D [dactinomycin], daunorubicin.

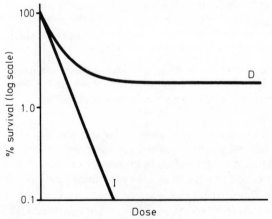

Figure 4.11 *Tumour colony-forming cells in culture*

In an advanced stage (many cells in G_O) some cancers respond to the use of cell-cycle phase-independent drugs first, both to reduce cell numbers and promote recruitment of cells into the growth phase of the cell cycle, thus rendering them susceptible to cell-cycle phase-dependent drugs. If exposure to cell-cycle phase-independent drugs is prolonged (say, > 2 cell cycles, about 48 hours in man) many normal cells will also be drawn out of G_O and killed.

Cell kinetic studies have provided a logical basis for the fact that high dosage intermittent combination therapy is the most effective treatment mode. Drugs and timings are selected which allow maximal tumour cell killing and minimal emergence of drug resistance.

PRINCIPAL SIDE-EFFECTS OF CANCER CHEMOTHERAPY

Immediate

Nausea and vomiting; relieved by *Metoclopramide* and other anti-emetics.

Delayed

(1)   Bone marrow depression: occurs 10–14 days after a single dose. Indicated by decrease in platelet and leucocyte counts (may lead to bleeding disorders, increased susceptibility to infection and even marrow aplasia).
(2)   Gastrointestinal tract disturbances – bleeding and diarrhoea.
(3)   Alopecia.
(4)   Neurotoxicity – especially with Vinca alkaloids.
(5)   Hepatic damage – may be due to toxic metabolites.
(6)   Teratogenicity.
(7)   Impaired growth in children.
(8)   Immune suppression – related to marrow depression and to a direct effect on lymphocytes and other 'immunocytes'. There is a low resistance to infection and may be a reduced immunological response against the neoplasia itself.

Many of the anticancer drugs (for example, *Azathioprine* and *Cyclophosphamide*) are also immunosuppressive agents useful in organ transplantation and for the treatment of certain autoimmune diseases such as systemic lupus erythematosus (single drugs and relatively low doses for longer periods).

Cyclophosphamide depresses mainly B-lymphocyte function as well as a population of suppressor T-cells. It can also be immuno-enhancing in some experimental situations, depending on the dose and time interval between drug and subsequent test antigen.

ANTIMETABOLITES

Most drugs in this category are closely related chemically to various essential endogenous compounds (for example, replacing –OH and –H in folic acid with –NH_2 and –CH_3 respectively produces *Methotrexate*).

Methotrexate inhibits dihydrofolate reductase (page 174) (affinity for this enzyme is 100,000 times that of folate). It is particularly prone to produce gastro-intestinal lesions. Given orally or iv its toxicity to normal cells can be lessened by concurrent administration of calcium folinate.

Fluorouracil and *Cytarabine* − (page 175).

Mercaptopurine (page 174) is metabolized in the liver by xanthine oxidase; this can be prevented by *Allopurinol* which is occasionally used to increase the cytotoxic action.

Azathioprine is a prodrug of *Mercaptopurine*(page 175); its main effect is depression of the immune response and it is reserved for this purpose.

ENZYMES

Colaspase (L-Asparaginase)

Some tumour cells have little asparagine synthetase and therefore must rely solely on extracellular sources of asparagine. Colaspase interferes by destroy-ing this aminoacid. It is utilized in certain acute leukaemias.

DRUGS AFFECTING DNA

Actinomycin-D is the most potent cytotoxic drug on a molar basis. It combines with DNA and prevents transcription to RNA. It is reserved for certain tumours, for example, teratoma of the testis.

Daunorubicin and doxorubicin have potent effects on bone marrow. They are effective in acute myeloid leukaemia: may damage cardiac muscle and produce latent cardiomyopathy. Recent animal studies indicate that selectivity can be enhanced by conjugation to DNA *in vitro.* The daunorubicin-DNA complex is endocytosed by tumour cells but not by cardiac cells. Lysosomal action intracellulary releases free drug capable of binding to tumour nuclear DNA, and preventing DNA replication and transcription. Procarbazine binds to DNA and promotes single strand breaks.

ALKYLATING AGENTS

Nitrogen mustards are all derivatives (different R-groups) of the basic structure given in *Figure 4.4.*

Mechanism of action − form ethyleniminium ions (page 175).

Mustine (R=CH_3) is given by iv injection only. It is the most effective member of the group but also the most toxic − usually used in combination with other agents.

Cyclophosphamide is a 'wide spectrum' antitumour drug given either by mouth or injection. It is a prodrug which requires activation by liver (mixed function oxidase, page 224) enzymes. A metabolite is irritant to the bladder causing cystitis (urine occasionally bloodstained). One of its active metabolites may denature cytochrome P_{450} thus impairing the biotransformation of various drugs including *Cyclophosphamide* itself.

Chlorambucil is the slowest acting nitrogen mustard and the treatment of choice in chronic lymphatic leukaemia. Orally active, it is considered by many to be a 'mild' agent but in the correct dosage is as toxic as *Cyclophosphamide* — particularly prone to produce thrombocytopenia.

Melphalan (R=L-phenylalanine) is usually reserved for myeloma and seminoma; there has been recent success in breast cancer (with other drugs); it is active orally.

Busulphan (a dimethanesulphonate derivative, not a N mustard). The least toxic of the alkylating agents (page 175). Platelet depression is unusual but it may produce marrow aplasia so frequent monitoring of the blood count is necessary. It is the treatment of choice for chronic myeloid leukaemia: active orally. Fibrosing alveolitis is a side-effect ('busulphan lung') peculiar to this agent.

Tumour cells may become resistant to alkylating agents with time, perhaps as a result of enhanced DNA repair mechanisms (animal studies indicate that agents which inhibit DNA repair processes, for example, *Caffeine* and *Chloroquine*, tend to lessen this resistance when given concurrently).

VINCA ALKALOIDS

These consist of two compounds with only a small difference in structure but different chemical and physical properties. Administration is by iv injection only.

Vinblastine — effective against Hodgkin's disease.

Vincristine — effective against acute lymphatic leukaemia.

Both drugs cause neurotoxic side-effects. This is probably due to their capacity to bind to tubulin and dissolve microtubules within various cells; they may inhibit axoplasmic flow.

HORMONES

The lympholytic action of glucocorticoids is exploited.

Specific hormonal therapy was introduced in 1939 by Huggins who treated prostate cancer with oestrogens. Tumours which respond are generally less anaplastic (that is, more highly differentiated) than those which do not. Often used in combination with other drugs because of undesirable effects on the immune response.

One-third of advanced breast cancers both possess oestrogen receptors (page 80) and remit in response to hormonal manipulation; for example, removal of ovaries, tamoxifen (page 83), removal of adrenals or, paradoxically, large doses of oestrogens or androgens (page 83).

RADIOTHERAPY

Radiotherapy is an extremely effective way of treating localized tumours: a second course of radical treatment cannot be given as this would damage normal tissues. Often used in combination with cytotoxic drugs.

^{32}P is as effective as *Busulphan* in chronic myeloid leukaemia (page 180). ^{131}I is the treatment of choice for elderly patients with thyrotoxicoses. It is selectively concentrated in the thyroid tissue (page 180) and therefore useful in the treatment of differentiated tumours of the thyroid gland.

ANTI-ANERGIC AGENTS AND IMMUNE STIMULANTS

Tumours bear tumour specific antigens which differ from host or 'self' antigens. These are recognized as 'foreign' by the functioning immune system leading to destruction of the neoplasm by the cellular immune response. This 'immuno-surveillance' concept of cancer therefore regards the immune system as impaired in malignant disease. The so-called 'anti-anergic' (anergy = no immune system response after exposure to antigens) agents (for example, levamisole) may restore the cellular (or T-lymphocyte) division of the immune response to normal. BCG and other microbial antigenic products are currently being investigated clinically in cancer patients in view of their capacity to heighten immune responsiveness. Recent evidence indicates that most immune stimulants act non-specifically by enhancing macrophage phagocytic activity. Much effort is now being directed to obtaining chemically defined immune stimulants derived from natural antigenic sources. One of the most promising is muramyl dipeptide which represents the smallest active molecule obtainable from bacterial cell wall peptidoglycans.

The interferons may also have therapeutic potential as anticancer agents.

5
Drug disposition and metabolism

AIMS

- To explain the entry of drug molecules into body tissues and their subsequent removal in terms of familiar physical, chemical and biological processes.
- To focus attention on the entry and removal of particular drugs which serve as type substances for broad groups with similar physico-chemical properties.

GENERAL PRINCIPLES – INTRODUCTION

Disposition is a comprehensive term which includes the processes of absorption, distribution and elimination.

Absorption is the entry of drug molecules into the blood via the mucous membranes of the alimentary or respiratory tracts or from the site of an injection.

Distribution is the movement of drug molecules between the water, lipid and protein constituents of the body.

Elimination is the removal of the original drug molecule from the body by excretion or by biotransformation (alteration of the structure of the molecule).

These processes are studied quantitatively in the science of 'pharmacokinetics' and together they determine the concentration of drug molecules at the site of drug action. The relationship between drug concentration and response is studied in 'pharmacodynamics'.

The processes of absorption, distribution and elimination are of critical importance in clinical medicine, pharmacy and toxicology. If they are ignored the patient suffers; toxic drugs may accumulate until the amount in the body is harmful or even fatal; useful drugs may give no benefit because the doses are too small to establish therapeutic concentrations; expensive and hazardous techniques may be used to remove drugs from patients after overdosage when the unaided physiological processes would have been adequate and safe.

Drug absorption

Most drugs are given as tablets or capsules. Advantages of these formulations include precise control of dose and chemical stability of drugs as dry solids. Two processes precede absorption.

Disintegration

Rate is determined by pharmaceutical formulation. Minimum standards are specified in pharmacopoeias. Sometimes disintegration is slow. Radiologists occasionally see intact tablets in lower small bowel. Conglomerations of *Aspirin* tablets can be recovered from stomach many hours after an overdose. Disintegration may be deliberately delayed by an 'enteric coating' which is soluble only at the higher pH of the intestine.

Solution

Rate depends on the particle size, the drug and the ambient pH, for example, *Aspirin* dissolves slowly at pH 1 (stomach) and more rapidly at pH 6 (duodenum/ jejunum). Once in solution the drug is available for absorption through the appropriate mucous membrane.

With certain drugs neither process is complete; 'bioavailability' is reduced.

SITES OF ABSORPTION

Small intestine

The small intestine is more important than the stomach because of its vastly greater area. The barrier to drug absorption consists of the following:

(1)   Bimolecular lipid sheet — 10 nm thick, with polar (hydrophilic) groups outside and non-polar (hydrophobic) groups inside. Chemical composition: lecithin, triglyceride, free fatty acid and cholesterol. Water-soluble drugs cannot penetrate because they are insoluble in the lipid. Lipid-soluble drug molecules or species of drug molecules penetrate readily by 'non-ionic diffusion'.

(2)   Water-filled pores (diameter about 1 nm) can be penetrated by water-soluble drugs if the molecules are small enough (MW < 100). Examples: Ethanol (MW = 46, page 239), urea (60), and the antibiotic *Cycloserine* (99).

(3)   Specific carrier systems. Active transport systems which exhibit substrate stereospecificity, saturability and competition between analogues; for example, L-aminoacids (*Levodopa, Methyldopa, Thyroxine*), antimetabolites (purines, pyrimidines), essential ions.

Note: Most drugs are absorbed by passive diffusion through the lipid sheet, few are small enough to diffuse through the water pores and few meet the structural requirements for active transport.

Other mucous membranes

(1) Buccal mucosa provides a convenient site for the administration of esters without their being exposed to gut and liver enzymes (for example, *Glyceryl trinitrate* [nitoglycerin] in the prophylaxis of effort angina).

(2) Bronchial mucosa provides a large surface area accessible to vapours and ultrafine droplets (aerosols).

Examples	*Effects*
Amyl nitrite	Relief of angina pectoris
Salbutamol	Relief of bronchial asthma
Pb	Poisoning of workers using oxy-acetylene cutters
Hg	Poisoning of dental nurses

(3) Nasal mucosa provides an inefficient (high proportion of dose is wasted) but convenient route of entry for relatively low MW peptides. They can be administered as a nasal spray thus avoiding exposure to gut peptidases.

Examples	*Uses*
Lypressin (ADH)	Diabetes insipidus
Oxytocin	Facilitates breast feeding

(4) Rectal mucosa provides a useful absorptive surface when the patient is vomiting or suffering local gastric side-effects.

Examples	*Uses*
Aminophylline suppositories	Bronchial asthma
Rectal *Diazepam*	Serial seizures in young children
Rectal tribromethanol	Seizures during labour
Indomethacin suppositories	Arthritis

Skin

(1) Healthy skin is a highly specialized protective envelope which prevents uncontrolled water loss and the entry of water-soluble compounds. However, many lipid-soluble drugs can enter and produce pharmacological effects.

Examples	*Effects*
Methyl salicylate	Salicylate intoxication
Camphor	Convulsions
Corticosteroid esters	ACTH suppression
Phenol	Acute renal failure

Infants and toddlers are specially vulnerable because of their high surface/mass ratio (*Table 5.1*).

Table 5.1

	Child (1 month)	*Child (5 years)*	*Adult*
Height (m)	0.50	0.90	1.80
Surface (m^2)	0.25	0.67	1.90
Weight (kg)	5.00	20.00	70.00
m^2/kg x 100	5.00	3.40	2.70

(2) Diseased skin (for example, extensive burns, wounds, eczema). In this case the water barrier is lost; even water-soluble drugs can enter and fatal accidents have resulted.

Examples	*Effects*
Tannic acid (on burns)	Acute renal failure
Sulphonamides	Crystalluria
Neomycin	Paralysis of respiration

Injection

(1) Intravenous (iv) — absorption is complete when injection is complete unless accidentally spilled outside the blood vessel.
(2) Intraperitoneal — rapid absorption by diffusion through large surface area; *Neomycin* causes respiratory paralysis when applied to the peritoneum in excessive dose.
(3) Intramuscular (im) — skeletal muscle has a rich capillary plexus. The capillary endothelium has large water-filled pores which are freely permeable even to water-soluble drugs of high MW. This route is the standard one for injections by nurses. Many antibiotics are given by this route (deltoid, gluteal and quadriceps muscles). The rate of absorption is proportional to the dose, the extent of dispersion and the rate of tissue blood flow. Exercise promotes absorption.
(4) Subcutaneous (sc) — tissues are poorly perfused especially in low cardiac output states (haemorrhagic shock, acute diabetic ketoacidosis). This is the standard route for self-injection (diabetics) — convenient sites are the upper arm, thigh and abdomen. Absorption is relatively slow even in healthy subjects and may be deliberately delayed by administration of sustained release formulations (for example, depot insulins).

SUSTAINED AND DELAYED RELEASE FORMULATIONS

Rapid dissolution of drugs may cause local damage to the gut mucosa (*Aspirin*, potassium, iron), or systemic side-effects due to a brief, high peak of concentration in the blood (*Digoxin*-induced nausea). Alternatively, the duration of drug response may be too short for practical day-to-day treatment (*Procainamide, Quinidine*). These problems are sometimes solved by producing pharmaceutical formulations which release the drug slowly or after a delay. Not all these formulations are justified but all are more expensive than the standard drug. A variety of techniques is employed.

Enteric coated tablets

The coating dissolves on reaching a non-acid medium. It is used to protect the drug from acid or to protect the stomach from the drug (for example, *Aspirin*, *Prednisolone*). The thicker the coating the slower the solution. Smoothly sustained release may be obtained by filling capsules with mixed granules having different solution rates. A thin or soluble coating to the granules gives immediate release. A thick or insoluble coating gives delayed release. Intermediate coatings give intermediate properties.

212

Wax matrix tablets

The drug (for example, *Ferrous sulphate, KCl*) is slowly leached out from the interstices of an insoluble wax sponge. Local high concentrations of potassium ion do not develop and intestinal ulcers are prevented. The exhausted matrix is excreted with the faeces.

Solution in oil

Ester of drug and long chain fatty acid (for example, *Fluphenazine* decanoate) dissolved in non-toxic oil. Drug very slowly diffuses out from an injection site over a period of weeks. Used for maintenance dosage in psychotic patients who otherwise fail to take prescribed treatment.

Soluble colloid complex in water

Drug is held in a micelle by weak, hydrogen bonds. Release from complex occurs slowly in the circulation after absorption (for example, *Iron dextran* given iv or im).

Suspension of insoluble complex

Complex between soluble drug and relatively inert molecule is almost insoluble. Soluble drug is slowly released from suspension at site of im or sc injection. Extends duration of action of *Benzylpenicillin* (*Procaine penicillin*) or insulin (*Protamine zinc* and *Isophane insulin*).

Suspension of crystals

Notably *insulin zinc suspension* — smallest particles (*Amorphous,* semi-lente) give most rapid absorption. Largest crystals (ultra-lente) give slowest absorption and longest duration of action. Mixture of *Amorphous:crystalline* of 3:7 (lente) spans 4–24 hours.

Note: Sustained release formulations contain more drug than would normally be given at one time. Therefore, release must not be erratic.

Distribution

Once a drug has entered the circulation, the rate and extent of its distribution depend on the relative arterial blood perfusion rates of different organs and the permeability characteristics of cell membranes towards different drug molecules.

In the special case of absorption from the gut, drug molecules are distributed first to the liver. When the drug is highly lipid-soluble it may be extensively metabolized on its 'first pass' so that only a small proportion of the dose reaches the systemic circulation unchanged (*Lignocaine*, page 247). Thus, incomplete absorption is not the only cause of reduced systemic bioavailability.

Haemodynamic factors

The whole of the right heart output (and therefore the 'absorbed' dose) is passed through the lungs to the left heart. The bulk of the absorbed dose is then carried rapidly to the 'vessel-rich' group of organs which receive about 80 per cent of the cardiac output at rest (brain, myocardium, liver, kidneys, adrenals and thyroid). During late pregnancy the uterus and placenta should also be included.

A few minutes after a drug is injected as an iv bolus it is relatively concentrated in these organs. Gradually, however, the drug becomes distributed more widely or 'redistributed' to skeletal muscle which has a relatively low blood flow at rest. More slowly still it reaches skin and adipose tissue and only very slowly indeed does it reach avascular structures such as tendon and cartilage.

Permeability factors

Arterial blood flow determines the rate at which a drug reaches the interstitial fluid of a given organ or tissue. The capillary endothelium presents no barrier to its passage. The rate of penetration into cells and across special tissue barriers is, however, dependent on the physical characteristics of the drug molecule. Highly water-soluble drugs (*Gentamicin*, page 231) behave like inulin, that is, they penetrate into cells slowly or not at all; conversely, highly lipid-soluble drugs (Thiopentone, page 236 and inhalational anaesthetics, page 240) penetrate so rapidly that the rate of entry into cells is limited solely by blood flow.

SPECIAL COMPARTMENTS AND SPECIAL BARRIERS

Blood brain barrier

In 1909, Goldman showed that trypan blue given intravenously did not stain the brain but the brain was stained after intrathecal injection. The barrier to entry may be thin astrocyte processes which envelop the capillary endothelium. The penetration of drugs is dependent on their lipid solubility and ionization.

Highly polar, water-soluble drugs (for example, *Gentamicin*, page 231 and quaternary ammonium salts, *Table 5.16*) penetrate slowly, if at all. Non-polar, lipid-soluble drugs (for example, Thiopentone, page 236) and inhalational anaesthetics, page 240) penetrate rapidly and drugs with intermediate solubility (for example, barbitone) penetrate at an intermediate rate.

The stronger an acidic drug (that is, the lower the pK_a) the smaller the concentration of unionized molecules and the slower the rate of penetration into brain; for example, *Salicylic* acid (pK_a 3, page 244) penetrates more slowly than

214

barbitone (pK_a 8). Similarly, the stronger a basic drug (that is, the higher the pK_a) the smaller the concentration of unionized molecules and the slower the rate of penetration into brain; for example, *Quinine* (pK_a 8) penetrates more slowly than aniline (pK_a 5). The penetration of acidic and basic drugs depends also on the lipid solubility of the unionized molecules. For example, *Adrenaline* has few CNS effects but the less polar Amphetamine (no $-OH$ groups) has marked CNS effects.

Several drugs are transferred from the CSF to the plasma across the choroid plexus against a concentration gradient. This mechanism resembles the transport system in the renal tubule.

Examples

Anions	*Cations*
Aminohippurate	*Pentolinium*
Benzylpenicillin	Tubocurarine
Probenecid	

This phenomenon impairs the effectiveness of the penicillins against bacterial infections within the CNS. As a consequence very large doses of these antibiotics are required.

Essential nutrients (amino acids, glucose, purines, pyrimidines) are actively transported into the CSF and brain. *Methyldopa* and *Levodopa* also enter by this means.

Eye

Anterior compartment

The conjuctiva, sclera, iris and ciliary muscle receive a moderate vascular supply but the cornea and lens are avascular. Drugs which exist in a relatively lipid-soluble form can penetrate to these structures and the aqueous humour from the conjunctival sac (for example, *Prednisolone* sodium phosphate, *Chloramphenicol, Atropine* and *Cocaine*).

Note: Benzylpenicillin is extruded from the aqueous humour as it is from the CSF.

Posterior compartment

The sclera, choroid and retina are moderately vascular but the vitreous humour is avascular. These structures are not penetrated from the conjunctival sac but only from the systemic circulation.

Placenta

There is direct contact between the maternal blood and the foetal (placental) tissues in primates. Several transfer mechanisms operate:

(1) Passive diffusion down a concentration gradient: examples O_2, CO_2, many drugs. Even highly polar water-soluble drugs like *Gentamicin* and

quaternary ammonium salts penetrate to the foetus slowly. *Tetracycline* penetrates and complexes with calcium in foetal bone (page 199). The antithyroid drug *Carbimazole* penetrates and can produce a neonatal goitre (page 262). Lipid-soluble drugs (for example, anaesthetics) penetrate readily and interfere with respiration in the newborn child. *Morphine* and related analgesics cause the same problem (page 147).

(2) Active transport, for example, aminoacids and glucose.

(3) Pinocytosis, for example, foetal red cells and maternal immunoglobulins.

Note: All drugs penetrate into the foetal circulation at some rate, slow penetration only protects the foetus if delivery is imminent. Anoxia and hypercapnia make the placental barrier more permeable to drugs.

Serous cavities (pleural, pericardial, peritoneal sacs and joint spaces)

In general, drugs enter and leave slowly down concentration gradients. Water-soluble drugs penetrate slowly and lipid-soluble drugs more rapidly. Acute inflammation facilitates the penetration of drugs but chronic inflammation with fibrosis impedes penetration.

Bones and teeth

Drug access is proportional to the local blood flow. Infection produces oedema, ischaemia and avascular necrosis so that only prompt treatment is effective. Certain drugs and ions complex with bone salt, especially in growing bone (for example, lead, fluoride and *Tetracycline*).

Skin and nails

Avascular and prone to fungal infection. *Griseofulvin* has an affinity for keratin precursor cells (page 180). Arsenic forms a stable complex with disulphide groups.

Abscess cavities

Acute abscesses are thin-walled, local blood flow is increased and antibiotics penetrate readily. Chronic abscesses have thick avascular walls and drugs do not penetrate. In acute otitis media the organisms are accessible but not in chronic otitis media. Vegetations on heart valves have a poor blood supply and big doses of bactericidal antibiotics are required to treat bacterial endocarditis.

BINDING OF DRUGS BY PROTEINS (and other macromolecules)

The drug-protein complex differs greatly from the free drug because the complex lacks pharmacological activity, cannot penetrate significant drug barriers (for example, cell membranes, blood brain barrier) and the drug in the complex is not directly available for biotransformation or ultrafiltration.

216

Sites of binding

(1) Plasma proteins, mainly albumin — well studied.
(2) Tissue proteins (ligands), for example, the concentration of Thiopentone by skeletal muscle is probably due to protein binding and solution in lipid.
(3) Tissue nucleic acids, for example, the antimalarial *Chloroquine* persists for months in liver cell nuclei (page 179).
(4) Gut lumen, glycoproteins impede drug absorption, lignins and celluloses are little studied.

Plasma albumin

Measurement: equilibrium dialysis, ultrafiltration. Measure: the free drug concentration (d) in plasma water and the total drug concentration in plasma. Calculate: the bound drug concentration (total — free).

The proportion of drug bound (β) depends on many factors:

(1) Physical conditions: temperature, pH, concentration and charge of ions (ionic strength). These alter the affinity constant (K_a) and the number of binding sites (n).
(2) Protein concentration (P): hypoalbuminaemia reduces the protein available for drug binding (nephrotic syndrome, intestinal malabsorption, hepatic cirrhosis).
(3) Nature of drug and its free concentration: binding important with fat-soluble (Thiopentone, page 236) and acidic drugs, page 242).
$\beta = 1/(1 + 1/K_a nP + d/np)$.

Acidic drugs

Only one or two specific binding sites are available on plasma albumin, therefore a wide variety of acidic drugs compete. Acidic drugs with high affinity displace acidic drugs with low affinity producing exaggeration of biological effects.

Examples

Displacing drugs	*Displaced molecules*
Phenylbutazone	*Warfarin*
Sulphadimethoxine	*Tolbutamide*
	Bilirubin

Determination of Affinity Constant (*Figure 5.1*).
r = Molar concentration of bound drug / molar concentration of albumin.
n = Maximum number of sites on albumin molecule.
d = Free drug concentration in plasma water.
K_a = Affinity constant
$r/d = K_a (n - r)$ Scatchard.
plot r/d against r
when $r/d = 0$, $r = n$ when $r = 0$, $r/d = K_a n$

217

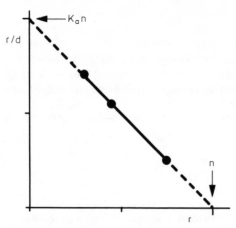

Figure 5.1. *Binding of phenylbutazone (MW 308) to human plasma albumin*

Plasma albumin concentration = 40 g/ℓ
MW   = 70,000
Molar concentration $^{40}/_{70}$ = 0.57 mmol/ℓ

Experimental results

Drug concentration (mmol/ℓ)			
Total	Free	r	r/d
0.175	0.004	0.30	70
0.265	.0.008	0.45	55
0.458	0.030	0.75	25

Extrapolation — when r/d = 0, n = 1.0 = binding sites per albumin molecule
— when r = 0, r/d = 100 = affinity constant

The dispositional significance of protein binding

Usually drug protein complexes dissociate rapidly with a half time ($t_{1/2}$) measured in mseconds. Active tubular secretion, for example, is not hindered. Thus, the complex represents a pharmacologically inert but readily available 'storage' form of the active drug. The reversible association smooths fluctuations in the concentration of free drug in the plasma water. This effect is lost when: (1) the drug is not bound (for example, *Gentamicin*); (2) the total albumin is low (hypoalbuminaemia, infants); (3) the binding sites are saturated (rapid iv *Diazoxide*, big doses of salicylate or *Phenylbutazone*).

The drug binding sites on plasma and tissue proteins effectively represent an extension of the volume (V) available for the distribution of the drug. If these are saturated the drug concentration in the body water increases and the pharmacological effect is increased but plasma concentration $t_{1/2}$ is reduced.

218

Conversely, those members of a series of similar drugs which are most highly protein bound are likely to have the longest $t_{1/2}$. Thus, the more protein bound sulphonamides are more persistent than *Sulphadimidine.*

Elimination

EXCRETION

Excretion of drugs is mainly by the kidney but also by other organs.

Kidney

The renal plasma clearance is the volume of plasma effectively cleared of drug by the kidney in unit time. The total drug clearance (CL mℓ/min) is the sum of the renal plasma clearance and clearance by biotransformation or by excretion through other organs, notably the liver.

The following factors determine the renal clearance of a drug.

The rate of its filtration at the glomerulus

This is itself determined by the glomerular filtration rate (GFR), the concentration of drug in plasma water and its effective MW.

The drug/albumin complex is not filtered, thus, drugs with a high affinity constant are filtered to negligible extent:

Examples	
Drug	*Proportion bound*
Phenylbutazone	0.98
Warfarin	0.97

The rate of filtration is not directly affected by the lipid solubility or by the degree of ionization of the drug.

Passive tubular reabsorption

Water and salt are removed from the filtrate in the renal tubules and drug molecules diffuse back into the peritubular plasma down a concentration gradient. The extent of reabsorption depends on the physical properties of the drug.

Highly polar water-soluble drugs (for example, *Gentamicin*, quaternary ammonium salts, oxidized drug metabolites and conjugates, page 231) are too large to penetrate the water pores of cells and have negligible solubility in the membrane lipids. There is little reabsorption and the renal clearance is a high proportion of the GFR. Drugs with intermediate polarity (for example, *Digoxin*, page 234) resemble the water-soluble drugs. Non-polar, lipid-soluble drugs (for example, Thiopentone, *Phenytoin* and the inhalational anaesthetics, page 236) are reabsorbed from the tubular urine almost completely. The renal clearance is therefore very small.

Acidic drugs (pK_a 2–8) (for example, *Salicyclic* acid) show pH-dependent excretion. The lipid-soluble species (acid) is reabsorbed but the charged, polar species (anion) is not. The maximum renal clearance is obtained at the maximum urine pH, usually 8 (*Table 5.12*). Basic drugs (pK_a 6–12) for example, *Lignocaine*) also show pH-dependent excretion. The lipid-soluble species (base) is reabsorbed but the charged, polar species (cation) is not. The maximum renal clearance is at the minimum urine pH, usually 5 (*Table 5.15*).

Active tubular reabsorption

This occurs for drugs which resemble essential metabolites (for example, L-amino acids, *Thyroxine, Methyldopa*). The active reabsorption of uric acid is inhibited by another acid *Probenecid* (page 319).

Tubular secretion

There are two distinct systems each with a low specificity. Each system shows competition and saturation kinetics. Compounds with a low rate of transport are the more effective inhibitors. The transport is often bidirectional.

(1) Anions
     Penicillins, *Probenecid*, thiazides and loop diuretics
     Salicylates, *Phenylbutazone*
     Drug conjugates, glucuronides
         Glycine conjugates (for example, salicyluric acid)
         Sulphates
(2) Cations (onium salts and strong bases)
     Choline
     Morphine
     Neostigmine
     Quinine

The renal clearance usually exceeds GFR and can be as large as the renal plasma flow (RPF). Clearance can exceed the RPF if drug in red cells is available for secretion.

Note: Protein binding: the drug/albumin complex usually dissociates very rapidly as free drug is secreted, so that the renal clearance is not reduced by the protein binding. Thus, although *Benzylpenicillin* is about 50 per cent bound the renal clearance approximates to the renal plasma flow. Competition: all drug transport by the tubules is continuously in competition with endogenous acids (for example, 5-hydroxyindoleacetic acid, page 110, steroid glucuronides) and bases (for example, cadaverine, putrescine).

Drug disposition in renal insufficiency

There is accumulation of unchanged drug or metabolites until the clearance of a small volume of plasma with a high drug concentration equals the rate of intake.

Water-soluble and intermediate drugs accumulate, for example, *Gentamicin* (toxic effects on inner ear and kidney, page 199), *Digoxin* (toxic effects on the heart, page 234).

Lipid-soluble drugs do not accumulate (for example, *Phenytoin*). The water-soluble hydroxylated metabolites do, however, accumulate and their effects may be clinically detectable.

Actively transported drugs show intermediate accumulation. Large doses of diuretics (for example, *Frusemide*) are sometimes given without evidence of systemic toxicity.

Peritoneal dialysis effectively removes drugs, especially if they are water-soluble, with a low MW and a low affinity for plasma albumin. This is a technique in which a solution is allowed to flow into the peritoneal cavity through a tube piercing the abdominal wall. The solution is retained for a chosen contact period then drained, discarded and replaced. Depending on the composition of the fluid, selected small molecules can be removed from the body. The technique can be used in patients with severe impairment of kidney function to increase the clearance of electrolytes, creatinine, urea, water and even drugs. The mean effective peritoneal clearance varies with the volume of fluid and the period of contact; it is always less than the healthy renal clearance.

Artificial kidney: plasma dialysis

This is a continuous flow dialysis system with a large surface area. The stream of blood from a cannulated artery is spread out in a thin film over a cellophane membrane in contact with a physiological salt solution.

All diffusible solutes exchange across the semi-permeable membrane. The blood is then returned to the body through a venous cannula. The salt solution (dialysis fluid) is continuously renewed from a reservoir. Exchange is accelerated by a counter current flow. The rate of removal of a drug by plasma dialysis is directly proportional to the concentration drop between plasma water and dialysis fluid. The proportionality constant is termed the 'dialysance'.

Application to severe drug intoxication   Plasma dialysis is effective for small, water-soluble drug molecules which are protein bound (for example, chlorate ion, ethylene glycol, barbitone) but ineffective for highly lipid-soluble drugs (for example, *Thiopentone*, *Phenytoin*) unless the dialysis fluid is replaced by a bath of non-toxic vegetable oil. Plasma dialysis is ineffective for drugs which are highly bound to the proteins of plasma (for example, *Phenylbutazone*) or to tissues (for example, *Digoxin*, page 234).

Blood may be pumped through columns of activated carbon particles for rapid clearance of lethal foreign compounds (for example, paraquat).

Liver

Drug molecules are transferred from the plasma in the hepatic sinusoids, via large pores between endothelial cells to hepatic cells and finally into bile.

Active transport systems exist for carbohydrates (for example, dextran, inulin, sucrose, Mannitol) and acidic compounds (for example, bile acids, bilirubin, iodine contrast media, sulphobromophthalein (bromsulphthalein, B.S.P.), glucuronide, glycine and sulphate conjugates, penicillins and phenolphthalein, page 243).

Note: Excreted compounds are often reabsorbed from the gut; they may be reexcreted by the liver to produce 'enterohepatic recycling' which partly accounts for the persistence of phenolphthalein and the phenothiazines. The reabsorbed drug or metabolite or conjugate is often finally excreted by the kidney.

Biliary obstruction and hepatocellular failure produce impairment of excretion.

Lungs

Drug molecules may diffuse across alveolar membrane, for example, volatile anaesthetics (page 240). Excretion in expired air may be obvious to smell but quantitatively insignificant (for example, *Ethanol, Paraldehyde*, thiols).

Saliva, milk, sweat, sebum

The amounts of drug excreted are small but relevant to breastfeeding (for example, anthracene purgatives) and to the treatment of acne (Oxytetracycline, page 320).

DRUG METABOLISM

Most lipid-soluble compounds are metabolized to more water-soluble products. The metabolism (biotransformation) of foreign compounds (xenobiotics) occurs mainly in liver, although kidney, adrenal cortex, lungs, placenta, skin and even lymphocytes may be involved to a small extent.

The enzyme system involved in biotransformation of xenobiotics is located in the smooth endoplasmic reticulum (microsomal fraction). It is termed the mixed function oxidase (MFO) or mono-oxygenase system and it utilizes O_2 and NADPH (the primary electron donor) and is relatively non-specific.

A major (terminal oxidase) component of the MFO system (*Figure 5.2*) is the haem protein cytochrome P_{450} (so-called because in the reduced state it will form a complex with CO which absorbs light at 450 nm). Cytochrome P_{450} is now known to be widespread in nature (including bacteria, yeasts and plants). It is also involved in the metabolism of several endogenous substances (for example, steroids of adrenal cortex).

In the biotransformation process one molecule of O_2 is utilized per molecule of compound metabolized (only one atom of the O_2 ends up in the (hydroxylated) product, however, hence the term 'mono-oxygenase' for the MFO).

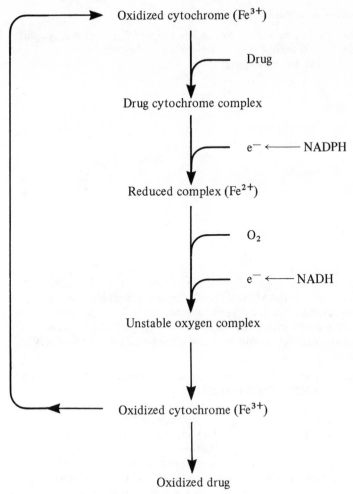

Figure 5.2 *Mixed function oxidase enzyme system of liver. Role of cytochrome* P_{450}

The MFO system is inducible; that is, after exposure to certain lipid-soluble substrates (notably *Griseofulvin, Phenobarbitone, Phenytoin* and *Rifampicin*) there is an increase in (1) enzyme (MFO) activity; (2) cytochrome P_{450}; (3) liver weight; (4) microscopically visible smooth endoplasmic reticulum.

As a result there is a decrease in $t_{1/2}$ of many other drugs (or the inducing drug itself, 'self-induction').

Certain agents may inhibit the MFO (for example, proadifen (SKF-525A) – clinically Disulfiram, *Sulthiame* and *Isoniazid* can inhibit the metabolism of *Phenytoin*).

Induction and inhibition of the MFO can lead to complex drug interactions (page 265)

The MFO can perform several biochemical reactions, aromatic and aliphatic hydroxylation, dealkylation, N and S oxidation and deamination.

The biotransformations occur in two phases (*Figure 5.3*).

Phase I — includes oxidations such as the addition of an OH group to a lipophilic part of the original compound. Phase I reactions generally produce a more water-soluble and less active compound.

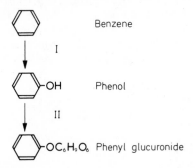

Figure 5.3

Phase II — conjugation reactions (usually with glucuronic acid but also with glycine, glutamine, glutathione and ethereal sulphate). The conjugation occurs at the site of a reactive group such as OH (added perhaps by a Phase I reaction). Following a Phase II reaction a compound is rendered much more water-soluble and totally inactive.

Some compounds (prodrugs) are converted to pharmacologically more active (or toxic) products by the MFO (Phase I reaction).

Examples

Inactive/less active	*Active/more active*
Cyclophosphamide	Alkylating derivative
Malathion	Malaoxon
Phenylbutazone	*Oxyphenbutazone*
Polycyclic aromatic hydro-carbons	Carcinogenic metabolites (which may be epoxide intermediates)
Phenacetin*	*Paracetamol*
*O-dealkylation	

A wide variety of biotransformations occurs and one drug can give rise to many products. More than 100 metabolites of *Chlorpromazine*, for example, have been postulated and many identified in human excreta. The relative proportions of different metabolites vary from species to species. Within the human species there is also genetically determined variation in drug metabolism. The best studied examples are N-acetylation (page 257) and the hydrolysis of choline esters (page 35) but there is also evidence that populations are heterogeneous with respect to the hydroxylation of drugs (for example, *Debrisoquine*). This topic has direct relevance to toxicology but in most instances the pharmacology of a particular drug metabolite has not been studied.

Model simulation of drug disposition

A stirred beaker of water which is continuously emptied and replenished by two identical pumps simulates the major processes of drug disposition. The rate and completeness of absorption are under the control of the operator when he injects a dose of the dye (for example, amaranth) into the beaker. This is then distributed throughout the volume of water in the beaker at a rate which is determined by the stirrer. Elimination from the beaker starts as soon as some dye has entered and is determined by the rate at which one pump removes coloured water and the other replaces it by clean water; that is, the rate at which the pumps 'clear' the water in the beaker.

It is characteristic of this model that the dye does not disappear at a steady rate. The higher the concentration the more rapidly does it fall; the decay is exponential and is conveniently described by a $t_{1/2}$.

This simple model describes adequately the handling of most drugs used in patients, although it is sometimes necessary to postulate more than one distribution compartment and an elimination process which can be saturated at high concentration. It will be used to illustrate the principles of pharmacokinetics (page 227) but it is first necessary to define terms.

Pharmacokinetic terms and equations

Pharmacokineticists who study the processes of drug handling in animals and man have evolved a series of common terms and equations.

D (mg) — dose of drug or mass in the body at a particular time.

k_a (h^{-1}) — absorption rate constant, reciprocally related to the time for 50 per cent absorption.

F — fraction of dose absorbed from site of administration.

V (ℓ) — distribution volume, size of conceptual compartment in which drug is distributed.

C_{pt} (mg/ℓ) — concentration in main/central/plasma compartment at time t (h) after the previous dose.

C_{po} (mg/ℓ) — zero time concentration in hypothetical state of complete absorption with no elimination, obtained by back extrapolation.

$$C_{po} = D/V \qquad\qquad (5.1)$$

CL (ℓ/h) — drug clearance, volume of fluid (blood, plasma or water) which would contain the mass of drug eliminated in unit time.

CL_{cr} (ℓ/h) — clearance of endogenous creatinine, useful measure of kidney function which approximates to glomerular filtration rate (GFR).

$t_{1/2}$ (h) – half time, time for C_{pt} to fall by one half or time for 50 per cent elimination.

$$t_{1/2} = 0.7\ V/CL \qquad\qquad (5.2)$$

k_d (h^{-1}) – elimination rate constant, reciprocally related to the time for 50 per cent elimination.

$$k_d = 0.7/t_{1/2} \qquad\qquad (5.3)$$
$$k_d = CL/V \qquad\qquad (5.4)$$

T (h) – interval between doses during a course of drug treatment.
$\overline{C}_{pss}$ (mg/ℓ) – mean plasma drug concentration when a steady state is attained.
FD/T (mg/h) – mean rate of drug input, which in steady state equals mean rate of drug output.

$$FD/T = \overline{C}_{pss} \times CL \qquad\qquad (5.5)$$

$\overline{D}_{ss}$ (mg) – mean total body drug in steady state.
$\overline{D}_{ss}/FD$ – accumulation index, mean total body drug relative to single dose.

$$\overline{D}_{ss}/FD = 1.44\ t_{1/2}/T \qquad\qquad (5.6)$$

dC_{pt}/dt ((mg/ℓ)/h) – gradient of concentration decay – first order kinetics

$$dC_{pt}/dt = -\ k_d\ C_{pt} \qquad\qquad (5.7)$$
$$C_{pt} = C_{po}e^{-k_d t} \qquad\qquad (5.8)$$

– saturable kinetics (Michaelis–Menten)

$$dC_{pt}/dt = -\ V_{max}\ C_{pt}/\ (K_m + C_{pt}) \qquad\qquad (5.9)$$

V_{max} ((mg/ℓ)/h) – maximum rate of decay of plasma concentration when elimination is saturated.
K_m (mg/ℓ) – plasma concentration at which elimination is 50 per cent saturated.
pK_a – acid dissociation constant, pH at which acid 50 per cent dissociated (Henderson–Hasselbalch)

$$pH = pK_a + \log (H\ \text{acceptor}/H\ \text{donor}) \qquad\qquad (5.10)$$

r – molar ratio of bound drug molecules to protein molecules.
n – total number of binding sites per protein molecule.
K_a (ℓ/mg) – affinity constant, reciprocal of free drug concentration at which half the available binding sites are occupied (page 217).
d (mg/ℓ) – concentration of drug free in the water of plasma.

$$r/d = K_a\ (n-r) \qquad\qquad (5.11)$$

$\lambda_{b/g}$ – partition coefficient for a volatile anaesthetic between blood (for example) and gas phases (page 240).

EXAMPLES

In these examples the amaranth model has been scaled up to the dimensions which might apply to a drug used in the treatment of an adult patient.

Example A

Obtain a sheet of two or three cycle semi-log graph paper and plot the time/concentration data (*Table 5.2*). The points lie on a straight line which cuts the concentration axis (C_{po}) at 33.3 mg/ℓ. Thus, the distribution volume (V) given by rearrangement of Equation 5.1 is 500/33.3 or 15 ℓ.

Table 5.2

Dose: 500 mg at zero time Time (h)	Concentration (mg/ℓ)		
	A	B	C
0.5	27.3	–	3.70
1	22.3	–	2.75
2	15.0	–	1.50
4	6.7	–	0.46
6	3.0	1.28	0.14
8	1.4	–	0.04
10	0.6	–	0.01
12	0.3	1.17	0.00
24	–	0.94	–
36	–	0.77	–
48	–	0.63	–

The concentration is observed to halve in 1.75 hours ($t_{1/2}$). Substitution into a rearranged form of Equation 5.2 gives a clearance (CL) of $0.7 \times 15/1.75$ or 6 ℓ/hour.

If the dose was repeated every 12 hours no accumulation would occur.

Assuming complete absorption (F = 1) the mean steady state concentration ($\overline{C}_{pss}$) from Equation 5.5. would be 6.9 mg/ℓ and the accumulation index from Equation 5.6 would be 0.21. That is, the average amount of drug present during a dosage interval in the steady state is about $\frac{1}{5}$ of a single dose.

Repeat this exercise for data sets B and C (answers on page 229). These three examples represent different patterns of drug disposition observed with drugs which have different physicochemical properties (A, page 232; B, page 234; C, page 248).

Pharmacokinetics and dosage regimens

Use of pharmacokinetics in therapeutics:

(1) Distinguishes between pharmacokinetics and pharmacodynamics (page 209) as a cause of an unusual degree of response to a drug.

(2) Concepts of pharmacokinetics are common to all drugs; thus, information gained about one drug helps in anticipating the pharmacokinetics of another drug.

(3) Pharmacokinetics often explains the manner of a drug's use and occasionally will suggest a more convenient or an improved dosage regimen.

(4) Pharmacokinetics often allows anticipation of the likely outcome following a therapeutic manoeuvre.

When prescribing a dosage regimen it is essential to consider the therapeutic index of the drug. This is the ratio, toxic dose or concentration : therapeutic dose or concentration. If the index is high, wide variation in dosage is tolerable. If it is low, however (*Gentamicin*, page 231 and *Digoxin*, page 234), the tolerable dosage regimen for an individual patient has narrow limits.

A second important consideration is the need for a loading or priming dose. When clinical circumstances demand an immediate drug effect it may be necessary to give a larger first dose (D_0) sufficient to yield a therapeutic concentration after distribution throughout the volume (V). The effect is then sustained by giving at intervals (T) a smaller maintenance dose (D_m) sufficient to keep pace with clearance (CL).

A third consideration is the $t_{1/2}$ which may be short (< 1 hour), moderate ($4-24$ hours) or long (> 24 hours).

If the $t_{1/2}$ is short and the therapeutic index is large (for example, penicillins, page 198) a very large dose is given at convenient intervals of 4, 6 or 8 hours $(D_0 = D_m)$. Despite the shortness of $t_{1/2}$ the effect persists long enough for a therapeutic response, yet each dose is completely eliminated before the next is given. When the index is small, however, it becomes necessary to give the drug by small, frequent doses (for example, *insulin* in ketoacidosis) or continuous iv infusion (for example, *Oxytocin* for induction of labour, *Lignocaine* for suppression of ventricular ectopic beats).

If the $t_{1/2}$ is moderate it is convenient to give half the initial dose every $t_{1/2}$ $(D_0 = 2D_m)$. There is then no accumulation (for example, *Co-trimoxazole* every 12 hours, *Tetracycline* every 8 or 12 hours *see Table 4.6*).

If the $t_{1/2}$ is long it is usual to use a 24-hour dosage interval (T). The theoretical maintenance dose corresponds with the proportion of the initial dose (D_0) which is eliminated during that time (equation 5.8 page 226).

D_m = amount at beginning (D_0) − amount at T $(D_0 e^{-kdT})$
$D_m = D_0 (1 - e^{-kdT})$

If $t_{1/2} \gg T$, $D_m = D_0 k_d T$. A patient receiving *Digoxin*, for example, may have a $t_{1/2}$ of 2 days.

$k_d = 0.7 / t_{1/2}$ = about 1/3 (equation 5.3, page 226)

Thus, a daily dose of 250 µg would correspond with a loading dose of 750 µg. Even if no loading dose were given the amount in the body would accumulate until the same steady or plateau state was attained. The mean plasma concentration $(\overline{C}_{pss})$ in this state is given by equation 5.5 (page 226) and the mean amount of drug in the body $(\overline{D}_{ss})$ by equation 5.6 (page 226). In the special case of continuous infusion the infusion rate (mg/hour) replaces FD/T in Equation 5.5.

228

The time to reach the plateau without loading dose in either case depends only on $t_{1/2}$ (*Table 5.3*).

Table 5.3

Time ($\times t_{1/2}$)	Plateau level (*percentage*)
1	50
2	75
3	87.5
3.3	90
4	93.75
5	96.87

The shorter $t_{1/2}$ the quicker the plateau is attained. There are no such entities as accumulating or non-accumulating drugs.

Answers to examples (*Table 5.4*).

Table 5.4

	A	B	C
D (mg)	500	500	500 (given)
C_{po} (mg/ℓ)	33.3	1.4	5
V (ℓ)	15	350	100
$t_{1/2}$ (h)	1.75	40.8	1.17
CL (ℓ/h)	6	6	60
T (h)	12	12	12 (given)
F	1	1	1 (given)
C_{pss} (mg/ℓ)	6.9	6.9	0.69
D_{ss}/FD	0.21	4.9	0.14

Note: This discussion of drug dosage regimens presupposes that absorption and elimination are 'first order' exponential processes and that distribution is rapid.

PARTICULAR EXAMPLES

It is the physicochemical properties, rather than the pharmacological actions of drugs, which determine how they are handled in the body. Five characteristic patterns of drug disposition will be described corresponding with five physico-chemical groups (*Table 5.5* and *Figure 5.4*).

Table 5.5

Groups	Examples
1. Water-soluble drugs	*Gentamicin*
2. Intermediate drugs	*Digoxin*
3. Lipid-soluble drugs	*Thiopentone*, *Phenytoin*, Inhalational anaesthetics
4. Acidic drugs (pK_a 2–8)	*Salicylic* acid
5. Basic drugs (pK_a 6–12)	*Lignocaine*

There are two major properties of a drug which determine how it is handled by the body.

(1) The degree of ionization of the drug molecules in solution. This is dependent on the pK_a of the drug, (that is, the pH at which half the drug molecules are ionized) and the pH of the fluid in which the drug is dissolved (Equation 5.10, page 226).

(2) The lipid solubility of the unionized drug molecules: this is often expressed as the partition coefficient between organic solvents and water.

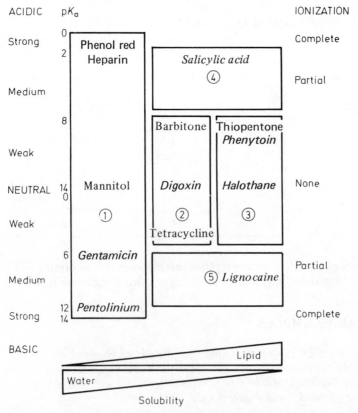

Figure 5.4 *Five physicochemical groups of drugs. In this diagram ionization increases when moving up (acidic) or down (basic) from the middle. The lipid solubility of the unionized molecule increases when moving from left to right*

230

Water-soluble drugs

EXAMPLES

(1) Highly ionized (strong) acids ($pK_a < 2$) which are almost 100 per cent ionized in all biological fluids.
Phenolsulphonphthalein (phenol red).
Drug conjugates: sulphates, glucuronides, glycine conjugates

(2) Drugs with multiple polar groups.
Polyhydric alcohols — Mannitol, sorbitol.
Sugars, mucopolysaccharides — *Heparin.*
Amino sugar antibiotics — *Streptomycin, Neomycin, Gentamicin.*
Polypeptide antibiotics — polymixins

(3) Highly ionized (strong) bases ($pK_a > 12$) which are almost 100 per cent ionized in all biological fluids.
Quaternary ammonium derivatives ($R_4N^+OH^-$).
   (*a*) Mono-onium compounds — atropine methonitrate, choline, Tubocurarine, *Neostigmine, Pyridostigmine, Benzalkonium* chloride, *Cetrimide.*
   (*b*) Bis-onium compounds — *Pentolinium,* pancuronium, Suxamethonium.

CHARACTERISTIC FEATURES

Resemble inulin

(1) Absorption from the gastrointestinal tract is negligible and injection is usually necessary for systemic effects.
(2) Distribution is restricted to the ECF.
(3) The drugs do not penetrate into CSF or brain.
(4) Binding to plasma proteins is not important except for some strong acids.
(5) Elimination is mainly by excretion of the unchanged drug in the urine. The drug usually enters the urine by ultrafiltration but many anions and cations are also actively secreted into the urine and the bile.

The disposition of the aminoglycoside antibiotic *Gentamicin* is representative of the group.

GENTAMICIN

This is a widely used antibiotic which is effective against Gram −ve bacteria including *Klebsiella pneumoniae* and *Pseudomonas aeruginosa.* It is important to understand how it it handled in the body because it has toxic effects on the inner ear and on the kidney. The amount of drug required to produce damage is only a little greater than the amount required to treat infection (low therapeutic index).

Chemistry

The antibiotic is a variable mixture of three very similar components giving an average MW of about 480. Each component consists of two substituted amino sugar molecules linked through an alicyclic base. There are several polar groups on the molecules (chiefly —OH) which make them readily soluble in water and insoluble in lipid or organic solvents.

Absorption

The drug is not absorbed from the gut and must be given by injection if a systemic effect is required. As with other drugs the rate of absorption from the site of injection is proportional to the local blood flow.

Distribution

The water-soluble antibiotic molecules cannot generally penetrate into mammalian cells. Therefore, like inulin, they are restricted to the ECF. The distribution volume (V) is about 15 ℓ in an adult as in example A (pages 227 and 229). Penetration across tissue barriers into brain, CSF, inner ear fluid, foetal circulation and sputum is slow.

Elimination

Excretion by the kidney is the major route and the clearance CL closely approximates to the GFR or creatinine clearance CL_{cr}. Since cells are not penetrated there is little opportunity for contact with intracellular enzymes and consequent biotransformation. Again the resemblance to inulin is strong.

Persistence and accumulation

When kidney function is normal the handling resembles example A and the average $t_{1/2}$ is about 2 hours. Thus, 8 hours after a dose more than 90 per cent ($50 + 25 + 12.5 + 6.25$) of that dose has been eliminated; the dose can therefore be repeated without accumulation.

Severe renal disease produces a very different state, however. A ten-fold reduction in CL, for example, causes a proportionate prolongation of $t_{1/2}$. It is then essential to scale down dosage in order to avoid accumulation and toxicity.

Plasma concentration and patient response

Concentration (C_{pt}) 1 hour after dosage must exceed 5 mg/ℓ for a therapeutic effect in septicaemia, for example, but can be as high as 12 mg/ℓ without causing toxicity.

232

Concentrations before dosage are more relevant to toxicity, however. Below 2 mg/ℓ there is little risk, but above 4 mg/ℓ the risk is high. If the trough concentration is high it is as if the tide never goes out; the relatively inaccessible compartment of the inner ear fluid therefore gradually fills up as would a leaky boat.

A mean concentration $\bar{C}_{pss}$ of 3–4 mg/ℓ represents a compromise avoiding inadequate peaks and excessive troughs.

Dosage requirements in renal disease

The daily dosage rate to maintain a desired $\bar{C}_{pss}$ is a linear function of CL_{cr}. It varies from about 20 mg/day (40 mg every 48 hours) in anuric patients to 480 mg/day (160 mg every 8 hours) in the normal. Thus, the daily dosage rate required to produce a given $\bar{C}_{pss}$ varies over a 24-fold range.

Dosage requirements in children

CL_{cr} and *Gentamicin* dosage requirements both regress with weight (or surface area) as the age scale is descended. The newborn is a special case, however; he has immature kidneys and CL_{cr} is about one-third of the value appropriate to his size. Since his ECF volume is relatively large the combined effect is a longer $t_{1/2}$ (Equation 5.2, page 226)

Renal excretion of water-soluble drugs

The principle that daily dosage rate for a given $\bar{C}_{pss}$ parallels CL_{cr} is generally valid for drugs which are not fat-soluble (rearrangement of Equation 5.5, page 226, demonstrates that dose rate per unit concentration has clearance units). Non-renal excretion is relatively unimportant for these drugs unless they have a high MW (> 800) when hepatic excretion becomes important.

Drugs with intermediate solubility

CHARACTERISTIC FEATURES

Not all drugs have extreme physical properties. Many are intermediate between the highly water-soluble aminoglycoside antibiotics and the highly lipid-soluble iv anaesthetics. *Digoxin* has been selected as an important example.

(1) Absorption from the gut is adequate for clinical use but is often not complete.
(2) Distribution is not restricted to the ECF; the drugs penetrate through cell membranes and into the intracellular water.

(3) Protein binding has an influence on the distribution and elimination of the drug.
(4) Elimination is predominantly by excretion of the unchanged drug in the urine; however, a proportion of the drug suffers biotransformation.

DIGOXIN

This drug has the invaluable effect of slowing ventricular rate in patients with atrial fibrillation and increasing the force of contraction in heart failure (page 275). The toxic dose (heart block, ectopic ventricular activity) is very close to the therapeutic dose, however; so there is little safety margin.

Chemistry

The relatively lipid-soluble steroid nucleus carrying two OH groups is linked to a highly water-soluble trisaccharide (three digitoxose units) by a glycosidic bond. This structure probably favours concentration at cell surfaces where the drug acts on Na^+/K^+ ATPase (page 275). The glycoside (MW 781) dissolves more readily in Ethanol than in water or other organic solvents.

Absorption

Usually administered by mouth in tablet form. Absorbed quickly but not completely. Dissolution standard − 75 per cent in solution within 1 hour. The fraction (F) absorbed is about 0.6 mean (0.4–0.8).

Distribution

Distributed throughout body water. Bound to protein in plasma (about 0.30) and probably in tissues. When distribution is complete most of the dose is located in skeletal muscle. *Digoxin* does not enter fat. V is much greater than bodyweight (about 5 ℓ/kg) because of the high 'capacity' of skeletal muscle. In this respect it is very different from *Gentamicin* (example B, pages 227 and 229).

Elimination

Excretion and biotransformation. Renal CL is approximately equal to CL_{cr}. Both glomerular filtration and tubular secretion contribute. Non-renal CL is about one-half the renal CL in normal subjects. Sugar molecules are split off and the steroid nucleus is further hydroxylated in the liver.

Total CL is greater than for the aminoglycosides but $t_{1/2}$ is much longer (1–2 days as in example B) because of the large V.

234

Persistence and accumulation

About one-third of dose excreted per day (page 228). *Digoxin* therefore
accumulates until the total body drug is about three times the single daily dose
(accumulation index = 3). This process is 90 per cent complete in about one
week ($3-4 \times t_{1/2}$, page 229). Once the steady state has been attained the total
body *Digoxin* fluctuates relatively little during the dosage interval (contrast
Gentamicin, page 232).

Plasma concentration and patient response

The concentration/time curve is biphasic because absorption is more rapid than
distribution. The brief high peak may be associated with nausea (CTZ, page 300)
but not with cardiac toxicity. The cardiac response parallels the hypothetical
concentration in a deeper tissue compartment. $\overline{C}_{pss}$ is probably the most relevant
concentration which approximates to C_{pt} at 6 hours.

A concentration of $1-2$ $\mu g/\ell$ is usually adequate to control the ventricular rate in
atrial fibrillation. However, a concentration above 2 $\mu g/\ell$ is associated with an
increased frequency of ventricular ectopic beats. The therapeutic index approaches
unity.

Dosage requirements in disease

The rapid attainment of a high therapeutic concentration (2 $\mu g/\ell$) requires iv
injection of $2 \times V$ μg or 10 μg/kg. V is approximately halved, however, in the
elderly and in those with severe renal impairment. Both these states are
associated with a relatively low skeletal muscle mass. Gradual accumulation
is usually preferred.

Daily dosage requirement for $\overline{C}_{pss}$ of $1-2$ $\mu g/\ell$ in the adult varies from 62.5 μg
(one paediatric/geriatric tablet) in the anuric to 500 μg in the patient with
normal kidney function. Dosage requirement approximately parallells CL_{cr}.

Table 5.6

	Digoxin	*Digitoxin*
Lipid solubility	Less	Greater
Intestinal absorption	$40-80$ per cent	$80-100$ per cent
Single dose	0.25 mg	0.10 mg
Binding to plasma albumin	$20-30$ per cent	> 90 per cent
Biotransformation	Limited	Hydroxylated (liver) products include *Digoxin*
Kidney	Glomerular filtration Tubular secretion	Filtration of unbound *Digitoxin* passive tubular reabsorption
Drug in urine	90 per cent as unchanged *Digoxin*	10 per cent as unchanged *Digitoxin*
$t_{1/2}$	$1-2$ days	$5-9$ days

Digitoxin and digoxin

There are important differences in the handling of these two cardiac glycosides which illustrate the differences between dispositional groups 2 and 3. The two drugs are compared in *Table 5.6*.

Lipid-soluble drugs

EXAMPLES

This group of drugs is large and includes many drugs which depress the CNS. They have in common a high oil (or organic solvent)/water partition coefficient. This group includes: (1) weakly acidic drugs ($pK_a > 8$), for example, Thiopentone and other iv anaesthetics, *Phenytoin* and other anticonvulsants; (2) virtually neutral drugs, for example, *Digitoxin*, many hypnotics and inhalational anaesthetics.

CHARACTERISTIC FEATURES

(1)   Absorption from the gut is usually rapid and complete unless chemically inactivated.
(2)   Initial distribution of the drug is very rapid. Characteristically the drugs enter tissues, including brain, at a rate which is limited by the flow of blood, not by the rate of diffusion through the cell membranes.
(3)   A large proportion of the drug is bound to plasma proteins and to intra-cellular proteins and lipids. The concentration of drug molecules free in the body water may be very small indeed.
(4)   The concentration of drug in the glomerular filtrate is also very small and the drug molecules are so lipid-soluble that they are reabsorbed from the renal tubule as quickly as the filtered water. Thus, the unchanged drug is not effectively excreted in the urine.
(5)   Some of the drugs in this group which have a high vapour pressure are excreted unchanged in the expired air.
(6)   In the liver, and to a lesser extent in other tissues, drugs of this group are oxidized to more polar metabolites which may be alcohols or phenols (Phase I, page 224).
(7)   Water-soluble metabolites resemble *Gentamicin* in their elimination. Many are conjugated with sulphate, glycine or glucuronic acid prior to excretion (Phase II, page 224).

THIOPENTONE — MW (acid) 242; $pK_a = 8$

This very short-acting barbiturate is used as the sodium salt at a dose of 150—500 mg. It is administered iv for the production of complete anaesthesia of short

236

duration or for the induction of sustained anaesthesia. Thiopentone, one of the most lipid-soluble barbiturates, is about 70 per cent bound to serum albumin by 'hydrophobic bonds'. The binding of barbiturates increases with lipid solubility (*Table 5.7*). Less than 1 per cent is excreted unchanged in the urine over 48 hours. Most is metabolized.

Table 5.7

	$CH_2Cl_2/water$	Proportion bound
Thiopentone	580	0.75
Pentobarbitone	39	0.35
Phenobarbitone	3	0.20
Barbitone	1	0.05

A single iv dose of Thiopentone can produce almost instantaneous anaesthesia that only lasts for about five minutes. Large doses cause respiratory arrest.

Pentobarbitone has a similar potency to Thiopentone (that is, approximately the same concentration in brain needed to produce anaesthesia). However, no dose of pentobarbitone will mimic the very short duration of action seen with Thiopentone. This short duration of action is not due to rapid metabolism but to rapid redistribution into skeletal muscle. After several hours, a substantial fraction of a single dose is located in fatty tissue. Consciousness returns whilst a high proportion of the original dose is still in the body. Repeated doses are cumulative.

The biexponential decay in plasma Thiopentone (due to rapid redistribution) suggests that its pharmacokinetics should be considered in terms of a two compartment (or more complex) model. Entry into various tissues (for example, brain and liver) is so rapid that it appears to be limited solely by the rate of blood flow. Multicompartment 'physiological models' have been devised for Thiopentone which employ known blood flow rates to principal anatomical regions. One relatively simple model of this kind comprises the following:

(1) Highly perfused central compartment or vessel-rich group of organs including brain, liver, myocardium, adrenals, kidneys and receiving about 4 ℓ/minute.
(2) Lean tissue compartment (mainly skeletal muscle) and receiving about 1 ℓ/minute at rest.
(3) Adipose tissue compartment receiving about 0.3 ℓ/minute.

Thiopentone is 'cleared' exclusively by metabolism from the central vessel-rich compartment; here the clearance concept is equally applicable as to the renal excretion of *Gentamicin* or *Digoxin.*

Computers are used to solve the numerous simultaneous equations involved in such complicated pharmacokinetic models. Some Thiopentone is metabolized to pentobarbitone (that is, the S is replaced by O). Both Thiopentone and its pentobarbitone product are further metabolized by the addition of an OH group to the longer hydrocarbon side-chain. The MFO system is responsible for this metabolism.

237

PHENYTOIN — MW (acid) = 252; $pK_a = 8.3$

This anticonvulsant is widely used in epilepsy at a daily dose of 200–500 mg of the sodium salt. It lacks the pronounced hypnotic action seen with barbiturates. It is poorly soluble in aqueous solutions (14 mg/ℓ) at pH < 7. The higher solubility in serum (75 mg/ℓ) is due mainly to extensive protein binding, about 90 per cent being bound to serum proteins *in vivo*. Concentrations in saliva and CSF are about 10 per cent of the serum concentration.

Phenytoin is extensively metabolized by the MFO, < 5 per cent appearing in the urine as unchanged drug. The glucuronide conjugate of the parahydroxylated product is the main metabolite in urine (that is, both Phase I and Phase II biotransformations, page 224).

Generally, *Phenytoin* serum concentrations < 10 mg/ℓ are only partially effective, whereas serum concentrations > 30 mg/ℓ are associated with toxic symptoms (for example, ataxia, dysarthria, nystagmus). Monitoring of serum concentration is desirable, since the relationship between serum concentration and daily dose is non-linear. There is a disproportionate rise in serum concentration with increase in dose as a consequence of the distinctive 'dose-dependent' pharmacokinetics of this drug. The $t_{1/2}$ increases with the dose or C_p. Therefore, the pharmacokinetics cannot be 'first order'. The elimination of *Phenytoin* from the body is best described in terms of Michaelis–Menten/enzyme/non-linear kinetics (Ethanol and *Salicylic* acid are eliminated similarly).

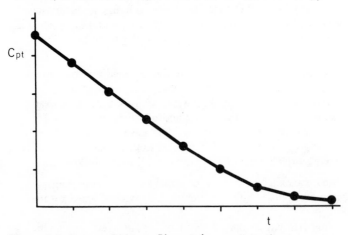

Figure 5.5 *Decay of plasma Phenytoin concentration*

The C_{pt}/t curve (*Figure 5.5*) appears to be biphasic: zero order (linear) at high concentration (> 30 mg/ℓ), first order (exponential) at low concentration (< 10 mg/ℓ).

The rate equation applicable to a single large dose is Equation 5.9 (page 226). This can account for both the apparent zero-order and first-order phases. At low serum concentration when $C_{pt} \ll K_m$ the equation reduces to a form analagous to a first order rate equation:

$$dC_{pt}/dt = -(V_{max}/K_m)\, C_{pt} = \text{constant} \times \text{concentration}$$

Conversely, at high serum concentration when $C_{pt} \gg K_m$ the equation reduces to a zero-order type of relationship:

$$dC_{pt}/dt = -V_{max} = \text{constant}$$

Clinical applications

Progressive but slow (increment every 2—4 weeks) increase in daily dose is appropriate until control of seizures is obtained or further increase is prevented by toxicity. Non-linear kinetics demands diminishing increments (*Table 5.8*). Reductions in dosage necessitated by mild intoxication require similar adjustments.

Table 5.8

$\bar{C}_{pss}$ (mg/ℓ)	Increment in daily dose (mg)
< 5	100
5—10	50
> 10	25

Individual differences in D_m/T for desired $\bar{C}_{pss}$ are not accurately predictable. Surface area is the best guide but this only accounts for a part of the variation. Daily dose/surface area (mg/day per m^2) is greater in children than adults.

Low CL_{cr} in patients with renal impairment reduces clearance of metabolites of barbiturates or *Phenytoin* but does not reduce the rate of biotransformation of unchanged drug. Protein binding is reduced in severe kidney disease and as a result the drug is metabolized more rapidly. The metabolites accumulate and can produce measurable effects, for example, CNS depression due to hydroxy-amylobarbitone.

ETHANOL CH_3CH_2OH

In a dispositional sense Ethanol (ethyl alcohol) belongs to group 3 (*Table 5.5*) but it is not a highly lipid-soluble drug. Its low MW (46) enables the drug to pass readily through the water-filled pores of the cell membranes which constitute the major barriers to drug distribution.

(1) Through the mucosae of stomach and jejunum it is rapidly and completely absorbed.

(2) Across the blood/brain barrier Ethanol equilibrates rapidly with plasma producing progressive general CNS depression varying from mild sedation to general anaesthesia and fatal respiratory depression (page 159). The effect of Ethanol on the brain depends not only on the plasma concentration (*Table 5.9*) but also on the direction in which the concentration is changing. The effect of a given concentration is greater when the concentration is rising and less when the concentration is steady or falling. The same is true for other CNS depressant drugs. This is termed acute tolerance.

Table 5.9

Plasma concentration mg/ℓ	Clinical state
500	Mild sedation
800	Legal driving limit
2000	Mild to moderate intoxication
4000	Severe intoxication
5000–8000	Death

(3) The distribution volume is the total body water.

(4) Hepatic parenchymal cells oxidize 90 per cent to acetaldehyde (alcohol dehydrogenase) and then to acetate (aldehyde dehydrogenase). Disulfiram inhibits aldehyde dehydrogenase causing acetaldehyde concentrations to rise (page 165). Above a certain plasma Ethanol concentration (C_p) elimination is 'zero order', that is, independent of C_p. The average maximum rate equals 10 mℓ/hour or 8 g/hour, that is, 200 mℓ beer or 20 mℓ whisky/hour. $t_{1/2}$ increases with C_p.

(5) Ethanol is reabsorbed from the renal tubule so that the urine concentration is only slightly greater than the plasma concentration. Thus, renal plasma clearance about equals the rate of urine flow. After small or moderate doses < 10 per cent of the dose is eliminated in the urine.

(6) Excretion in expired air occurs but represents < 1 per cent of the dose.

INHALATIONAL ANAESTHETICS

In general, the response to a drug is considered to be a function of the concentration in the biophase (fluid in intimate contact with receptors). In the particular case of the volatile anaesthetic, however, response is a function of tissue (brain) 'tension' not concentration. Since these agents are highly lipid-soluble the vessel-rich group of organs behaves as a continuum. Thus, brain tension, arterial blood tension and alveolar air partial pressure are almost equal (that is, brain tension = alveolar concentration). The alveolar concentration necessary for anaesthesia varies with the potency of the anaesthetic.

Potency

A potent anaesthetic produces minimal surgical anaesthesia at a low concentration or partial pressure in the alveolar air (mac per cent v/v). Contrast the potent Halothane (0.8) with the impotent N_2O (> 80). The amount of anaesthetic required to attain the required brain tension is dependent on solubility.

Solubility

The greater the solubility (λ), the greater the amount of anaesthetic (D) which must be dissolved in a mass (m) of tissue to attain the necessary tension

(T^1): solubility = concentration (tissue) / concentration (gas): $\lambda = (D/m)/T^1$: $T^1 = D/(m \times \lambda)$ compare $C_{po} = D/V$ (Equation 5.1, page 225), that is, $(m \times \lambda)$ is the 'gas equivalent volume' of the tissue just as V is the 'plasma equivalent volume' of the body. Contrast ether ($\lambda = 12$) with N_2O ($\lambda = 0.5$).

Minimal dose for anaesthesia

Potency and solubility are correlated variables (page 159). The dose is smaller with the highest potency (lowest mac) and the lowest solubility (lowest λ, *Table 5.10*). Ether too soluble and N_2O too impotent.

Cyclopropane, Halothane and trichloroethylene each represent practical combinations of λ and mac.

Table 5.10

Anaesthetic	λ (blood/gas)	mac (percentage)	$\lambda \times$ mac
Ether	12	2	24
Trichloroethylene	9.2	0.2	1.8
Halothane	2.3	0.8	1.8
Nitrous oxide	0.5	>80	>40
Cyclopropane	0.5	8	4

Kinetic models — multiple compartments as described for Thiopentone

(0)   External air
(1)   Central rapidly equilibrating
      functional residual lung capacity less dead space + blood volume $\times \lambda$ (blood/gas) + mass of 'highly perfused organs' $\times \lambda$ (tissue/gas) adds up to the gas equivalent volume.
(2)   Lean (skeletal muscle)
      mass $\times \lambda$ (muscle/gas).
(3)   Fat (adipose tissue)
      mass $\times \lambda$ (fat/gas).
      Clearances for transfer between compartments are dependent on ventilation and perfusion
      $0 \leftrightarrow 1$ elimination or uptake = alveolar ventilation.
      $1 \leftrightarrow 2$ muscle blood flow $\times \lambda$ (blood/gas).
      $1 \leftrightarrow 3$ fat blood flow $\times \lambda$ (blood/gas).

Note: Adipose tissue (10 kg, high λ) represents an enormous gas equivalent volume but has a low blood flow. Therefore, in the short term, transfer of anaesthetic is unidirectional. Fat uptake and liver metabolism are almost equivalent.

Induction

Time from onset to minimal anaesthesia is dependent on the rate of rise of

241

tension in the central compartment. It is rapid when the inspired partial pressure and alveolar ventilation are high, bodyweight is small and the anaesthetic is poorly soluble but potent.

Recovery

Time from cessation of administration to recovery is dependent on the rate of fall of tension in the central compartment.

It is rapid when the inspired partial pressure is zero and alveolar ventilation is high, bodyweight is small, the anaesthetic is poorly soluble and the duration of exposure was short. Unequilibrated muscles represent a sink unless blood flow is impaired by shock. The converse applies. Anaesthetic washing out of muscles after long exposure delays recovery.

Acidic drugs (pK_a 2–8)

Acidic drugs have similar modes of absorption, distribution and elimination but widely diverse pharmacological actions.

EXAMPLES

(1) Analgesic, anti-inflammatory drugs: *Phenylbutazone, Aspirin, Indomethacin* produce analgesia due to peripheral and CNS effects and reduction of inflammation.
(2) Oral anticoagulants: *Warfarin*, nicoumalone are competitive antagonists of vitamin K which inhibit the biosynthesis of clotting factors.
(3) Penicillin antibiotics: important penicillins and some vulnerable bacteria, for example, *Benzylpenicillin, Penicillin V (Str. pneumococcus), Ampicillin (E. coli), Cloxacillin (Staph. aureus), Carbenicillin (Pseudomonas aeruginosa)*. Penicillins are bactericidal and bacteriostatic but relatively non-toxic to the host.
(4) Sulphonamides: *Sulphamethizole*, sulphadiazine (*E. coli*, Meningococcus) are selectively bacteriostatic. Host side-effects exist and several have been usefully exploited (*Table 5.11*).
(5) *Phenobarbitone* is the only common barbiturate with pK_a significantly < 8. It produces general CNS depression and specific anticonvulsant effects.

Table 5.11

Systemic effects	Specially derived 'sulphonamides'
(a) Inhibition of carbonic anhydrase	*Acetazolamide*
(b) Inhibition of tubular sodium reabsorption	*Bendrofluazide*
(c) Inhibition of thyroxine biosynthesis	*Carbimazole*
(d) Potentiation of endogenous insulin	*Tolbutamide, Chlorpropamide*

(6) Uricosuric agents: *Probenecid* and *Sulphinpyrazone* increase rate of urinary excretion of uric acid, lower the plasma urate and reduce crystallization in connective tissues.

(7) Diagnostic radio-opaque compounds are usually acidic. They are used, for example, in pyelography (X-ray examination of the upper urinary tract) and cholangiography (of the gall bladder and bile ducts). Radio-opacity is due to the high atomic number of iodine. Selective concentration is due to carrier mediated transport.

All these drugs with diverse pharmacological properties are acids (donors of H ion). We can arrange them in order, the strongest at the top, the weakest at the bottom (*Table 5.12*).

Table 5.12

| Drug | pK_a | Concentration ratio $(A^-):(HA)$* | | | |
		Stomach pH 3.0	Urine (acid) pH 5.0	Plasma pH 7.4	Urine (alk) pH 8.0
Benzylpenicillin	2.8				
Salicylic acid	3.0	1:1	10^2:1	10^4:1	10^5:1
Probenecid	3.5				
Aspirin	3.6	0.3:1	25:1	10^3:1	10^4:1
Aminohippurate	3.9				
Phenylbutazone	4.3	0.01:1	5:1	10^3:1	10^3:1
Sulphadiazine	6.5	10^{-4}:1	10^{-2}:1	10:1	30:1
Acetazolamide	7.1				
Phenobarbitone	7.4	10^{-5}:1	10^{-3}:1	1:1	4:1

* Calculated from Equation 5.10 (page 226).

CHARACTERISTIC FEATURES

(1) Most acidic drugs are present mainly as the uncharged acid (HA) at pH 3. The acid (HA) is the more lipid-soluble form; thus, conditions in the stomach are favourable to absorption but surface area is small.

(2) In the plasma acidic drugs are present to a large extent as the charged anions (A^-). The anions of different acidic drugs compete for binding sites on plasma albumin and for active secretion into bile and urine.

(3) The plasma clearance (CL) varies inversely with the extent of reabsorption from the renal tubule. If the urine pH is high, the drug in the urine is present mainly as the anion (A^-), non-ionic diffusion is discouraged and *CL* is high. Increase in *CL* causes a corresponding reduction in $t_{1/2}$.

Note: (1) Importance of urine pH when measuring daily excretion of acidic compounds. (2) Use of forced alkaline diuresis in acute poisoning by salicylates or *Phenobarbitone.*

SALICYLIC ACID (O-HYDROXYBENZOIC ACID)

Salicylic acid is used as an anti-inflammatory agent to treat, for example, painful swollen joints. It is usually administered in the form of *Aspirin* (acetylsalicylic acid) but this is rapidly hydrolysed within the body ($t_{1/2}$ 15 minutes) to give acetate and *Salicylic* acid.

Physicochemical Properties

pK_a 3, Soluble in water and organic solvents.

Absorption

Drug in solution is rapidly absorbed primarily from the small intestine.

Dosage form

Conventional tablets give rapid and complete absorption. Enteric-coated tablets give erratic and incomplete absorption. Large doses give slow fractional absorption. There is a dissolution problem. Salicylates are poorly soluble at low pH.

Distribution

Salicylic acid enters cells by non-ionic diffusion. Distributed throughout total body water and binding sites on plasma albumin and tissue protein. At high salicylate doses plasma concentration approaches molar concentration of albumin (0.6 mmol/ℓ), binding sites are saturated and there is a disproportionate rise in free drug concentration.

Metabolism and disposition kinetics (*Table 5.13*)

The process of conjugation becomes saturated in the therapeutic dose range and the $t_{1/2}$ is dose dependent (*Table 5.14*). *Salicylic* acid displays the same non-linear kinetics as *Phenytoin* and Ethanol. There is saturation of metabolizing enzymes and also of binding sites.

Table 5.13

Fate		*Metabolite*	*Urine (percentage)*
Conjugated (Phase II) with	Glycine	Salicyluric acid	45—55
	Glucuronic acid	Acyl glucuronide	7—12
	Glucuronic acid	Phenolic glucuronide	15—25
Hydroxylated (Phase I)		Gentisic acid	<3
Excreted unchanged (low dose)			5—25

Table 5.14

Dose (g)	$t_{1/2}$ (hour)
0.3	2.3
1	6
10	19
overdose	<35 (untreated)

Accumulation kinetics

Within the therapeutic range dosage increase produces a disproportional increase in $\overline{C}_{pss}$ and the time to reach steady state, for example, doubling the dose (1.5–3 g/day) in one experimental subject produced a 4-fold $\overline{C}_{pss}$ increase (30–120 mg/ℓ).

Renal clearance – increases with pH and urine flow

CL increases about 4-fold with unit rise in urine pH. Renal excretion is a minor pathway at low concentration but a major pathway at high concentration (for example, intoxication). This explains the effective use of alkaline diuresis in salicylate intoxication.

Plasma salicylate and patient response

< 300 mg/ℓ: therapeutic – analgesic, anti-inflammatory, antipyretic effects. Side-effects include bleeding from gastric erosions (hypoprothrombinaemia and reduced platelet stickiness may contribute), tinnitus and deafness at maximum therapeutic concentrations and even bronchospasm (idiosyncrasy).

300–750 mg/ℓ: mild to moderate intoxication is manifest as hyperventilation, respiratory alkalosis, sweating, tachycardia, salt and water depletion. Toxicity increases with time. 500 mg/ℓ at 48 hours after overdose may represent severe intoxication.

> 750 mg/ℓ: severe intoxication is manifest as impaired utilization of pyruvate and lactate, metabolic acidosis, convulsions, circulatory arrest and renal failure. Treatment is by correction of salt and water depletion and by alkaline diuresis.

Basic drugs (pK_a 6–12)

Basic drugs have similar modes of absorption, distribution and elimination but widely diverse pharmacological actions.

EXAMPLES

(1)   Narcotic analgesics: *Morphine* and *Pethidine* (antagonist *Naloxone*) reduce especially the reactive component of pain also produce euphoria, addiction and respiratory depression.

(2)   Local anaesthetics: *Cocaine, Procaine* and *Lignocaine* stabilize the membrane potential and inhibit the propagated action potential in peripheral nerve.

(3)   Anti-arrhythmic drugs: *Lignocaine, Procainamide* and *Quinidine* inhibit ectopic rhythms in the heart.

(4)   Ganglion stimulants: Nicotine.

(5)   Antimuscarinic drugs: *Atropine,* hyoscine.

(6)   Adrenergic neurone blocking agents: *Guanethidine, Bethanidine, Debrisoquine, Reserpine.*

(7)   Anticholinesterases: *Physostigmine.*

(8)   Sympathomimetic amines: direct − NA, *Adrenaline, Isoprenaline*; indirect − Amphetamine, *Ephedrine.*

(9)   Antagonists of sympathomimetic amines: Phenoxybenzamine, Phentolamine, *Propranolol.*

(10)   Neuroleptics: Phenothiazines (*Chlorpromazine, Promethazine*); control of psychotic states, schizophrenia, delirium tremens.

(11)   Anxiolytics: *Diazepam*: anxiety states, bereavement, neurosis.

(12)   Tricyclic antidepressants: *Imipramine* and *Amitriptyline* elevate mood in endogenous depression.

(13)   Analeptics: *Nikethamide* promotes wakefulness and coughing in patients with acute exacerbations of chronic bronchitis.

(14)   Antihistamines: *Mepyramine, Chlorpheniramine.*

All these drugs with diverse pharmacological properties are bases (acceptors of H ion); we can arrange them in order, the strongest (high pK_a) at the top and the weakest (low pK_a) at the bottom (*Table 5.15*).

pK_a

Whatever the pharmacological action, the disposition of the basic drug is determined, in part, by its pK_a.

Henderson−Hasselbalch equation

Acid form:

$$pH = pK_a + \log [(A^-) / (HA)]$$

General form (Equation 5.10, page 226):

$$pH = pK_a + \log [(H \text{ acceptor}) / (H \text{ donor})]$$

Base form:

$$pH = pK_a + \log [(R.NH_2) / (R.NH_3^+)]$$

246

Table 5.15

| Drug | pK_a | Concentration ratio $(B^+H):(B)$ | | | |
		Stomach (acid) pH 3.0	Urine pH 5.0	Plasma (alk) pH 7.4	Urine pH 8.0
Guanethidine	11.7	$10^9:1$	$10^7:1$	$10^5:1$	$10^4:1$
Adrenaline (amine group)	9.9				
Isoprenaline (amine group)	9.9				
Amphetamine (amine group)	9.9	$10^7:1$	$10^5:1$	$10^3:1$	$10^2:1$
NA (amine group)	9.8				
Atropine	9.6				
Promethazine	9.1				
Procaine, Mepyramine	8.9				
Lignocaine	8.7	$10^5:1$	$10^4:1$	$10:1$	$4:1$
Quinine, Quinidine	8.6				
Morphine, Cocaine	8.0				
Physostigmine	8.0				
Nalorphine	7.9				
Diamorphine	7.8				
Reserpine	7.5	$10^4:1$	$300:1$	1.1	$0.3:1$
Pilocarpine	6.9				

CHARACTERISTIC FEATURES

(1)   Basic drugs exist almost entirely as the non-diffusible cation at pH 3; conditions do not favour absorption from stomach.

(2)   The concentration of total drug (cation plus base) in urine is greatly increased when the urine pH is reduced from 8 to 5 (*Table 5.15*).

(3)   When excretion is a major factor in elimination (for example, Amphetamine, *Quinine*), the plasma concentration $t_{1/2}$ is shortened if the urine is made acid.

Notes: (1) Urine pH should be controlled when estimating excretion rates of basic compounds. (2) The use of forced acid diuresis in severe poisoning by Amphetamine or *Quinine*.

LIGNOCAINE

This is one of the most widely used anti-arrhythmic agents in coronary care units. It has particular value in the treatment of ventricular arrhythmias.

Plasma concentration and effect

Generally ineffective below 1.5 mg/ℓ; frequency and severity of toxicity increase above 6 mg/ℓ.

Physicochemical properties

pK_a 8, limited solubility in water (7 mg/ℓ) but very soluble in organic solvents.

Absorption

Rapid ($t_{1/2}$, about 15 minutes) and complete from all sites except gut (discussed later). More rapidly absorbed from an alkaline environment. Rapidity of absorption greatest from highly perfused tissues.

Distribution

Volume of distribution (dose independent) is about 120 ℓ/70 kg. The drug lies mainly outside plasma in lung, kidney, brain, muscle and adipose tissue: 60 per cent of the drug in plasma is bound but not to albumin (presumably globulin). Displacement is an unlikely phenomenon. It is so lipophilic that membranes are no barrier to penetration. The rate of tissue uptake is a function of organ perfusion. This explains the rapid onset (about one minute) and termination (about 20 minutes) of CNS and cardiac effects following a therapeutic bolus dose (1 mg/kg). It also explains the size of the 'reservoir' in muscle after prolonged administration.

The arterial plasma decay curve after iv bolus is biexponential as with Thiopentone. The peak amount (percentage dose) in the rapidly equilibrating compartment is established almost immediately. This then decays due to: (1) muscle uptake; (2) biotransformation; (3) slow uptake into fat.

Metabolism and disposition kinetics

The hepatic MFO removes one or both ethyl groups (N dealkylation). Both products are biologically active. Aromatic C hydroxylation also occurs and hydrolysis of the side-chain at amide position.

Clearance, availability and $t_{1/2}$ (example C, pages 227 and 229)

CL is almost exclusively by hepatic metabolism and is very high (1 ℓ/min/70 kg) approaching liver blood flow (1.5 ℓ/min/70 kg). High hepatic extraction (70 per cent) explains the low bioavailability (30 per cent) of oral *Lignocaine* (often called the 'first pass effect'). Because metabolites are active, however, the oral dose is more effective than the low availability suggests.

Infusion via the portal vein demonstrates that low systemic availability after oral dose is not due to incomplete absorption. Changes in liver perfusion affect clearance. Dosage requirements, are diminished in diseases causing depressed hepatic metabolism (cirrhosis) and circulatory function (congestive heart failure).

Although CL is high, $t_{1/2}$ is not excessively short (1–2 hours) because V is large. There is a long delay (3–5 × $t_{1/2}$) between initiation of an infusion and attainment of the plateau concentration, therefore a bolus dose is given. Renal clearance depends on filtration, secretion and reabsorption which is extensive. Reabsorption is reduced when urine is acid. Acidification, however, has no major effect on the elimination kinetics of *Lignocaine* because renal excretion is a minor pathway of elimination.

Contrast Amphetamine

Urine pH	$t_{1/2}$ (hour)
5	5
7	16

Effect of pH on pharmacological activity of bases, for example, local anaesthetics

(1) The penetrating form is the unionized base. *Procaine* (pK_a 8.9) is more fully ionized at pH 7.4 than is *Cocaine* (pK_a 8), thus, *Cocaine* penetrates conjunctiva more readily to produce corneal anaesthesia. *Cocaine* buffered at pH 5 is less effective than *Cocaine* buffered at pH 7.4 when applied to rabbit cornea.

(2) The pharmacologically active form is the cation. A nerve trunk ceases to conduct at a critical *Procaine* concentration (pH 7) but conduction returns at the same *Procaine* concentration when the pH is raised to 9.5. Many basic drugs produce their pharmacological effects in the cationic form (for example, anticholinesterases, ganglion blocking drugs).

Table 5.16

	R_4N^+ (onium salt)	R_3N^+H (tertiary amine)
Water-soluble		
Lipid-soluble		R_3N
Disposition		
Intestinal absorption	Slow, incomplete	Rapid, complete
Distribution	ECF	Total body water
Biotransformation	No	Yes
Kidney	Glomerular filtration: tubular secretion	Glomerular filtration: passive tubular reabsorption
Pharmacological actions		
(1) Antimuscarinic	More active	Active
(2) Neuromuscular blockade	Definite	Negligible
(3) Ganglion blockade	Definite	Slight
(4) CNS	No effect	Excitement, delirium, convulsions

Note: Similar changes demonstrated for N-methyl iodide derivatives of following alkaloids (**Strychnine, *Codeine, Morphine,* Nicotine**) by Crum-Brown and Fraser (1868).
(1) Loss of characteristic CNS effects
(2) Reduction of toxicity
(3) Development of neuromuscular blockade

Quaternary ammonium derivatives

When a tertiary amine like *Atropine* is converted into the corresponding onium salt a highly polar compound results and there are important changes in pharmacological properties (*Table 5.16*).

Summary

The drugs discussed illustrate important pharmacokinetic phenomena of direct relevance to therapeutics.

Gentamicin — distribution volume, $t_{1/2}$, clearance, accumulation, steady state, dosage adjustment in renal impairment.

Digoxin — effect of tissue binding on $t_{1/2}$, therapeutic index, principles of dosage regimens.

Thiopentone, *Phenytoin,* inhalational anaesthetics — biexponential decay, redistribution, MFO system, hydroxylation followed by conjugation, inhibition and induction, non-linear kinetics, Michaelis—Menten equation, multicompartment systems, tension, solubility, gas equivalent volume, potency.

Salicylic acid — pK_a, effect of pH on ionization, non-ionic diffusion, dose-dependent $t_{1/2}$, pH-dependent urinary excretion, plasma protein binding, carrier mediated transport, competition.

Lignocaine — high extraction, first pass effect, active metabolites, bioavailability, absorption from different sites, infusion.

6
Applied pharmacology

AIMS

- To provide a stimulus to revision of pharmacological actions and their mechanisms.
- To present information on some BNF drugs which are missed by the themes chosen for the bulk of the book.
- To provide insight into the pathophysiology of disease and thus a framework for the rational use of drugs in treatment.
- To introduce some more to the language of medicine.
- To satisfy the craving which students of pharmacology clearly show for an understanding of the uses of drugs.

Since this is not a textbook of medicine it is neither possible nor desirable to attempt a general coverage of disease.

We have adopted certain criteria for the inclusion of disease states and forms of therapy. A disease state should be a chronic condition of relatively common occurrence with the patient either ambulant or being treated at home. Alternatively, it should be the kind of condition for which pharmacists are often asked to advise. Since many proprietary preparations are advertised for self-medication we have attempted to guide the reader through the jungle of 'over the counter' prescribing so that logical and relevant advice can be given.

Abuse of drugs

Drug abuse is the taking of, or recommendation to take, a drug or a dose of drug different from that advised by authoritative medical opinion.

In addition to the well publicized aspects of drug dependence, drug abuse also involves such practices as excessive self-medication with proprietary preparations (for example, weak analgesics, vitamins, cold 'remedies'), the bulk addition of antibiotics to animal foodstuffs in factory farming, over-prescribing and mis-prescribing by the medical profession, the unnecessary sale of 'nostrums' by pharmacists and much else.

In lecture notes such as these so many facets cannot be covered. The following points are intended to provide some factual information and to encourage discussion.

DEPENDENCE

Dependence is defined in terms of the consequences of stopping drug taking. If the consequences are psychic or mental (for example, craving, behavioural changes), this is psychic or mental dependence (habituation). Drugs which cause psychic dependence include Nicotine (as in tobacco) centrally acting sympatho-mimetics (*Amphetamines, Ephedrine*) and cannabis.

If the consequences are physical, this is physical dependence (addiction). Only two groups of drugs cause physical dependence:

(1) Narcotic analgesics (page 149) — withdrawal syndrome includes diarrhoea, abdominal cramps, sweating, vomiting.
(2) Non-specific depressants (page 166) — withdrawal syndrome includes EEG changes, confusion, disorientation, convulsions.

The severity of the syndrome depends both on the drug and on the frequency of drug taking. *Diazepam* or *Ethanol* can take years of regular consumption before dependence is detectable, *Diamorphine* requires a few days. Withdrawal after six consecutive injections of *Diamorphine* may produce only a mild syndrome — that after one year may be fatal.

The molecular mechanism of dependence is unknown. Any theory must explain tolerance (which is a prerequisite of dependence) and the nature of the with-drawal syndrome.

The following should be regarded as a model rather than actual mechanism of action (*Figure 6.1*).

Consider a part of the brain in which there is a balance between an excitatory and an inhibitory transmitter (E and I). Assume the drug (D) of dependence acts as a mimic of transmitter I. The balance is altered to a state of inhibition or depression as a result of the primary effect of the drug.

If the drug effect persisted, the body would try to compensate and a method of compensation could be to increase excitatory activity. This could be by an increase in E (as shown), or by receptor proliferation or other mechanisms of supersensitivity. The balance is restored although the drug is still present (tolerance). If the drug is withdrawn a new imbalance occurs which must produce symptoms opposite to those of the drug (the withdrawal syndrome). It will then require some time (during treatment) before the biological adaption reverts back to normal.

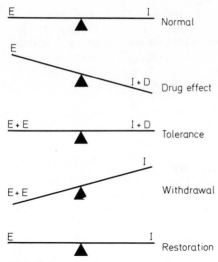

E ——————— I Normal

E ——————— I + D Drug effect

E + E ——————— I + D Tolerance

I ——————— Withdrawal
E + E

E ——————— I Restoration

Figure 6.1

Two other points are pertinent:

(1) There is a grey area between psychic and physical dependence; character-istics are best defined for each drug group.
(2) Man is a creature of habit. Dependence can occur to almost anything done habitually. A person accustomed to walking round the block before retiring will not sleep so well (a behavioural response) if deprived of the habit. Linked to this is dependence on an environment (social dependence) which can be a very potent behavioural influence.

THE DRUG LAWS

An assortment of laws control the availability, prescribing, storage and labelling of drugs in the UK.

The Misuse of Drugs Act (1971) covers the most publicized drugs of abuse. The drugs listed in the Act are known as Controlled Drugs and are narcotic agonists, *Cocaine*, hallucinogens (LSD, mescaline, page 153), cannabis preparations, centrally acting sympathomimetics (amphetamines, some other anorectics) and methaqualone (a barbiturate-like depressant chemically unrelated to barbituric acid).

(1) The above drugs are grouped into three classes (A, B and C) dependent on abuse potential; *Morphine* is more rigidly controlled than *Codeine*.
(2) Control of a drug may vary dependent on formulation; morphine injection is in Class A, *Kaolin* and *Morphine* mixture is exempt.
(3) The classification has little pharmacological basis — the barbiturates are absent from, and the cannabis constituents included in, the same class as the highly addictive *Diamorphine*.

DRUG DEATHS

About 3000 people die as a consequence of self-poisoning each year in England and Wales (accidentally or intentionally) – this is about half the number of people who die on the roads. Since more than one drug usually appears on the death certificate, it is difficult to establish precise poisoning figures. *Table 6.1* shows approximate numbers.

Table 6.1

Total (acute) deaths in England and Wales (1974)	3,000
Deaths due to barbiturates	1,600
Aspirin	200
antidepressants	200
anxiolytics	50
Ethanol	35
narcotic analgesics	30
paraquat	20

Appearance in the list is a function of both toxicity and availability.

If chronic poisoning is considered, tobacco, which causes cardiovascular and lung damage, puts all other drugs in the shade (estimated 60,000).

INCIDENCE OF DEPENDENCE

Again, incidence is a function of availability. Ethanol is responsible for the greatest incidence of physical dependence (300,000), narcotic analgesics the least (2500). It is difficult to place a figure on the barbiturates since prescribing habits are changing. Individual surveys would imply a number several fold greater than the incidence of narcotic addiction.

Before 1960 the number of known narcotic addicts in the UK remained constant at about 300. During the 1960s there was a massive increase which levelled at 2500 followed by a sharp increase in the early 1980s to 3800.

SOME POINTS FOR DISCUSSION

Drugs have always been a part of society. Many primitive societies revolved around (usually hallucinogenic) drug cults (religions). Ethanol was established in Roman and Greek cultures and has remained so in those that succeeded them throughout Europe and the Americas. Cannabis is established in some Asian societies. Because drugs are a part of society, drug laws cannot always be rational (some would argue that tobacco should be banned and Ethanol put on prescription, or even controlled).

Medication with legally obtained drugs occurs on a vast scale. Sales of anti-pyretic analgesics suggests a national intake of one tablet per person per day.

Twenty-five million prescriptions for anxiolytics are dispensed each year (assume about 60 tablets or capsules per prescription).

It is estimated that half the number of prescription items are unnecessary (over-prescribing).

The likelihood of a patient taking a preparation as instructed is remote (non-compliance) : 5 per cent of all prescriptions are not even dispensed. The more complicated the instructions, the greater the non-compliance. This can have serious consequences in certain conditions (notably epilepsy, page 301). Bacterial resistance can be encouraged by erratic taking of antibiotics.

The influence of drug promotion (advertising, representatives) on doctor's prescribing in western countries becomes dominant a few years after qualification, by which time the cost of such promotion roughly equals the cost of medical education. Whilst the volume of medical information (biased and unbiased) is indeed vast, the existence of concise independent assessments of new drugs such as *Prescribers' Journal* and *Drug and Therapeutics Bulletin* simplifies the problem of keeping up to date.

Ignorance (not only on the part of the lay public) remains one of the most important contributions to drug abuse. People fail to appreciate that drugs are more or less selective poisons. Lay people would categorize Strychnine as a poison, *Penicillin V* as a medicine, *Diamorphine* as a drug and Ethanol as none of these. Cannabis has appeared in all categories. This lack of respect for drugs as poisons contributes much to drug abuse and is also at the root of many well-meant irresponsible habits such as handing over prescribed drugs to neighbours (irrespective of disorder or drug) or children (parent's anxiolytics for child's examinations). This is the province of health education. The pharmacist is in an ideal position to act as a health educator (though often not involved to the extent he should be). The general practitioner is regrettably seldom interested.

Toxicity

This is the name given to the undesired, detrimental effects of a drug. All drugs are toxic to all individuals if large enough doses are given, but toxic effects often occur after reasonable therapeutic doses and this section aims to summarize the mechanisms responsible. Toxic reactions can be subdivided into two categories: (1) those arising from the normal pharmacology of the drug; (2) those arising because of an abnormality (idiosyncrasy) in the recipient.

EXTENSION OF NORMAL PHARMACOLOGY

Features

The toxic response is part of the drug's normal, but not necessarily its main, action. Its size, and therefore severity, depends on dose and is neither

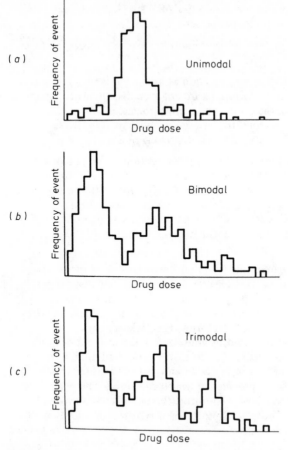

Figure 6.2

qualitatively nor quantitatively unusual. Treated population displays unimodal frequency distribution of toxic response, that is, all individuals will show the response to some extent and if the number of individuals showing toxicity (frequency) is plotted against minimal toxic dose, a smooth, continuous, bell-shaped curve, with a single peak (mode) is obtained (*Figure 6.2a*). This kind of distribution arises because sensitivity to the drug is the result of the expression of many genes (multifactorial). Many examples of this kind of toxicity appear throughout the book.

IDIOSYNCRATIC RESPONSES

These arise because the individual is different from the general population, either quantitatively (hypersensitive) or qualitatively. Idiosyncratic responses can be further subdivided into three groups: (1) drug allergy; (2) genetically determined differences; (3) reactions the mechanisms of which are as yet unknown.

Drug allergy

Characterized by a group of similar qualitatively unusual responses involving an antigen-antibody reaction, after a previous uneventful exposure (of which the patient may be unaware), for example, asthmatic reaction to *Aspirin*, anaphylactic reaction to penicillins, haemolytic anaemia due to *Methyldopa*. The mechanisms by which drugs induce allergic responses are poorly understood, but in most cases the drug molecules themselves are too small to induce antibody formation. However, these small molecules behave as haptens and form complexes with proteins which then induce the formation of antibodies directed against the particular hapten and its close chemical relatives.

Genetically determined idiosyncrasies

When abnormal responsiveness to a drug is determined by the expression of a single allele (for example, the synthesis of an atypical enzyme) the frequency distribution curve will be discontinuous, that is, multimodal (*Figures 6.2b* and *6.2c*), the phenotype of each individual depending on the genetic contributions of his parents.

Autosomal recessive (*Figure 6.3*)

(1) *Isoniazid* acetylation. In North America and Europe about 50 per cent of the population inactivate *Isoniazid* slowly. This is due to the occurrence of an abnormality in the gene responsible for directing the synthesis of the acetylating enzyme. The atypical enzyme acetylates *Isoniazid* more slowly than the normal enzyme. There are three possible genotypes – those with two normal genes (that is, rapid-rapid), those with one abnormal gene and one normal gene (that is, slow-rapid or rapid-slow) and those in whom both genes are of the slow type (that is, slow-slow). These genotypes give rise to two phenotypes – slow acetylators and rapid acetylators (*Figure 6.3*). When given to slow acetylators at dose rates suitable for rapid acetylators, *Isoniazid* may accumulate to toxic concentrations, usually resulting in polyneuropathy. Other drugs which are acetylated and which therefore accumulate in patients with the atypical acetylation enzymes include *hydralazine* (page 281), *Phenelzine* and *Sulphamethizole*.

(2) In hereditary methaemoglobinaemia, NADH methaemoglobin reductase is absent. This enzyme does not inactivate any drugs but it is the main route for regenerating haemoglobin from methaemoglobin. Consequently, the methaemoglobinaemia produced by certain oxidizing drugs (for example, nitrites, nitrates, sulphonamides) is severe and prolonged in individuals with this condition.

Autosomal autonomous (*Figure 6.3*)

Suxamethonium occasionally produces unduly prolonged apnoea, necessitating artificial ventilation, as there are atypical forms of the enzyme ChE (page 35). Like slow *Isoniazid* acetylation, atypical ChE is due to an abnormality in a single gene. In heterozygotes the trait is partially expressed so that there are individuals with intermediate ChE activities (trimodal frequency distribution curve, *Figure 6.2c*). The dibucaine test identifies individuals with the atypical form of ChE — the enzyme in blood from normal subjects is more easily inhibited by cinchocaine [dibucaine] than is the atypical enzyme.

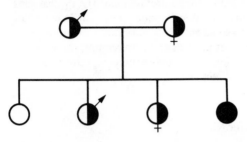

Autosomal recessive	Normal	Normal	Normal	Affected
Autosomal autonomous	Normal	Partially affected	Partially affected	Affected
Autosomal dominant	Normal	Affected	Affected	Affected
X-linked autonomous	Normal	Affected (inherited from mother)	Partially affected (inherited from father)	Affected

Genotype:

○ Normal – normal (homozygous for normal gene)
● Affected – affected (homozygous for affected gene)
◐ Normal – affected
      or   (heterozygous for affected gene)
   Affected – normal

Figure 6.3

Autosomal dominant (Figure 6.3)

(1) In the rare condition of malignant hyperthermia an exposure to a general anaesthetic (or possibly to *Suxamethonium* together with a general anaesthetic) causes a rapid rise in body temperature, muscle rigidity and loss of cellular K^+. Death is common (about 60 per cent of cases).

(2) Impaired *Debrisoquine* hydroxylation is also transmitted as an autosomal dominant trait.

(3) Hereditary porphyria is a condition in which sufferers have a disturbance in their haem synthesis pathway. They are generally free from symptoms but acute attacks, which involve abdominal pain, neuritis, psychosis and the excretion of large amounts of porphyrins, can be triggered by drugs, especially the barbiturates, but also by *Griseofulvin*, gonadal steroids,

sulphonamides, oral hypoglycaemics and *Phenytoin*. Attacks are sometimes fatal. The common step in drug-triggered attacks is induction of the enzyme δ-aminolaevulinic acid synthetase.

X-Linked autonomous (Figure 6.3)

People with glucose-6-phosphate dehydrogenase deficiency (page 188) are sensitive to *Nitrofurantoin* and sulphonamides, as well as to the anti-malarial *Primaquine*.

Multifactorial

Another example of a drug triggering an attack in a susceptible person is the precipitation of an acute attack of gout by thiazide diuretics in individuals with a genetic predisposition to the disease — there is clear evidence of a herditary component in gout but it is not a simple trait carried by a single gene (that is, it is multifactorial).

Idiosyncrasy of unknown origin

The fatal aplastic anaemia induced by *Chloramphenicol* (page 200); for a list of other drugs which can produce aplastic anaemia *see* page 315.

Developmental toxicity

HUMAN DEVELOPMENT

Development *in utero* can be conveniently separated into three stages: (1) pre-implantation; (2) embryonic; and (3) foetal (*Figure 6.4*).

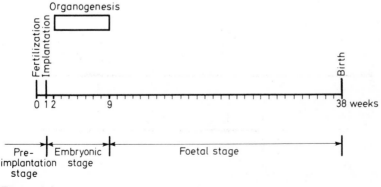

Figure 6.4

Pre-implantation stage

Fertilization (fusion of haploid oocyte and spermatozoon) occurs in the oviduct to form a zygote. This progressively divides to form a ball of cells (morula). A blastocyst is formed soon after the morula has passed into the uterus. This blastocyst embeds in the endometrium.

Embryonic stage

Implantation occurs one week after fertilization or about three weeks after the commencement of the last menstrual period, and pregnancy will not usually be confirmed until some four weeks after implantation. In the human, organogenesis starts soon after implantation. During this stage differentiation of cells is occurring and primordia of organ systems are being formed.

Foetal stage

By about nine weeks after conception, the major organ systems have been formed. Foetal development consists of growth in size, finer differentiation and functional maturation. Some development of major organ systems occurs during this stage, for example, major brain growth occurs around birth in the human, after birth in the rat. Obviously, much human development takes place after birth.

DEVELOPMENTAL TOXICITY

Developmental toxicity is the study of factors and mechanisms producing abnormalities of development. Possible adverse effects of drugs on development include the following:

(1) Embryonic or foetal death.
(2) Major structural malformation.
(3) Growth retardation.
(4) Functional defects.

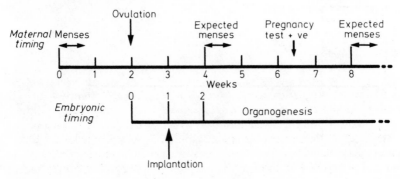

Figure 6.5

260

The nature of the effect produced will principally depend on: the drug itself; the time of administration in relation to the stage of development. For example, Thalidomide produced limb deformities (phocomelia) and internal organ deformities. The critical period was 3—5 weeks after conception. Thalidomide used towards the end of pregnancy had no effect on development. Rubella (German measles) virus has its most profound effect in producing heart and eye deformities over the same period. A comparison of maternal and embryonic timings is shown in *Figure 6.5*. Any restriction of the use of a drug during pregnancy should apply to all women of reproductive age.

DRUG EFFECTS ON DEVELOPMENT

Androgens

There are several stages of sexual development and some can be modified by drugs:

Genetic sex

The normal female has XX chromosomes and the normal male has XY chromosomes. This is determined at fertilization.

Gonadal sex

The normal female has ovaries and the normal male has testes. Oogonia and spermatogonia derive from common primordial germ cells. Differentiation is determined by chromosomes and unaffected by ovarian hormones. Gonads form about five weeks after conception. Oocytes are formed only from 8 to 24 weeks after conception in the foetus. Spermatogenesis begins after puberty.

Hormonal sex

Males produce mainly testosterone and females mainly 17-β-oestradiol and progesterone from their gonads.

Phenotypic sex

Primordia of reproductive tracts are two duct systems — present in both genetic males and females. In genetic males, Wolffian duct development is actively stimulated by local foetal testosterone to produce epididymides, vasa deferentia and seminal vesicles. Another local hormone (structure unknown) from foetal testis actively inhibits growth of the Mullerian duct. In genetic females it is lack of this hormone which allows growth of the Mullerian ducts to form oviducts, uteri and part of vagina. Primordia develop about eight weeks after conception. Therefore, exogenous androgens (and progestogens with androgenic activity) can stimulate abnormal tract development in genetic females. Cyproterone acetate (an androgen antagonist, page 88) will antagonize normal tract development in genetic males (animal studies).

External sexual primordia are very sensitive to androgens in the foetus; they form about 12 weeks after conception. Androgens (and progestogens with androgenic activity) can produce excessive growth of clitoris in genetic females.

Hypothalamic sex

The anterior pituitary gland of the male secretes FSH and LH in an acyclic pattern. In the female it secretes FSH and LH in a monthly cyclic pattern. Animal studies suggest the pattern is determined in the hypothalamus of the foetus by the presence of androgen (male type) or absence of androgen (female type). It is uncertain whether exogenous steroids can modify the pattern in the human.

Anticonvulsants

The incidence of malformations (mainly cleft lip and palate and congenital heart defects) in neonates of epileptic women treated with *Phenytoin* plus *Phenobarbitone* is three-fold higher than in the general population. Animal studies suggest this is more probably due to the *Phenytoin.* It is essential, however, that anticonvulsant therapy in pregnancy be continued.

Antineoplastic drugs

Present antineoplastic drugs show only a narrow degree of selective toxicity towards neoplasms relative to normal cells. These drugs act particularly on rapidly proliferating cells and could be expected to produce embryotoxicity and foetotoxicity (page 205). The group includes antimetabolites such as *Methotrexate* and *Mercaptopurine*, and alkylating agents such as *Cyclophosphamide, Chlorambucil* and *Busulphan.* If used during the first trimester ($\frac{1}{3}$) of pregnancy, miscarriages or malformations frequently, but not inevitably, result. Following their use in the second and third trimester growth retardation often occurs.

Antithyroid drugs

Neonatal hypothyroidism and even cretinism is possible but is rarely seen following the use of antithyroid drugs such as *Carbimazole* (page 91). Thyroid gland enlargement present at delivery is usually temporary.

Mercury salts

Some organic mercury salts in late pregnancy can produce cerebral palsy.

Stilboestrol

Use of high doses of *Stilboestrol* in pregnancy has led to the development of a type of vaginal carcinoma in a small proportion of postpubertal offspring.

Tetracyclines

Tetracyclines are readily deposited, by calcium chelation, in developing teeth and bone in the third trimester and postnatally leading to discoloration and occasionally hypoplasia (page 199).

Warfarin

There is an association between *Warfarin* use and a variety of structural malformations including facial deformities and optic nerve atrophy, and perhaps mental retardation. Excessive 'moulding' of the skull during delivery has produced intracranial bleeding.

Ethanol

There are several reports of a higher incidence of growth retardation, microcephaly, limb and heart deformities and mental deficiency in the offspring of chronic alcoholic mothers. Deficiency of maternal diet probably contributes.

General anaesthetics

A higher incidence of spontaneous abortions and deformities in the offspring of females who work in operating theatres is presumed to be due to general anaesthetics.

Tobacco smoking

This is associated with smaller neonates and a higher incidence of perinatal complications.

The justifiability of treating a pregnant woman with a drug having one of these adverse effects depends on: (1) the nature and incidence of the effect; (2) the severity of the disease; (3) the therapeutic value of the drug to the mother.

Adverse drug interactions

An undesirable response to a drug (toxicity, side-effect) is a frequent occurrence both in hospital and in general practice. The outcome of such a response depends on a number of factors, for example, the severity of the toxic effect, the intrinsic lethality of the disease for which the drug is prescribed, whether the response is dose related or idiosyncratic.

Thus, the dangers associated with dose-related bone marrow depression in the chemotherapy of leukaemia with cytotoxic drugs (page 205) are accepted, but the risk of an idiosyncratic aplastic anaemia with *Chloramphenicol* (page 200) prescribed for minor infections is not. The chance of an adverse response to a drug is greater if the drug is taken for a prolonged period, or if more than one drug is prescribed. Many patients receive multiple drug therapy and one component may modify the activity of another, either enhancing or reducing potency. Such an interaction may be beneficial, for example, antihypertensive drugs in combination, but this chapter is concerned with the problems posed by two or more drugs acting simultaneously to cause an unwanted response, that is, an adverse drug interaction. The Boston Collaborative Drug Surveillance Program has collected quantitative information on nearly 10,000 patients admitted to medical wards. These patients received 83,000 drug exposures (that is, 8.3 different drugs per patient on average) with 3600 adverse responses to drugs reported by the trained monitors. Of these responses, 234 were attributed to adverse drug interactions of which there are three basic types: (1) between drugs having similar pharmacological effects; (2) between drugs having opposing pharmacological effects; (3) where one drug interferes with the disposition of another.

Pharmacodynamic interactions (types 1 and 2) are in most instances predictable; for example, Ethanol increasing the sedative effect of antihistamines, benzo-diazepines, antidepressants, *Carbenoxolone* (page 271) increasing the urinary K^+ loss with thiazide or loop diuretics (page 104), *Aspirin* in high doses reducing prothrombin concentrations further in patients on *Warfarin* (page 118), Muscarinic antagonists preventing the increase of gut motility due to *Metoclopramide* (page 301), anti-inflammatory agents antagonizing antihyper-tensive drugs.

Of the adverse interactions reported by the Boston Surveillance Programme, 230 were of type 1 or 2. The remaining four cases were dispositional interactions (type 3) which could have occurred at various points in the life history of a drug from manufacture to elimination.

DISPOSITIONAL OR PHARMACOKINETIC INTERACTIONS

Occurring before administration of the drug to the patient and mediated by reduced bioavailability

(1)   Due to an additive in the formulation of a tablet or suspension, for example, calcium phosphate used as a filler in *Tetracycline* capsules.

(2) When incompatible drugs are mixed in a syringe or solution for iv infusion, for example, *Carbenicillin* and *Gentamicin, Phenytoin* and glucose (5 per cent w/v) solution.

Interference with absorption of a drug

(1) By forming an insoluble complex, for example, antacids and iron salts with tetracyclines (page 199).
(2) By altering gastric emptying — the peak blood concentration is affected with total absorption usually unchanged. Absorption from liquid formulations is little affected. Food has a variable effect, opiates and tricyclic antidepressants (atropine-like) slow gastric emptying.
(3) By preventing the formation of lipid micelles, for example, fat soluble vitamin absorption with *Neomycin* or cholestyramine.

Competition for binding sites on albumin

The effect of an interaction at this site is short-lived because the displaced drug is metabolized and a new steady state is achieved with elimination equal to the dose ingested, that is, the same effect is achieved at a lower total drug concentration in plasma. These transient changes are only important for very highly protein-bound drugs with a low therapeutic index, such as *Warfarin* and *Tolbutamide*; in both cases the displacing drug also interferes with metabolism (*see below*). For example, *Phenylbutazone* with *Warfarin*, sulphonamides with *Tolbutamide* (page 217).

Alteration of drug metabolism

Stimulation of drug metabolism

A number of factors increase the rate at which endogenous (steroids) and exogenous (xenobiotics = drugs, foodstuffs) substances are metabolized (detoxified) by hepatic microsomal oxidation (Phase I reactions, page 224). The capacity for detoxification is greater in smokers, alcoholics (without advanced cirrhosis), in those exposed to hydrocarbons and in patients taking a wide variety

Table 6.2

Inducing agents	Drugs undergoing oxidative metabolism
Rifampicin	Oral contraceptives (1)
Phenobarbitone	*Warfarin* (1)
Phenytoin	*Paracetamol* (overdose) (2)
Ethanol	Doxycycline (1)
Griseofulvin	Glucocorticoids (1)
Dichloralphenazone	

of lipid-soluble drugs. This increased rate of drug oxidation is due to enzyme induction, a process involving synthesis of more microsomal enzymes and co-enzymes, for example, cytochrome P_{450}. Drugs differ in their capacity to cause induction, which is non-specific, that is, oxidation of drugs other than the inducing agent is promoted.

Table 6.2 lists drugs which induce MFO and those whose oxidative metabolism is thereby increased. Consequences are: (1) More rapid inactivation – more drug is needed for the desired therapeutic response. If the inducing agent is discontinued the rate of oxidation will slow and the drug may accumulate to a toxic concentration. (2) More rapid activation – toxicity arises from the more rapid production of the active drug; the duration of action is shortened.

Inhibition of drug metabolism

(1) Some drugs are administered because the desired therapeutic response is mediated by inhibiting the metabolism of endogenous or exogenous substances. The administration of other drugs, in their presence, can then produce an adverse response; for example, MAO inhibitors with *Pethidine* and indirect sympathomimetics *Allopurinol* with *Azathioprine* or *Mercaptopurine* Disulfiram with *Phenytoin*.

(2) The metabolism of some drugs is inhibited in an unpredictable manner by others. Dosage reduction is usually all that is needed but changing to a different drug may be desirable; for example, *Metronidazole* or *Chlorpropamide* with Ethanol (page 165), *Phenylbutazone* and *Chloramphenicol* with *Tolbutamide*, *Phenylbutazone* with *Warfarin, Isoniazid* with *Phenytoin*.

Uptake into the noradrenergic neurone

The active transport of released NA back into the adrenergic neurone is a site of competitive drug interaction, for example, either tricyclic antidepressants or *Ephedrine* (page 48) : (1) prevent the antihypertensive action of noradrenergic neurone blocking agents (*Guanethidine, Bethanidine* and *Debrisoquine*) (page 54) or; (2) potentiate NA or *Adrenaline* administered with a local anaesthetic (page 55).

Competition for renal excretory mechanisms

Most drugs are eventually filtered and excreted by the kidney, the 'purpose' of Phase I and Phase II reactions being to increase water solubility (polarity). (Some large molecules are excreted in the bile where competition is unimportant.) Active tubular secretion of anions and cations is a potential site for interactions of therapeutic relevance; for example, *Aspirin* with *Methotrexate*.

Acute poisoning

THE PROBLEM

In adults, acute poisoning is commonly deliberate and self-inflicted with the object of harming the patient or manipulating somebody else. It is typically a problem of Western Europe and North America; less frequent in countries with a peasant economy and Roman Catholic religion. A small proportion of such patients (< 20 per cent) have serious psychiatric disease. The annual incidence of hospital admission is about 1:1000 population and annual deaths (England and Wales) about 3000: 80 per cent of these deaths occur outside hospital — mortality amongst hospital admissions is < 1 per cent.

In children acute poisoning is an accidental result of oral exploration and is commonest in boys aged 1.5—2.5 years, social class IV, with several preschool siblings. There is a high incidence of ingestion (probably similar to adult figures) but poisoning (measurable harmful effects) is uncommon and death rare (< 30/year).

DRUGS INVOLVED

Adults: hypnotics, anxiolytics, antidepressants, minor analgesics, anticonvulsants. Children: random selection of ingestable items in the environment — anything from iron salts to weedkiller, contraceptive tablets to antifreeze.

PRINCIPLES OF MANAGEMENT (NOTE THE ORDER OF PRIORITIES CAREFULLY)

(1) Establish and maintain a clear airway: remove debris (vomit, mucus, dentures), suck away secretions, consider providing an oropharyngeal airway, endotracheal tube or tracheostomy.

(2) Ensure adequate ventilation: tidal volume > 400 mℓ and minute volume > 4 ℓ/minute for adults, by mechanical means if necessary (too little leads to hypoxaemia, too much to alkalosis and hypotension).

(3) Supress convulsions provoked by drugs (for example, *Aspirin*, antidepressants) unless they cease with adequate ventilation.

(4) Fluid — two objectives for iv fluid therapy: (*a*) Expansion of circulating blood volume, restoration of venous return and cardiac output, for example, isotonic saline solution (0.9 per cent w/v) and isotonic glucose solution (5 per cent w/v) or plasma. Overdosage with CNS depressants may be an indication for measurement of central venous pressure to prevent salt and water overload. (*b*) Water and salt replacement — 1 ℓ of isotonic saline solution + 1 ℓ of isotonic glucose solution per day.

(5) Decontamination: the stomach may be emptied by gastric lavage in a conscious adult, a child can be made to vomit with 10—20 mℓ *Ipecacuanha* paediatric emetic draught [syrup of ipecac]. Avoid gastric lavage or induction of vomiting in an unconscious patient, aspirate gastric contents

only. Activated charcoal 10—30 g in suspension in 100—200 mℓ water may be introduced to bind unabsorbed drug (for example, *Digoxin*, barbiturates, alkaloids). Other binding agents are more suited to other toxic agents, for example, *Desferrioxamine* for iron salts and Fuller's earth for paraquat. Decontamination procedures have a low efficiency; for example, 30 minutes after an experimental overdose the yield by vomiting or lavage averages only 20—30 per cent.

(6) Identification. Tablet identification may be difficult with old/white/ discoloured preparations. The National Poisons Information Service provides useful data on the content of household cleaners, bleaches, weed-killers, solvents. The hospital biochemistry service can assist with assessment of severity of poisoning by *Aspirin, Paracetamol* and iron salts; severity tends to increase with serum drug concentration.

(7) Assisted elimination of the poison is seldom required — if the top priorities (1- 4) are followed hepatic metabolism and renal excretion will eliminate the toxic agent without special assistance.

SPECIAL CASES

Salicylate poisoning in an adult

Alkaline diuresis increases the clearance of salicylate four-fold for each unit pH rise. High urine pH may be obtained by iv *Acetazolamide* (page 105) and isotonic (1.4 per cent w/v) *Sodium bicarbonate*, 2 ℓ in 4 hours.

Phenobarbitone poisoning

Two-fold increase in clearance can be obtained if urine pH is raised above 8 — achieved by replacing iv isotonic *Sodium chloride* by *Sodium bicarbonate*. Dialysis procedures (peritoneal and haemodialysis) are seldom required except when the intoxication produces acute kidney failure.

Specific antagonists are only available for a few drugs (*Table 6.3*).

Table 6.3

Drug	Antagonist	Mechanism
Iron salts	*Desferrioxamine* [deferoxamine]	Chelation
Lead salts	*Penicillamine*	Chelation
Narcotic analgesics	Nalorphine	Partial agonist
(*Morphine*, etc.)	*Naloxone*	Antagonist
Mercury salts	Dimercaprol	Chelation
Organophosphorous	*Atropine* and	ACh antagonist
anticholinesterases	Pralidoxime	Cholinesterase reactivation
Paracetamol	Acetylcysteine	Reduction of oxidized glutathione

SUMMARY

(1) Progress in the management of acute poisoning has been achieved by the more effective support of vital functions (respiration and circulation). Assisted elimination and drug antagonism have only a limited importance.

(2) Since mortality in hospital is so low, further reduction of total mortality can only be achieved by removal of social causes of self-poisoning and by more restricted availability of lethal drugs (for example, barbiturates).

(3) The introduction of the safer benzodiazepines as hypnotics and anxiolytics has helped to reduce the mortality associated with self-poisoning.

Gastrointestinal complaints

PEPTIC ULCERATION

Definition

Localized loss of mucosa, submucosa and smooth muscle layers of the stomach (gastric ulcer) or of the duodenum (duodenal ulcer).

Symptoms and diagnosis

Pain in upper part of abdomen, usually midline. Gastric ulcers are characterized by poor appetite, weight loss and pain often aggravated by food. Duodenal ulcers are characterized by exacerbations and remissions of heartburn and nausea, often relieved by food and antacids. Bleeding may occur which can lead to anaemia (page 312). Further diagnosis requires radiography and endoscopy.

Complications

Sudden and severe bleeding. Leakage of gastric contents into abdomen and so peritonitis. Narrowing of outlet of stomach.

Aetiology

Hydrochloric acid (HCl) and pepsin are not the primary cause of ulcers but ulcers are aggravated or perpetuated by these secretions. Patients with gastric ulcer usually have normal or reduced acid secretion. The cause of gastric ulcer is uncertain but it may be due to bile regurgitation which damages the mucosa and renders it susceptible to the action of HCl. In duodenal ulcer patients, both nocturnal resting secretion and stimulated acid secretion are increased. There may be a familial component to the causation of duodenal ulceration.

Aims of treatment

(1) To relieve symptoms.
(2) To hasten healing.

Most treatments are directed at reducing acid secretion or its effects.

General therapeutic measures

Determine that a gastric ulcer is not malignant. Rest may enable gastric and duodenal ulcers to heal more rapidly but is not essential. Symptoms are reduced by small meals, stopping smoking and avoiding Ethanol and any food which makes the symptoms worse. The use of anti-inflammatory analgesics should be reduced to a minimum. There is a large spontaneous cure rate for gastric and duodenal ulcers, but both are likely to recur periodically.

Symptomatic therapy

(1) Antacids may be used intermittently for the symptomatic management of pain. They do not alter the rate of healing except at high dosage. Antacids are the mainstay of treatment of duodenal ulcers and are beneficial for gastric ulcers. They are weak bases which neutralize HCl so the pH of the luminal contents becomes > 4 and pepsin is inactive (*Figure 6.6*). The use of antacids promotes gastrin secretion so that the acidity and volume of gastric secretion is increased. It is difficult, therefore, to take antacids in quantities sufficient to maintain a pH of 4. The action of antacids is brief due to their rapid removal from the stomach and duodenum.

Sodium bicarbonate has a rapid but brief action. It can alter ECF pH to give a metabolic alkalosis and alkaline urine. It is not, therefore, suitable for use in large doses and is not used on its own.

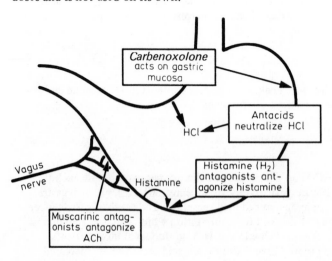

Figure 6.6

270

Magnesium hydroxide and *Aluminium hydroxide* have a moderate rate of onset and duration of action. Little Mg^{2+} or Al^{3+} is absorbed. Mg^{2+} is laxative and Al^{3+} is constipative.

Aluminium hydroxide is also absorbent.

Magnesium trisilicate has a slow onset and relatively prolonged action. On reaction with HCl it forms a hydrated silicic acid which is an absorbent.

(2) Muscarinic antagonists (for example, *Propantheline, Dicyclomine, Mebeverine*) inhibit vagally mediated acid secretion and motility (*Figure 6.6*). They are useless in gastric ulcer and of limited value in duodenal ulcer. Unwanted effects include inhibition of salivation, urinary retention and the possibility of precipitating an attack of glaucoma (page 9).

Therapy which promotes healing

(1) Liquorice derivatives: *Carbenoxolone* is synthesized from glycyrrhetinic acid which is extracted from liquorice root. *Carbenoxolone* does not alter gastric acid or pepsin secretion. It promotes the healing of peptic, especially gastric, ulcers (*Figure 6.6*). It has local anti-inflammatory actions and systemic effects like aldosterone (page 98) — sodium and water retention and potassium loss leading to oedema, hypertension and hypokalaemia. Potassium supplements may be needed. It should be used as a short course of treatment of 4–6 weeks only. *Spironolactone* (aldosterone antagonist) interferes with *Carbenoxolone* healing of peptic ulcers.

(2) Histamine (H_2 receptor) antagonists (for example, Cimetidine): histamine is involved in the final common pathway of stimuli which cause acid and pepsin secretion. Cimetidine (page 110) reduces fasting and stimulated acid and pepsin secretion by antagonizing the action of histamine (*Figure 6.6*). It is very effective in promoting healing of gastric and duodenal ulcers. The possibility of periodic recurrence of duodenal ulcers remains.

(3) Surgery may be used if simpler treatments fail to relieve pain or there are dangerous complications (for example, continued or recurrent haemorrhage). It involves removal of part of the stomach and reconnection with the duodenum or jejunum. Also selective division of the vagal nerve supply to the antrum of the stomach may be performed, thus reducing or abolishing the neural component of acid secretion.

Surgery is not lightly undertaken as there is a 2–4 per cent mortality following partial gastrectomy. Vagotomy alone has about 0.5 per cent mortality. Anaemia may follow gastrectomy due to malabsorption of iron or loss of intrinsic factor secretion. Jejunal ulcers can be a sequel to gastrojejunostomy.

ULCERATIVE COLITIS

Definition

Severe, chronic inflammation of the mucosa of the colon, usually involving the rectum.

271

Symptoms and diagnosis

If the disease is confined to the rectum, constipation may be the dominant feature. More commonly, bloody diarrhoea is the main symptom. Pain is only occasionally a symptom. Continued diarrhoea can lead to dehydration, malnutrition and severe emaciation. Loss of blood may give anaemia. Dilatation of the colon and perforation may occur.

Aetiology

Unknown, possibly an autoimmune disease in which a component of the mucous membrane is rejected. Bacterial infection may then be involved.

General therapeutic measures

Modify the diet — but it may be difficult to combat malnutrition without contributing to symptoms. Parenteral rehydration and feeding may be necessary.

Symptomatic treatment

(1) Constipative drugs; treatment of diarrhoea.

(2) Glucocorticoids are used for the treatment of attacks but they do not remove the underlying cause. Their other effects preclude their use as maintenance therapy.

(3) *Sulphasalazine* is useful for maintenance therapy to reduce the frequency and severity of relapses. The effect is due to the anti-inflammatory action of the metabolite 5-amino-salicylic acid which is released in the colon by bacterial deconjugation.

Surgery

Removal of the affected part which may include the rectum, with the consequent need for an ileostomy (artificial opening of small intestine through front of abdomen). This can enable return to an active life.

DIARRHOEA

Aetiology

In the small intestine the contents are liquid. The caecum and the proximal colon absorb Na^+, K^+ and Cl^- and the bulk of the water. The distal colon absorbs Na^+ in exchange for K^+, this process being influenced by aldosterone. Water is absorbed so producing soft, but not watery faeces. If the time in the colon is too short or there is excess water present due to damage to the small intestinal mucosa, or if there is inflammation of the colon resulting in incomplete water absorption, then diarrhoea is produced. There is often over-activity of the propulsive muscles of the tract with low activity of 'mixing' waves.

Causes (with examples)

(1) Viruses (gastroenteritis) especially in children.
(2) Bacteria (bacterial food poisoning) usually due to heat-stable toxins (Staphylococcus, *E. Coli*) but can be infective (Salmonella, bacillary dysentery).
(3) Protozoa or Metazoa (amoebic dysentery, worm infestation).
(4) Irritant chemicals including drugs.
(5) Allergic reactions.
(6) Emotion.
(7) Disturbances of endocrine system (hyperthyroidism).
(8) Malabsorption syndromes (lactose intolerance in neonates).
(9) Organic disease of gut (diverticular disease, ulcerative colitis, neoplasm).
(10) Consequence of gut surgery.

Specific treatment

The underlying disorder should be diagnosed and treated.

General therapeutic measures

Many episodes of diarrhoea, especially viral and bacterial, are short-lived and self-limiting. Not eating but taking plenty of liquid for 24 hours will often terminate the diarrhoea and prevent dehydration. Severe diarrhoea (especially in infants, elderly people or in tropical climates) may lead to dehydration needing replacement with iv *Sodium chloride* and *Dextrose injection.*

Symptomatic treatment

(1) Narcotics (for example, *Morphine*, *Codeine* and Diphenoxylate, page 148). These decrease the propulsive intestinal contractions and increase the tone of colonic muscles and sphincters, allowing increased water absorption. Diphenoxylate displays slight selectivity for constipative actions versus central actions and may be useful for long-term, non-infective diarrhoea in adults.
(2) Absorbents (for example, *Kaolin* and *Chalk*). These are said to absorb bacteria and toxins. They are commonly used with *Morphine.*
(3) Bulk-forming agents (for example, bran and *Methylcellulose*) adsorb water so solidifying stools in diarrhoea.
(4) Antibiotics have no place in self-limiting viral or bacterial toxin-induced diarrhoea. Their use can be complicated by bacterial or fungal superinfection (page 200).

CONSTIPATION

Aetiology

If the passage of contents through the colon is unduly prolonged there is greater water absorption, therefore constipation.

Causes

(1) Diet containing too little residue.
(2) Prolonged bed rest.
(3) Habit.
(4) Organic disease of colon (for example, carcinoma, strictures, diverticular disease).
(5) Drug-induced (for example, narcotics, page 148, muscarinic antagonists, page 33 or aluminium-containing preparations, page 271).
(5) Endocrine disorders (for example, hypothyroidism).

If faeces stagnate and harden, straining will produce haemorrhoidal veins (piles) which may prolapse and thrombose. Painful defaecation may make constipation worse.

Specific treatment

Underlying disorder should be diagnosed and treated.

General therapeutic measures

Well balanced diet with roughage. Exercise. Knowledge that frequency of defaecation is very variable. Establish habitual time for defaecation.

Symptomatic treatment

Laxatives: chronic use of laxatives is contraindicated. Defaecation is promoted by increased colonic or small intestinal propulsive motility and altered electrolyte transport — the exact mechanism of action is unknown for most drugs. One classification is as follows:

Bulk-forming laxatives (for example, bran, Methylcellulose)

Swell in water to form gel which maintains hydrated, soft faeces. The bulk promotes peristalsis. The onset of action is slow (about 24 hours).

274

Emollient laxatives

These act by direct softening of the faeces. Dioctyl sodium sulphosuccinate — a lowering of surface tension may explain action. Liquid paraffin [mineral oil] — probably retards water absorption. It can reduce absorption of vitamins A and D.

If it gains access to the lungs it can cause lipid pneumonitis. *Glycerol* suppositories act by softening faeces.

Saline laxatives *(for example, Magnesium hydroxide*, Magnesium sulphate and Sodium sulphate)

Salts that are poorly absorbed from the digestive tract retain water by osmosis; peristalsis is increased indirectly. There is a fairly rapid onset of action (2—3 hours). An enema of Sodium phosphate and Sodium acid phosphate [biphosphate] acts as a saline laxative.

Stimulant laxatives

Their predominant action may be stimulation of intestinal motility, directly or reflexly and all cause intestinal cramps. The effective dose varies considerably from patient to patient. They act about 8 hours after taking. The diphenyl-methane group (Phenolphthalein and *Bisacodyl*) are, in part, absorbed, conjugated in liver, excreted in the bile and deconjugated by bacteria in the colon to exert their action. There is also the anthraquinone group (*Senna* and *Cascara*). Bacteria in the colon metabolize these drugs to the active aglycones.

Ideal mode of action. Reflex tachycardia occurs but this can be controlled with antagonists at β-adrenoceptors.

Status
Cardiac glycosides

Digoxin and Digitoxin are members of this naturally occurring group of drugs (foxglove). Each glycoside consists of an aglycone (steroid nucleus giving pharmacological activity) attached to sugar molecules. The pharmacokinetics of this group are described on page 233.

DIRECT ACTIONS ON CARDIAC CELLS

The digitalis glycosides inhibit the Mg-dependent Na^+/K^+ ATPase which is located within the cardiac cell membrane and regulates the cellular Na^+ and K^+ concentrations. Inhibition of this enzyme results in Na^+ accumulation within and K^+ loss from the cells. K^+ loss effectively lowers the membrane potential with two consequences: (1) in some cells action potential propagation (and generation) is inhibited resulting in transmission block, especially in the AV node (useful in atrial fibrillation, page 64); (2) in other cells, especially in the bundle of His, automaticity is increased and ventricular arrhythmias are produced (page 61). These can be treated with *Lignocaine* or *Phenytoin*(page 63).

K^+ depletion (for example, diuretic therapy and secondary hyperaldosteronism) enhances these actions and may lead to the development of fatal ventricular arrhythmias.

Perhaps the most important therapeutic action of the cardiac glycosides is their ability to increase the force of myocardial contraction in the failing heart (*see below*). Although not firmly established, this action may also result from inhibition of Na^+/K^+ ATPase. The build up of Na^+ which occurs within the cardiac muscle cells as a result of the inhibition of this enzyme may allow more Ca^{2+} to enter the cell with each action potential, thus producing a more powerful contraction (page 278). This improvement in myocardial work effectively offsets the processes which result in the development of heart failure (*see below*).

INDIRECT ACTIONS ON CARDIAC CELLS

The cardiac glycosides augment vagal activity which slows the heart and summates with their direct AV nodal blocking actions.

TOXICITY

The cardiac glycosides have a very low therapeutic index. All their actions can be regarded as 'toxic' but in some instances (for example, heart failure) these can be exploited to the benefit of the patient.

Nausea, anorexia and vomiting are all early features of cardiac glycoside toxicity. Later, cardiac arrhythmias supervene; any pathological arrhythmia can be imitated by *Digoxin* toxicity, but ventricular tachycardia and fibrillation terminate the sequence. Blurred vision and disturbances of colour vision are also produced.

Heart failure

DEFINITIONS

An abnormality of the heart interfering with its efficiency as a pump.

Pathophysiological definition

Depression of the (Starling) curve relating cardiac performance to the ventricular filling pressure.

Clinical definition

An inadequate cardiac output causing breathlessness at rest or on exertion (pulmonary congestion), salt and water retention (oedema) and fatigue, confusion, renal failure (underperfusion of tissues).

TREATMENT

General measures include the treatment of the precipitating factor, for example, infection (page 191), anaemia (page 312), thyrotoxicosis (page 91), cardiac arrhythmia (page 60), fever.

There are three aims of therapy:

Reduce cardiac work

Rest from physical activity. If obese, restrict calorie intake. Treat hypertension (page 279). Decrease ventricular end-diastolic pressure (*see below*). Relieve distress and severe dyspnoea of acute pulmonary oedema with *Morphine* iv which also promotes venous pooling and reduction of venous return.

Decrease pulmonary congestion and peripheral oedema

Pulmonary oedema occurs when the pulmonary capillary pressure exceeds the osmotic pressure exerted by the plasma proteins (principally albumin). Urgent reduction of pulmonary congestion required. Sit patient up. Administer 60 per cent O_2 (MC mask (Polymask), 6 ℓ/minute, O_2). Give iv *Aminophylline* for its bronchodilator, vasodilator and +ve inotropic effects (*see below*). Give a loop diuretic such as *Frusemide* (page 104) for its potent rapid onset of action, steep dose-response curve and possible direct effect on pulmonary veins before diuretic action. Pulmonary venous congestion causes breathlessness by decreasing pulmonary compliance at venous pressures below those producing pulmonary oedema. In the longer term diuretic therapy is indicated − start with a thiazide such as *Bendrofluazide* (page 104) which has a shallow dose-response curve. If the response is inadequate change to a loop diuretic (*Bendrofluazide* 10 mg = *Frusemide* 40 mg). Response may be impaired by failing to restrict dietary salt intake.

Pathophysiology of oedema

Decreased cardiac output activates both the baroreceptor reflex (increased sympathetic activity produces tachycardia and peripheral vasoconstriction) and the renin-angiotensin-aldosterone system (NaCl and water retention with K^+ and H^+ loss, effect of secondary hyperaldosteronism on distal tubule). The retained fluid increases the circulating blood volume but is also sequestered by gravity to give oedema of lower limbs. Potassium supplement (for example, KCl slow) is needed when loop and thiazide diuretics are prescribed for heart failure; the K^+ losing action of these diuretics summates with the secondary hyperaldosteronism (contrast with essential hypertension in which K^+ supplements are not essential when a thiazide is prescribed, page 280). K^+ sparing diuretics are *Spironolactone* (an aldosterone antagonist), *Amiloride* and *Triamterene* (page 105). *Spironolactone* is best used in combination with a loop diuretic in patients resistant to the latter — secondary hyperaldosteronism is often the cause of the poor diuretic response. Stop K^+ supplements when adding *Spironolactone* or another K^+ sparing diuretic, and never use these drugs together (risk of hyperkalaemia).

Increase cardiac output

Low cardiac output is commonly due to myocardial ischaemia (coronary artery disease). The capacity for increasing the cardiac output (contractility) is greatest with valvular heart disease, atrial fibrillation or hypertensive heart disease.

Digoxin

Digoxin increases myocardial contractility (+ve inotropic effect) which allows the cardiac output to be maintained at a lower ventricular filling pressure.

It slows the ventricular rate in atrial fibrillation thus allowing a longer diastolic filling time which reduces pulmonary congestion. It has a narrow therapeutic range - the toxic dose (nausea, heart block, ectopic ventricular beats) is very close to the therapeutic dose, especially if there is K^+ depletion. A loading dose may be given, succeeded by a once daily maintenance dose. Dosage reduction is imperative in the elderly and others with renal impairment (page 235).

Aminophylline

This has a +ve inotropic action and potentiates (via cAMP, page 288, *Figure 6.7*) agonists at β-adrenoceptors (increased sympathetic activity sustains cardiac output in heart failure).

INTRACTABLE SEVERE HEART FAILURE

In addition to the above therapy, venesection or tourniquets on one limb at a time and either: (1) an iv infusion of a +ve inotropic drug (dopamine, *Salbutamol*, *Isoprenaline*); or (2) a vasodilator drug (iv infusion of sodium nitroprusside, sublingual *Glyceryl trinitrate*).

Intermittent +ve pressure ventilation with +ve end expired pressure; aortic balloon pump, open heart surgery with valve replacement and cardiac transplantation are measures used with variable success.

Hypertension and antihypertensive drugs

Hypertension is a complex disease characterized by a resting diastolic blood pressure (BP) > 90 mm Hg. Ten per cent of the population in 'developed' countries may be hypertensive.

CLASSIFICATION OF THE DISEASE

Hypertension is classified in two ways: (1) aetiology; (a) primary (essential) hypertension (90 per cent) cause unknown, (b) secondary hypertension (10 per cent) cause known, for example, kidney disease, adrenal cortical or medullary tumours, pregnancy (toxaemia). (2) Severity (diastolic BP); (a) mild (90−105 mm Hg), (b) moderate (105−120 mm Hg), (c) severe (> 120 mm Hg).

CONSEQUENCES OF HYPERTENSION

Patients with mild, moderate or severe hypertension have few, if any, symptoms. However, life insurance statistics clearly show that hypertensive patients die earlier, are more likely to suffer heart and renal failure and are more likely to become blind or have a stroke. The disease may progress to a malignant stage when death will occur within a few months without adequate drug therapy. Patients with malignant hypertension show general vascular damage, proteinuria, retinal haemorrhages and papilloedema (oedema of the optic nerve head).

ANTIHYPERTENSIVE TREATMENT

In patients with secondary hypertension, treatment of the cause (for example, surgical removal of tumour) produces a cure. In the 90 per cent of patients with essential hypertension, antihypertensive drugs are used to lower the diastolic BP. This can be shown to prolong life and reverse to some extent any pathological changes which have already occurred.

THE IDEAL ANTIHYPERTENSIVE DRUG

Objective

Lower the diastolic BP so that physiological control mechanisms (increased heart rate and contractility, salt and water retention via secondary hyperaldosteronism) cannot overcome the reduction (revise the physiology of BP maintenance and control).

Method

Since BP = cardiac output × peripheral resistance, diastolic BP can be lowered either by reducing cardiac output or peripheral resistance (or both).

Reduction in cardiac output

This can be achieved by (1) interfering with the cardiac sympathetic supply, (2) dilating veins with consequent reduction in central venous pressure.

Neither mechanism is ideal, since the blood supply to vital organs may be reduced, perhaps precipitating their failure.

Reduction in peripheral resistance

This can be achieved by (1) interfering with the sympathetic control of resistance vessels which, together with dilatation of capacitance vessels, results in postural (orthostatic) and postexertional hypotension (fall in BP on standing up or after exercise, leading to dizziness and fainting), (2) dilating resistance vessels directly without involving sympathetic nerves. This is probably the best method at present available.

ANTIHYPERTENSIVE DRUGS

Vasodilators

Bendrofluazide and Chlorthalidone

Bendrofluazide and *Chlorthalidone* are diuretics (page 104) of the thiazide type or close chemical relatives. Once daily administration is adequate for *Bendrofluazide* and *Chlorthalidone*. Lowering of BP is achieved in two ways: (*a*) by the diuresis which initially lowers plasma volume. After 1–2 weeks, the plasma returns to its previous volume but the fall in diastolic BP is maintained by: (*b*) a direct dilator action on peripheral arterioles not involving sympathetic nerves.

Status

Ideal mode of action. The antihypertensive effect is only adequate for mild hypertension but this group can be useful with other antihypertensive types. No postural hypotension.

Toxicity

Hypokalaemia (low blood K^+ concentration but K^+ supplements are rarely necessary), hyperuricaemia (raised blood uric acid concentration), hyperglycaemia (raised blood sugar concentration).

Hydralazine

Hydralazine has a direct dilator action on peripheral blood vessels.

Status

Ideal mode of action. Reflex tachycardia occurs but this can be controlled with antagonists at β-adrenoceptors.

Toxicity

Headache, systemic lupus erythematosus (only occurs with high doses (in slow acetylators, page 257) which are unnecessary if *hydralazine* is prescribed with an antagonist at β-adrenoceptors and a thiazide diuretic).

Diazoxide

Diazoxide is a close chemical relative to the thiazide diuretics but with no diuretic action; indeed, it inhibits their diuresis. Like the thiazides, it has a direct dilator action on peripheral arterioles.

Status

Rapid. Ideal mode of action but side-effects restrict its use to hypertensive emergencies (*see below*).

Toxicity

Hyperglycaemia, salt and water retention, gout.

Sodium nitroprusside

Cardiac output is not increased. Used in hypertensive emergencies (*see below*).

Antagonists at β-adrenoceptors (page 51)

Propranolol and Oxprenolol

These have been found clinically to possess antihypertensive actions. Possible modes of action are: (*a*) reduction in cardiac output (not often observed); (*b*) interference with central control of BP; (*c*) inhibition of renin release; (*d*) re-setting of baroreceptors.

Each one has some experimental evidence in its favour.

Status

Apparently ideal (any reduction in cardiac output is an advantage in angina pectoris and hyperthyroidism). Useful in conjunction with a thiazide to enhance the action of the latter. There is no postural hypotension.

Toxicity

Cardiac failure (in predisposed patients), bronchospasm, impaired peripheral circulation and increased heart block.

Toxicity

Other drugs interfering with noradrenergic transmission

Guanethidine, Bethanidine and Debrisoquine (page 42).

Status

Non-ideal (postural and postexertional hypotension, reduced cardiac output, fall in central venous pressure).

Toxicity

Moderate. Diarrhoea, sodium retention (therefore always use with a thiazide diuretic), failure of ejaculation.

Antagonists at α-adrenoceptors, for example, Prazosin

Reserpine

The action of **Reserpine** in depleting all noradrenergic neurones of NA is described in detail on page 41. In addition, central monoaminergic neurones are also depleted (page 130).

Status

Non-ideal (postural hypotension, reduced cardiac output, sedation).

Toxicity

Severe depression with suicide.

Centrally acting drugs

Clonidine

Clonidine acts within the CNS possibly by virtue of partial agonist activity at presynaptic (page 42) α-adrenoceptors reducing the number of efferent impulses to peripheral sympathetic nerves.

Status

Non-ideal. Postural hypotension is mild. Dry mouth, sedation/clinical depression. Hypertensive crisis on sudden withdrawal, fatalities have occurred. If recognized can be treated with an antagonist at α-adrenoceptors. Used in conjunction with thiazides to minimize side-effects and enhance action of the latter. Useful in low dosage for the prevention of migraine (page 294).

Reserpine (*see above*)

Methyldopa

A major component of the antihypertensive action of *Methyldopa* (page 42) is exerted in the CNS. The final overall effect is a reduction in the number of efferent impulses to peripheral sympathetic nerves.

Status

Non-ideal (postural hypotension and reduced cardiac output). Combine with thiazides.

Toxicity

Mild to moderate. Tiredness − clinical depression, sodium retention, Coombs' test +ve and, rarely, haemolytic anaemia (page 315).

Propranolol (*see above*)

Ganglion blocking drugs

Pentolinium (*page 30*)

Status

Rapid. Non-ideal (severe postural hypotension, reduced cardiac output, fall in central venous pressure).

Toxicity

Severe. General ganglion blockade (dry mouth, blurred vision, paralysis of intestinal movement, urinary retention).

SELECTION OF AN ANTIHYPERTENSIVE DRUG

The ideal treatment for hypertensive patients involves dilating peripheral resistance vessels without affecting their sympathetic nervous control. Thiazide diuretics are very useful and they do not produce a reflex compensatory tachycardia. However, their action is mild and some patients fail to respond. The solution probably lies in the administration of a combination of agents − initially *Bendrofluazide*, followed by an antagonist at β-adrenoceptors and *hydralazine* if necessary. In this way, effective control can be achieved with the utilization of low doses of each drug and the consequent minimization of side-effects. This last factor is particularly important in persuading asymptomatic patients to persevere with life-long drug therapy. Patient compliance can be improved by simplifying dosage requirements, for example, once or twice daily administration of drug combinations.

PARENTERAL TREATMENT OF HYPERTENSIVE EMERGENCIES

Hypertensive emergencies are rare, but if the diastolic BP is > 150 mm Hg or if left ventricular failure, cerebral haemorrhage or cerebral oedema (hypertensive encephalopathy) is associated with a diastolic BP > 120 mm Hg immediate reduction of BP is required. In toxaemia of pregnancy, and after cardiovascular surgery, parenteral antihypertensive therapy may be urgent at a lower diastolic BP.

Management

Specific therapy should be instituted, for example, O_2, *Frusemide, Aminophylline* and *Morphine* for pulmonary oedema; *Phenytoin* for fits in eclamptic toxaemia or hypertensive encephalopathy.

Parenteral antihypertensive drug therapy

(1) *Diazoxide* is the drug of choice — 300 mg iv given over 15 seconds. Rapid injection is necessary to overcome high-affinity binding to plasma albumin. The hypotensive action of *Diazoxide* is maximum within 15 minutes and is sustained for up to 12 hours by which time oral therapy with other drugs will have become effective. *Diazoxide* may need to be continued and *Frusemide* in high doses will then become essential because of salt retention.

(2) Sodium nitroprusside is the most potent and predictable antihypertensive agent available. It is immediately effective with a very brief duration of action and so must be administered by iv infusion. It directly vasodilates capacitance as well as resistance vessels, and is particularly useful if cardiac failure is present or likely.

(3) Hydrallazine is not predictably effective in hypertensive emergencies because of reflex cardiac stimulation with an increase of cardiac output which offsets the hypotension. Its use is inadvisable in patients with angina. The cardiac effects of increased sympathetic activity can be suppressed by *Propranolol*. With renal impairment hydrallazine may be preferred because renal blood flow is better maintained than with other hypotensive agents.

PHAEOCHROMOCYTOMA

This is a tumour of chromaffin cells (for example, adrenal medulla) which secretes catecholamines and may cause a hypertensive emergency, especially when the tumour is being handled during surgical removal. This problem can be avoided by the following: (1) Interfering with normal catecholamine synthesis with α-methyltyrosine which competes with tyrosine for the rate-limiting enzyme in catecholamine synthesis — tyrosine hydroxylase. Side-effects are due to depletion of catecholamines within the brain — sedation, coarse tremor (dopamine). (2) Antagonizing effects of released catecholamines: (*a*) Phenoxybenzamine pretreatment for several days before surgery to allow restoration of a normal circulatory blood volume — this reduces the risk of large fluctuations in BP during and after surgery; (*b*) *Propranolol* to reduce the β-adrenoceptor-mediated effects of catecholamines.

Angina of effort

A crushing pain in the chest (retrosternal) referred to the left arm, neck or jaw and precipitated by exertion. This is typical of myocardial ischaemia due to atherosclerosis of the coronary arteries. This degenerative process develops in all individuals who indulge in the modern western life-style characterized by: (1) overnutrition; (2) a low roughage diet; (3) a sedentary job; (4) sedentary leisure pursuits.

Atherosclerosis is the consequence of the deposition of a lipid material beneath the endothelium of arteries (atheroma) which become thickened and calcified (sclerotic) and impede the flow of blood (ischaemia). Ischaemia is not an inevitable consequence of coronary atherosclerosis but atheroma is undoubtedly the principal factor underlying myocardial ischaemia with obesity, hypertension, cardiac arrhythmias, valvular heart disease and anaemia as important contributory factors. Myocardial infarction — necrosis of an area of the heart — develops when the blood supply to that area is completely interrupted.

Angina pectoris is due to reversible myocardial ischaemia which occurs when the activity of the heart increases and the supply of oxygenated blood is inadequate to sustain the metabolic needs of the increased myocardial work load. This concept of supply and demand is important and, in atrial pacing experiments, a critical threshold of O_2 consumption can be established, above which angina can be precipitated. Ischaemia can also be detected by recording the electrocardiogram and observing depression of the ST segment.

MYOCARDIAL WORK

The work and O_2 consumption of the heart are directly related to: (1) the heart rate; (2) the peripheral resistance (and BP); (3) ventricular diastolic filling pressure ('venous return'); (4) cardiac contractility; (5) plasma free fatty acid concentrations.

Cardiac work may be increased when no external physical work is performed, for example, watching television, arguing. Increased sympathetic activity can increase heart rate and BP separately or together. Such adrenergic (sympatho-adrenal) stress may precipitate angina at rest in susceptible patients and these attacks last 5—15 minutes. In contrast, angina of effort rarely lasts longer than three minutes if the exertion is lessened or stopped.

TREATMENT

Prevention of coronary atherosclerosis — avoid risk factors

(1)   Nutrition: (a) avoid obesity; (b) take high fibre diet; (c) treat severe hyperlipidaemia.
(2)   Maintain physical fitness.
(3)   Do not smoke cigarettes.

Prophylaxis of angina

(1) Remove contributory factors, for example, anaemia, hypertension, heart failure, obesity, thyrotoxicosis.
(2) Reduce cardiac work.

There are two ways in which myocardial O_2 consumption can be decreased during exertional or emotional stress — vasodilator therapy and β-adrenoceptor blockade.

Vasodilator therapy

Ischaemia is a most potent stimulus for increasing tissue perfusion, and atherosclerotic arteries are not capable of dilatation. Coronary blood flow is unchanged or reduced by *Glyceryl trinitrate* given for angina. Vasodilatation of capacitance veins and resistance vessels other than in the coronary circulation accounts for the therapeutic efficacy. Cardiac preload (ventricular diastolic filling) and afterload (diastolic BP) are lowered by reductions in venous return and peripheral resistance. Cardiac work and myocardial O_2 consumption are decreased despite a rise in heart rate.

Glyceryl trinitrate (1) is the drug of choice for preventing angina of effort, (2) onset of action within two minutes, (3) duration of action up to 20 minutes, (4) chew tablets for rapid sublingual absorption (page 211).

Glyceryl trinitrate absorbed from the stomach and intestine is completely metabolized in its first passage through the liver. Slow release tablets and longer acting nitrates are ineffective and may make a patient tolerant to sublingual *Glyceryl trinitrate.* This has not discouraged the pharmaceutical industry from marketing such preparations. *Glyceryl trinitrate* is no better than placebo in reducing the duration of established angina of effort but is of value for longer lasting attacks occurring at rest.

Side-effects due to vasodilatation (headache) or reduced cardiac output (fainting) are dose-related.

Sustained concentrations of *Glyceryl trinitrate* may be required for prolonged angina and can be achieved by applying the drug as an ointment. Iv infusion of sodium nitroprusside is an alternative.

β-Adrenoceptor blockade

Heart rate, cardiac contractility and BP rise during exercise and stress. *Propranolol* and other antagonists at β-adrenoceptors (page 51) prevent increases in these determinants of myocardial O_2 consumption and are most effective in angina with up to 70 per cent of patients gaining benefit. Therapeutic efficacy is related to antagonism at cardiac β-adrenoceptors and not to the quinidine-like activity (page 62) or the intrinsic sympathomimetric (partial agonist) activity possessed by some antagonists at β-adrenoceptors. The dose of *Propranolol* should be increased until relief is obtained or until the resting heart rate is reduced to 55—60 beats per minute. Administration once or twice daily has proved satisfactory.

In patients with congestive heart failure, the stores of NA in cardiac adrenergic neurones are depleted. Antagonists at β-adrenoceptors can precipitate severe cardiac failure.

A recent approach to decreasing O_2 consumption during exercise involves the calcium antagonist nifedipine. This drug inhibits the flow of Ca^{2+} into the myocardial cell and decreased myocardial contractility and O_2 consumption. It will exacerbate left ventricular failure.

Asthma

DEFINITION

Periodic attacks of breathlessness due to reversible increase in the resistance to airflow through the airways within the lungs.

ANATOMY AND PHYSIOLOGY

Revise the mechanism of quiet breathing. *Note:* In quiet breathing expiratory muscles (abdominal, shoulder girdle) and accessory inspiratory muscles (neck, shoulder girdle) are not used.

Revise the system of branching airways. At each airway branch, the sum of the cross-sectional areas of the daughter bronchi is $>$ that of the parent. Gas flow through tubes — in large airways flow is rapid and turbulent and resistance is large because total cross-sectional area is small. In small airways flow is slow and laminar and resistance is smaller because total cross-sectional area is larger. The effects of bronchoconstriction or dilatation on changes in resistance to flow are greater in smaller airways which possess less cartilage. Changes in resistance to flow are most significant in small bronchi exceeding 2 mm in diameter where excessive mucus secretion can contribute to obstruction.

Origin of increased resistance to flow: (1) material partly obstructing lumen (viscid mucus); (2) swelling of mucous membrane (oedema); (3) reduction in circumference (bronchoconstriction — shortening of circumferentially arranged bronchial smooth muscle).

Note: A 15 per cent shortening of smooth muscle cells (15 per cent reduction in radius, diameter and circumference) can cause a 400 per cent increase in resistance to flow.

AETIOLOGY

Extrinsic

Atopy is an inherited predisposition to develop immunoglobulin E (IgE) antibody in response to various antigens (allergens). An early onset (below the age of 30 years, often in childhood), previous history of other atopic (allergic) diseases (hay-fever, eczema, food allergy) and a family history of these disorders suggest atopy.

The commonest allergens identified are house-dust mite, pollens, animal dander (scales of hair or feathers) and moulds. Pollens are seasonal. Asthma may develop as part of a general anaphylactic reaction (for example, drug hypersensitivity).

Intrinsic

Later onset, no history of atopy, often smoker or ex-smoker, attacks usually precipitated by viral or bacterial infection, for example, exacerbation of chronic bronchitis.

Non-specific factors

Hyperreactive airways in asthmatics (test with inhalation of histamine or *Carbachol*) therefore dust, irritant fumes, exercise, cold air, dry air, emotion, coughing, forced expiration, anti-inflammatory analgesics and *Propranolol* may precipitate attack.

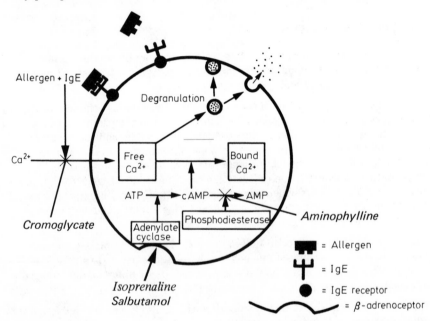

Preformed mediators
Histamine
factor of anaphylaxis

Newly formed mediators
Kinins
SRS-A
5-Ht
Prostaglandins

Vagal reflex mediator
ACh

Effects
Irritation of vagal afferents
Bronchoconstriction
Mucus secretion
Mucosal oedema
Eosinophilia

Figure 6.7

PATHOGENESIS OF EXTRINSIC ASTHMA

Production of the sensitized state

At some time before the first attack a sensitizing exposure to allergen occurs. Certain immunocompetent cells (lymphocytes and plasma cells capable of responding to the antigen) located in the lymphoreticular organs (thymus, spleen, bone marrow, lymphoid tissues) detect the allergen, proliferate and secrete antibodies to it into the circulation. This type of antibody is called IgE and has a high affinity for the cell membranes of mast cells and basophil leucocytes.

Production of tissue anaphylaxis (*Figure 6.7*)

In a sensitized individual allergen combines with the specific IgE antibody attached to the mast cell surface inducing a change in its membrane and a complex series of reactions culminating in degranulation (*Figure 6.7*).

Degranulation: allergen—IgE combination makes the membrane more permeable to Ca^{2+} which causes the release of intracellular calcium (regulated by cAMP concentrations). This leads to aggregation of microtubules with movement of granules (vesicles) to membrane and extrusion of preformed mediators and synthesis of other mediators. These produce tissue anaphylaxis with narrowing of lumen of airway by: (*a*) contraction of bronchial smooth muscle; (*b*) secretion of mucus from bronchial mucosa; (*c*) local vasodilatation; (*d*) increased permeability of mucosal capillaries giving oedema.

DIAGNOSIS

Clinical symptoms

'Short of breath' and 'tight chest' are typical descriptions of the dyspnoea (lit difficulty in breathing) of asthma which is related to the increased work of breathing due to airflow obstruction and lung overinflation (collapse of airways in expiration).

Overinflated chest, prolonged expiration and wheezing, use of accessory muscles of inspiration and muscles of expiration (that is, hard work).

Investigation

Spirometry: indicating airflow obstruction — forced expired volume in one second (FEV_1) and vital capacity decreased, peak expiratory flow rate decreased (use Wrights Peak Flow Meter or Peak Flow Gauge).

Lung volume increased: chest X-ray, helium dilution, whole body plethysmography.

Increased airways resistance which can be by 200—300 per cent without symptoms if change is gradual.

Sputum analysis for eosinophils.

Skin testing for immediate hypersensitivity (prick tests).

Arterial blood gas analysis. PaO_2 is low in proportion to the severity of the attack — note delay in recovery after treatment. $PaCO_2$ is usually below normal so normal or raised values indicate progressive respiratory failure.

TREATMENT

Prophylaxis

(1) Avoid allergen; especially by environmental control of the house-dust mite, for example, by damp dusting, having only man-made fibre materials in the bedroom, ban pets.

(2) Hyposensitization: a long series of allergen injections, starting with minute doses and increasing gradually, in order to develop a high titre of blocking IgG antibodies which will neutralize the allergen and prevent combination with IgE. Sometimes useful for seasonal asthma.

(3) Sodium *Cromoglycate* is inhaled as a finely divided powder using an insufflator ('Spinhaler'). It suppresses the release of mediators from sensitized mast cells challenged with allergen. It is of no value when administered after the challenge but is useful in exercise induced asthma.

(4) Anti-inflammatory steroids (for example, oral *Prednisolone*, inhaled *Beclomethasone*, iv *Hydrocortisone*) are very effective treatments but can produce side-effects (page 100); therefore, use as low a dose as possible, change to inhaled steroid and try alternate morning steroid therapy (allows normal growth in children and pituitary/adrenal gland suppression is avoided).

Symptomatic bronchodilatation and inhibition of mediator release

(1) Directly acting sympathomimetics (page 46).
   (a) Selective agonists at β-adrenoceptors of bronchial smooth muscle. *Salbutamol* or terbutaline: aerosol, nebulized, iv and oral. Long-acting because not metabolized by COMT. Side-effects (for example, tremor, tachycardia) are rare with low doses administered by aerosol but common with the larger doses used orally and by nebulization in prolonged severe acute asthma.
   (b) Non-selective agonists at β-adrenoceptors. *Isoprenaline* aerosol, short duration of action. *Orciprenaline* aerosol and oral. Side-effects (for example, tachycardia) are common.
   (c) Agonists at α- and β-adrenoceptors. *Adrenaline* aerosol and sc. Ventricular fibrillation is a hazard if given iv.

(2) Indirectly acting sympathomimetics: *Ephedrine* was the only orally effective sympathomimetic for asthma but the high incidence of side-effects (wakefulness, urinary retention, hypertension) indicate that it should not now be used.

(3) Methylxanthines (page 152) : phosphodiesterase inhibitors, non-specific smooth muscle relaxants. Theophylline is complexed to increase water solubility. *Aminophylline* oral, iv, suppositories. Side-effects (for example, nausea, vomiting, cardiac arrhythmias, convulsions) are related to blood concentrations and dose.

(4)   Parasympatholytics: inhibit reflex bronchoconstriction (page 11) :
        aerosol, therefore local action, atropine methonitrate, ipratropium.

Note: Antihistamines are of little value in asthma because the local concentration
of histamine in the bronchi is so great and because other mediators are important
in the pathogenesis. Drugs contraindicated in an asthmatic attack: respiratory
depressants — narcotics (for example, *Morphine*), sedatives (for example,
Diazepam, barbiturates) and antagonists at β-adrenoceptors (for example.
Propranolol). Extreme caution must guide the use of even 'cardioselective'
antagonists at β-adrenoceptors (page 51) in patients with asthma.

PROLONGED SEVERE ASTHMA (status asthmaticus)

This requires admission to hospital. Bronchodilator aerosol therapy is ineffective
(perhaps as a result of inadequate dosage). Often the patient is too breathless
to speak and has too great an obstruction to airflow to wheeze. Tachycardia
> 130/minute with pulsus paradoxus (marked decrease in pulse amplitude and
systolic BP during inspiration). Dehydration.

Estimate arterial blood gases and monitor peak expiratory flow rate.

(1)   Immediate treatment: *Aminophylline* (5—6 mg/kg, slowly iv),
        Hydrocortisone sodium succinate (3 mg/kg iv) and nebulized *Salbutamol*
        (5—10 mg, 4 hourly). Oxygen, humidified, for example, Ventimask 35
        per cent (> 60 per cent inspired concentration damages lung).

        Correct dehydration. If the patient deteriorates intermittent +ve pressure
        ventilation and bronchial lavage may be necessary.
(2)   After initial improvement — oral *Prednisolone* and continue nebulized
        Salbutamol. Effects on mediator release from mast cells may be most
        important at this stage. Physiotherapy — to dislodge plugs of tenacious
        mucus.
(3)   Reduce dose of *Prednisolone* gradually to zero (or low maintenance
        dosage). Reintroduce pressurized aerosol bronchodilator and Sodium
        Cromoglycate. This return to maintenance therapy should start in hospital.

PHYSICS OF AEROSOL ADMINISTRATION, INSUFFLATION
AND NEBULIZATION

Large particles (about 10 μm impact on the wall where the airstream changes
direction due to their momentum. Most remain in nose and throat and are then
swallowed (> 80 per cent). Retention (in patient) good, penetration (into lungs)
poor.

Small particles (about 0.5 μm) diffuse in air (Brownian motion) and so settle
slowly on wall. Most are exhaled again. Penetration good, retention poor.

Intermediate particles (about 2 μm) sediment giving maximum retention in lungs
but most in alveoli rather than airways. Retention is maximized by deep slow
inhalation and delayed exhalation. Pressurized aerosols use Freon propellant
which must evaporate to liberate small drug particles. If this has not happened
by the time the throat is reached drug is impacted there and swallowed.

EPIDEMOLOGY OF ASTHMA

1—2 per cent of population suffer: 1245 died in 1971 in the UK of whom 187 were below the age of 34 years. In most, death was sudden and unexpected. Between 1961 and 1967 a dramatic increase in deaths certified as due to asthma occurred. In the 10—14 year age-group this increase was eight-fold. Since then the epidemic has waned but we have not returned to the pre-1961 low death rate.

Hypotheses for origin of epidemic

(1) Altered nature of disease.
(2) Toxicity of propellant in pressurized aerosols.
(3) Toxicity of drug in pressurized aerosols (*Isoprenaline*).
(4) Excessive use of a pressurized aerosol — especially if it failed to relieve the attack.
(5) Inadequate anti-inflammatory steroid therapy.

Headache and migraine

HEADACHE

Headache is a common symptom and is usually due to: (1) muscular spasm — the tension headache; (2) referred pain, for example, from cervical spondylosis (arthritis), sinusitis, glaucoma, or errors of refraction. Within the cranium only large blood vessels and the lining of the inside of the skull have receptors for pain, the brain itself does not. The tissues of the scalp are sensitive to pain (for example, blood vessels); (3) vasodilatation is responsible for the headache associated with migraine, histamine, *Glyceryl trinitrate* and systemic infections. Contrary to popular belief, headache is not a feature of essential hypertension.

Treatment

Wherever possible the underlying cause should be identified so that specific and effective therapy can be instituted, for example, for meningitis, cerebral tumour, depression. If intracranial pathology is suspected narcotic analgesics should not be given because the associated respiratory depression raises intracranial pressure via hypercapnia and may disturb consciousness. Simple analgesics should be the first treatment for headache. Proprietary, over-the-counter, preparations usually contain *Aspirin, Paracetamol* or *Codeine.* Singly or in combination, these drugs are adequate for all types of moderate headache. Double-blind controlled trials have shown that 500—1000 mg of *Paracetamol* and *Aspirin* are equipotent as antipyretics and analgesics and are as effective as *Codeine* (30 mg), *Dihydrocodeine* (30 mg) and dextropropoxyphene (65 mg). Increasing the dose of these drugs does not provide further analgesia but should prolong the duration of action at the expense of increased toxicity, for example, gastric irritation with *Aspirin*, constipation with *Dihydrocodeine*, drowsiness with dextropropoxyphene. The use of an anxiolytic, for example, *Diazepam*, may occasionally be warranted if stress is an important causative factor. Which analgesic a doctor or a patient chooses is usually based on habit and not on recognized prescribing considerations (apart from the risk of gastric mucosal ulceration with salicylates although modern formulations of soluble *Aspirin* are much less hazardous). In the UK very frequently prescribed analgesics are dextropropoxyphene plus *Paracetamol* (Distalgesic) and *Dihydrocodeine* (DF118) and their trade names do not make it apparent that an opiate is being prescribed so that constipation or drowsiness may not be recognized as side-effects. Dextropropoxyphene is equally popular in America where controlled trials have failed to demonstrate its superiority over *Paracetamol.* Factors other than intrinsic therapeutic value are responsible for the commercial success of dextropropoxyphene.

MIGRAINE

Migraine is a familial disorder characterized by recurrent attacks of headache, widely variable in intensity, frequency and duration, and is often associated with neurological disturbances. The classical syndrome comprises: (1) a prodromal phase, in which visual disturbances are common, for example, blind spot (scotoma), scintillating lines accompanied by drowsiness, nausea and vomiting; (2) the headache which is usually unilateral and throbbing.

All the above characteristics are not present in each attack or in each patient.

The cause of migraine is unknown but instability of intracranial and extracranial blood vessels is responsible for the manifestations of the disease. This abnormality of vasomotor control is of pharmacological interest because 5-HT has been implicated in its pathogenesis, and drugs which mimic or antagonize 5-HT are of value in the prophylaxis of migraine. The effects of 5-HT on the cardiovascular system are complex but intracarotid infusion causes constriction of the temporal artery and scalp pallor, both of which occur in the prodromal phase. The other prodromal features are due to cerebral vasoconstriction. In contrast, extracranial vasodilatation is responsible for the throbbing headache.

Normally, 5-HT is confined to platelets but during an attack a factor in the plasma activates the release of 5-HT from platelets. Tyramine-containing foods, for example, cheese and Chianti precipitate attacks in susceptible patients and the headache associated with ingestion of these foods by patients on MAO inhibitors shows features of migraine. A higher premenstrual incidence of migraine in women may be related to a decrease of platelet MAO activity after ovulation. Prostaglandins released from activated platelets promote aggregation, further release of 5-HT and a lowering of the pain threshold in vessel walls. The lateralization of many migrainous headaches is unexplained.

THERAPY

Based on the above considerations, a number of approaches might prove of value in the prophylaxis of migraine and in the treatment of an acute attack.

Prophylaxis

(1) Remove factors triggering the disorder, for example, avoid stressful situations — psychotherapy, anxiolytic (*Diazepam* or *Propranolol* which can also reduce the effects of increased sympathetic activity); withdraw offending foodstuffs and Ethanol. Inhibit ovulation.

(2) *Methysergide* is a derivative of ergot and an antagonist of 5-HT at D receptors (page 111). However, on vascular smooth muscle *Methysergide* mimics the vasoconstrictor action of 5-HT. It is not effective in the treatment of the vasodilatation and headache but does reduce the frequency of attacks. A serious toxic effect of continued treatment with this drug is retroperitoneal fibrosis which may not become symptomatic until irreversible changes have occurred. It is therefore reserved for the prophylaxis of frequent incapacitating migraine.

Other compounds with similar actions are cyproheptadine and pizotifen which are less effective. An increase in appetite and drowsiness are side-effects of these drugs.

(3) *Clonidine* is useful in hypertension (page 282) but at lower doses reduces the sensitivity of vascular smooth muscle to various vasoconstrictor and vasodilator stimuli. Side-effects are less troublesome than with the antagonists of 5-HT, but the drug should not be discontinued abruptly.

(4) Inhibition of prostaglandin synthesis with *Aspirin* (600 mg bd) has been shown to reduce the frequency of headache in migrainous patients by more than 75 per cent.

Treatment of acute attack

It would appear rational to use agents which can cause vasoconstriction of scalp vessels to treat the headache.

(1) *Ergotamine* is the most reliable agent for relief, but to be maximally effective it must be given parenterally (0.25 mg im or sc) before the vasodilator phase. *Ergotamine* suppositories are also used (formulated with *Caffeine* which may enhance absorption). To overcome the erratic absorption from the gut a pressurized aerosol delivering a metered dose of micronized *Ergotamine* is available. A maximum of six doses in one day has been recommended. The drug is highly toxic, causing vomiting and diarrhoea, convulsions and severe vasoconstriction leading to paraesthesia and gangrene (cf St.Anthony's fire of ergot poisoning due to fungal contamination of rye). It is contraindicated in patients with vascular disease, thrombophlebitis, hepatic or renal disease and during pregnancy. It is doubtful whether in equieffective doses dihydroergotamine is any less toxic than *Ergotamine.*

(2) A sympathomimetic amine such as *Ephedrine* is occasionally effective.

(3) Prevent cerebral vasoconstriction — inhalation of 5 per cent CO_2 in oxygen abolishes scotomata and subsequent headache but this is impractical for most patients.

(4) Analgesics such as *Aspirin* (prophylaxis) or *Codeine* will have some palliative effect if taken early in the vasoconstrictor phase.

(5) For nausea and vomiting an anti-emetic by suppository ensures its absorption, for example, *Prochlorperazine, Metoclopramide* (page 301).

(6) If drowsiness is a problem *Caffeine* is a cerebral stimulant and is often a constituent of compound analgesic preparations.

Mental disorders and drugs which alleviate them

Psychological illness is common, manifest as disturbance of emotion, behaviour or thought and conventionally classified as neurosis or psychosis (page 132).

NEUROSIS

Neurosis is usually recognizable as an exaggeration of a normal behavioural trait, for example, anxiety state, reactive depression, but may occasionally be moderately severe, for example, agoraphobia, obsessions/compulsions, cardiac hypochondriasis. Environmental factors are often causative, and patterns of neurotic behaviour are easily learned in childhood.

Treatment

Psychotherapy

To help patients obtain insight into their problems.

Supportive measures

To alleviate environmental stress.

Drug therapy

Not a substitute for psychotherapy or supportive measures — anxiolytics used occasionally and intermittently.

The prognosis is usually good.

PSYCHOSIS

This is a disabling mental illness which prevents a normal private or social existence, for example, schizophrenia, mania, endogenous depression, dementia. Various biochemical abnormalities within the brain have been postulated as causing schizophrenia with none proven. Monoaminergic : cholinergic imbalance is proposed in manic depression. Organic degeneration of the cerebral cortex results in dementia.

Treatment

(1) Admission to hospital is often required, to protect patients and their families (compulsory admission sometimes necessary).
(2) Drug therapy — neuroleptics if disturbed or aggressive; antidepressants if depressed.
(3) Psychotherapy — to prevent institutionalization and to provide rehabilitation.

The prognosis is variable depending on severity and chronicity.

ANXIOLYTICS   *Chlordiazepoxide*
Diazepam.

Today the benzodiazepines are the principal anxiolytics (page 163) having replaced barbiturates which are much more sedative and dangerous in overdose. In the 1960's the advertising strategy of the pharmaceutical industry promoted a syndrome to the medical profession and to the public. The typical patient was an overanxious housewife with young children, unable to cope with her lot, exhibiting physical manifestations of sympatho-adrenal overactivity. This syndrome was alleged to respond dramatically to the first benzodiazepine, *Chlordiazepoxide* — 'a sedative anticonvulsant with marked taming effects in vicious animals'. Anxiety neurosis became respectable, *Chlordiazepoxide* fashionable and more potent analogues were introduced, for example, *Diazepam*, lorazepam. Many doctors and patients are convinced of the anxiolytic efficacy of these drugs. Other doctors view them as nostrums, safe in overdosage, which in controlled clinical trials have regularly failed to provide greater benefit than placebo for neuroses.

Selection of a benzodiazepine

Each benzodiazepine possesses all the properties of the group with minor differences in relative potency. Some effects are readily demonstrable in man, for example, sedation, suppression of paradoxical sleep, safety in overdosage and anterograde amnesia. Others such as appetite stimulation and relaxation of voluntary muscle (an effect mediated by depression of spinal synaptic transmission) are less so. The clinical use of individual drugs is determined solely by the marketing strategy of the pharmaceutical industry with onomatopoeia seeming to play an important role. Thus, *Nitrazepam* was promoted as a sedative, clonazepam as an anticonvulsant.

Most benzodiazepines (except lorazepam, oxazepam and temazepam) have an active metabolite with a prolonged elimination phase ($t_{1/2} > 24$ hours). Administration once daily is therefore appropriate, preferably at night to prevent insomnia due to anxiety. In the elderly, metabolism is less efficient ($t_{1/2}$ up to

90 hours) with cumulation leading to confusion, ataxia, drowsiness and incontinence.

NEUROLEPTICS

Phenothiazine (page 140) derivatives are powerful neuroleptics of value for:
(1) agitation complicating psychoses; (2) organic confusional states; (3) suppression of hallucinations and delusions; (4) modification of aggressive behaviour.

Miscellaneous effects

(1)   Potentiation of all non-specific cerebral depressant drugs (Ethanol, general anaesthetics and hypnotics).
(2)   Potentiation of drugs with hypotensive action by blockade of peripheral α-adrenoceptors.
(3)   Potentiation of narcotic analgesics.
(4)   Anti-emetic, for example, concomitant use with narcotic analgesics.
(5)   Anti-vertigo, for example, *Prochlorperazine* by suppository (because of associated nausea and vomiting) in vestibular (Ménière's) disease.
(6)   Alteration of temperature control.

Unwanted effects

(1)   Drowsiness, especially with parenteral *Chlorpromazine.*
(2)   Hypotension, especially with parenteral *Chlorpromazine.*
(3)   Cholestatic jaundice (intrahepatic obstruction) due to idiosyncratic response (not dose related), especially to the less potent phenothiazines *Chlorpromazine* and *Promazine.* This risk is sufficient to advise against prescribing these drugs casually as sedatives.
(4)   Extrapyramidal disorders. (*a*) Parkinsonism (hypokinesia, rigidity and tremor) is dose-related and more common with chronic administration of the potent *Trifluoperazine* and Perphenazine. Patients on high doses may need prophylactic therapy with, for example *Benzhexol* (note peripheral anticholinergic side-effects). (*b*) Acute dystonic responses occur in the young on first exposure to the drug and may be mistaken for tetanus. They subside spontaneously. (*c*) Tardive dyskinesia occurs in patients chronically taking phenothiazines. It is of delayed onset (tardive) and may be irreversible. The disorder involves bizarre movements (dyskinesia) of limbs, head, face and tongue. The cause is not understood although proliferation of dopamine receptors has been suggested.

Other preparations

Depot injections of specially formulated neuroleptics have been used to improve patient compliance. Butyrophenone derivatives are particularly potent, for example, *Haloperidol*, and necessitate antiparkinsonism prophylaxis. *Haloperidol* is useful in the treatment of acute mania.

ANTIDEPRESSANTS

Elevation of mood is the aim of antidepressant therapy which should also motivate the patient and relieve associated anxieties, insomnia and restlessness. Failure to recognize depression may result in inappropriate prescription of a benzodiazepine which will aggravate the condition.

The biochemical basis of depression may be related to a functional loss of mono-amines in the brain (page 129).

Early treatment used amphetamine-like agents for mild and ECT for severe depression. The important developments depended on fortuitous clinical observations of mood elevation: (1) with the antituberculous drugs *Isoniazid* and especially iproniazid which was shown to be a MAO inhibitor; (2) with *Imipramine* (a tricyclic compound) on trial as a neuroleptic in schizophrenia which was later shown to inhibit re-uptake of NA (page 54)

Clinically useful antidepressants interact with the disposition, metabolism or function of one or more monoamines. Differences relate to varying modes of action and side-effects.

MAO inhibitors

The clinical usefulness of this group is limited by its many adverse drug and food interactions. *Phenelzine* is most used because of acute stimulant effects and relative freedom from side-effects. Acetylator phenotype does not influence clinical response.

Precautions

Instructions must be given to avoid ingestion of tyramine-containing foods (cheese, yeast and meat extracts, yoghurt, Chianti) and administration of indirect sympathomimetics (Amphetamine, *Ephedrine*, decongestants).

Tricyclic antidepressants should not be administered concurrently with a MAO inhibitor because of a similar interaction. Occasional patients, however, only respond to such a combination prescribed in cautious dosage.

Tricyclic antidepressants

The onset of antidepressant effect is delayed for some days after the start of treatment possibly for pharmacokinetic reasons (cumulation), and possibly because this is the time course of the synthesis or breakdown of a neuronal constituent, the equilibrium of which is altered by the drug or its effects. Because of considerable variability in the disposition and metabolism of this group of drugs, start with a dose (especially in the elderly, to avoid toxicity, for example, dizziness due to hypotension, peripheral anticholinergic effects) increasing at weekly intervals.

Suicidal tendencies necessitate admission to hospital because of the delay in therapeutic effect. Overdosage can be fatal (respiratory depression, cardiac arrhythmia).

Imipramine is the first choice in endogenous depression but ECT may occasionally be needed for a rapid effect. *Amitryptyline* is more sedative and is suitable if agitation or insomnia are problems. Recent pharmacokinetic studies have shown that once daily administration is adequate. The sedative effect is turned to advantage by taking the drug at night, and dose-related anticholinergic side-effects (dry mouth, blurred vision) do not obtrude during sleep.

Newer antidepressants which are not tricyclic are claimed to have fewer peripheral anticholinergic side-effects and to be less likely to affect the cardiovascular system (page 136).

Endogenous depression may be one pole of the dipolar manic-depressive psychosis. Recovery from depression may be followed by pathological elevation of mood with acute mania. Suppression of such swings of mood can be achieved with *Lithium* carbonate. Toxicity can be avoided by regular monitoring of blood concentrations.

Nausea, retching and vomiting

EMETICS

The output of the medullary emetic centre, which lies laterally in the reticular formation, near the solitary tract, passes: (1) to high centres to be perceived as the sensation of nausea; (2) by parasympathetic outflows to the gut (relaxation of the cardiac or oesophagogastric sphincter) and salivary glands (secretion); (3) by somatic efferent pathways to the expiratory muscles of respiration and postural muscles.

The reflex, as a whole, cannot be usefully modified by treatment directed at these varied outputs.

The emetic centre itself can be depressed, not by specific therapies, but by any CNS depressant drug in doses sufficient to cause profound sedation (for example, general anaesthetics, Ethanol, barbiturates and non-barbiturate hypnotics and sedatives, phenothiazines and *Morphine*).

All therapeutically useful anti-emetic drugs seem to act on the input circuitry of the emetic centre. The inputs are of four origins (at least) as follows:

(1) Psychic: bombardment from higher centres generated by, for example, the sight, sound and smell of someone else vomiting.
(2) Gastrointestinal afferents: excited by, for instance, pharyngeal mechanical stimulation, irritation or disease in the gut.
(3) Motion: which is only partly of vestibular (labyrinthine) origin, a significant part is visual and disagreement between the visual and proprioceptive versions of the position of the body in space is a particularly potent cause.

(4)   Chemical: a great variety of chemical emetics exert their actions, like
Apomorphine (the principal research tool in this area, page 148) on the
CTZ. This is a discrete patch of neural tissue in the floor of the posterior
part of the fourth ventricle, which is also very vascular and permeable
(no blood brain barrier shields this part of the CNS from blood-borne
influences). Most drugs can cause nausea and vomiting as a part of their
acute toxicity but this action is a prominent feature of, or has been studied
experimentally for, the following:

Adrenaline, dopamine and *Levodopa*.
The ergot alkaloids (for example, *Ergotamine* and *Ergometrine* [ergonovine].
The narcotic analgesics (for example, *Morphine* and *Pethidine*).
Nicotine and *Pilocarpine*.
Emetine, both pure and as a constituent of *Ipecacuanha*.
Oestrogens (and the high oestrogen situation of early pregnancy).
Cardiac glycosides (for example, *Digoxin*) — the CTZ is the site of their
    early emetic action.
Salicylates.
Radiation (especially of the abdomen) — the CTZ mediates the emesis seen
    soon after the irradiation.
The radiomimetics (for example, alkylating agents).
The disease states of uraemia (renal failure) and carcinomatosis (disseminated
    carcinoma; vomiting may be due to hypercalcaemia).

In contrast, rather few chemicals are known to induce emesis by exciting gastrointestinal afferents:

Intragastric copper sulphate (which also has a central action once absorbed) is the
principal research tool.

A gastrointestinal peripheral component operates for *Ipecacuanha* and salicylates
and in the late nausea and vomiting after irradiation.

The role of enterotoxins produced by the infecting organisms of gastroenteritis
cannot at present be localized to the gut or the CTZ.

The late emetic effect of cardiac glycosides seems to be exerted on other (perhaps
cardiac) afferents.

ANTI-EMETICS

As with coughing, clinical situations in which vomiting is serving a protective
function should not be suppressed by drugs. In most clinical situations, however,
emesis serves no useful purpose — early pregnancy, travel sickness, postoperative,
migraine, radiotherapy, cancer chemotherapy and drug therapy (for example,
Morphine).

Motion sickness

Hyoscine (page 33) is most effective, though sedative and producing all the
expected atropine-like side-effects. Better tolerated (though still sedative) but less
effective are some antihistamines (for example, *Cyclizine*, *Promethazine*,
Dimenhydrinate and *Mepyramine*). The neural pathway carrying vestibular

impulses to the emetic centre actually passes through the CTZ, though its neurones are not those excited by Apomorphine and other chemical triggers. These two pathways converge on the emetic centre later. Not surprisingly, the drugs effective in motion sickness are effective in middle ear disease and to a lesser extent in Ménière's disease. They have some effect postoperatively (or postanaesthetic) and in the vomiting of early pregnancy. The narcotics are much more emetic in ambulant than bedridden patients and this (vestibular) component is countered by the drugs for motion sickness.

Other conditions

In most other situations the phenothiazines (*Chlorpromazine, Trifluoperazine*) are effective, notably postoperatively, in radiotherapy, uraemia, carcinomatosis and pregnancy. In pregnancy drugs should be avoided if at all possible (page 259). They are also very effective against Apomorphine, ergot alkaloids, sympathomimetics and *Levodopa* and at high doses against cardiac glycosides and narcotic analgesics.

The principal side-effects are drowsiness, sedation, orthostatic hypotension, extra-pyramidal (parkinsonian) symptoms and obstructive jaundice. *Trifluoperazine* and *Prochlorperazine* are more potent than *Chlorpromazine* both as an anti-emetic and in their CNS side-effects but less so at peripheral α-adrenoceptors.

Metoclopramide, an antagonist at dopamine receptors, is a new anti-emetic (a relative of *Procainamide*) with peripheral (increased gastric emptying, reduced reflux) and central anti-emetic actions. It has been found effective in the vomiting associated with migraine, pregnancy, Ménière's disease, motion sickness, narcotics, radiotherapy and postoperatively, but not against radiomimetics. It shows extrapyramidal side-effects, worse in children, which summate with those of phenothiazines. It causes prolactin release (galactorrhoea).

Epilepsy

Many otherwise healthy, alert and intelligent people suffer from epilepsy. The incidence in the UK and North America is about 7:1000 population. It is usually manifest as a sudden loss of consciousness or seizure.

Epilepsy is caused by cerebral neuronal membranes which have unstable permeability characteristics; this results in erratic polarity changes and spontaneous firing at high frequency. The location of this 'ectopic focus' determines the type of seizure.

CLASSIFICATION OF SEIZURES

Generalized

(1)   Grand mal or tonic/clonic: prodromal state, aura, loss of consciousness, skeletal muscle contraction — first sustained (tonic), later repetitive (clonic), relaxation, sleep.

301

(2) Petit mal or absence attacks: transient vacancy, 10–15 seconds duration, few motor features, characteristic 3 Hz spike and wave on EEG. Mainly restricted to childhood.

Focal or partial

(1) Temporal lobe or psychomotor: hallucinations, déjà vu, pallor, complex movements or behaviour patterns, automatism.
(2) Focal motor or jacksonian: local onset, progression, may become generalized, transient paresis.

Serial seizures

These occur under special circumstances precipitated by acute infection (febrile convulsions) in the child, by pregnancy (increased clearance of anticonvulsant drugs) or by abrupt withdrawal of drugs (Ethanol, barbiturates, anticonvulsants) – constitutes an acute medical emergency, especially when consciousness is not regained between seizures (status epilepticus).

CAUSES OF EPILEPSY

All the above clinical types can be caused by a variety of pathologies:

(1) Cryptogenic (idiopathic): usually no specific pathology is found.
(2) Symptomatic: tumour, angioma, ischaemia or haemorrhage, abscess, fever (children), posttraumatic scarring, meningitis, encephalitis.
(3) Drugs: acute poisoning with antidepressants, Nicotine, *Atropine,* Strychnine, salicylate, *Nikethamide* or acute withdrawal of, for example, barbiturates, Ethanol. Certain drugs increase the likelihood of seizures when used at conventional doses in predisposed patients, for example, antidepressants, glucocorticoids, phenothiazines.
(4) Metabolic causes: hypoglycaemia, insulin, hypocalcaemia, alkalosis, hypocapnia, anoxia, water intoxication, uraemia, hepatic encephalopathy.
(5) Electroconvulsive therapy.
(6) Hypertension: hypertensive encephalopathy, eclamptic toxaemia.

ELECTROPHYSIOLOGY

Hughlings Jackson (born 1835) – 'a sudden, excessive, rapid and local discharge in the grey matter of the brain'.

The discharge originates in an abnormal focus. Single cells in the focus give intermittent bursts of high frequency (> 100 Hz) spikes. These have been detected by microelectrodes. The abnormal high frequency discharge can be detected on the EEG, but it is clinically silent unless it spreads into surrounding areas of normal brain tissue:

(1) Factors which encourage spread are the drug and metabolic factors which can precipitate an epileptic attack (*see* Causes, above).

(2) Factors which discourage spread are factors which can suppress epilepsy and prevent clinical attacks: (*a*) anticonvulsant drugs (membrane stabilizers) do not abolish the abnormal focus which remains detectable on the EEG, but they raise the threshold of surrounding normal brain; (*b*) carbonic anhydrase inhibitors (raise brain PCO_2, lower brain pH).

TESTS IN PATIENTS

Will a new drug produce fewer fits when added to the existing therapeutic regimen of a patient with poor control of epilepsy? Will it prevent fits in new patients with fewer side-effects (for example, sedation, ataxia, anaemia) than existing drugs?

GENERAL PRINCIPLES OF MANAGEMENT

(1) Record frequency and severity of attacks with co-operation of patient and relatives. Without this record you can have no measure of the efficacy of treatment.
(2) One seizure does not constitute epilepsy. Do not rush into drug treatment.
(3) Get the best out of one drug before adding another. Simplest regimen is the best (*Table 6.4*).
(4) Twice daily dosage is adequate. Avoid tablets at work. When one dose is forgotten patient should take a double dose at the next occasion.
(5) Do not make frequent changes in dosage. About two weeks are required for accumulation to attain a new steady state. Several weeks or months may be required to determine if improvement has occurred. Never stop drugs suddenly or withdrawal fits/status epilepticus may ensue.
(6) Monitor serum concentration when appropriate.
(7) After two years free from attacks an attempt can be made to wean patient off drugs.
(8) Seek a remediable underlying cause particularly in late onset epilepsy.

USE OF ANTICONVULSANT DRUGS

Available drugs (this list is selective)

Phenytoin, relatively selective, excessive doses produce dysarthria, nystagmus and ataxia but not general CNS depression. Acne, gum hyperplasia and hirsutism occur and are particularly unacceptable in the female. There is an increased tendency to macrocytic anaemia due to folate deficiency in otherwise predisposed patients and an increased frequency of hair lip and cleft palate in progeny of mothers. Hazards of uncontrolled seizures and alternative drugs must be weighed against this. Aggravation of vitamin D deficiency is unproven.

Carbamazepine — chemically related to tricyclic antidepressants — may particularly benefit patients with psychotic features complicating temporal lobe epilepsy. Active metabolite (epoxide) complicates interpretation of serum concentration. Popular second drug but considered first-line drug by many neurologists particularly when treating young women. Effective in 'shooting' pains, for example, trigeminal neuralgia, phantom limb (*Phenytoin* also). Adverse effects include drowsiness, dizziness, hypersensitivity states — marrow depression rare.

Sodium *Valproate* — introduced recently, less knowledge of long-term hazards. May potentiate the inhibitory transmitter GABA by inhibiting its enzymic inactivation — few recognized side-effects apart from heartburn, hair loss, obesity and occasionally thrombocytopenia. Unusual in being effective against both grand mal and petit mal — potentiates concurrently administered *Phenobarbitone* by inhibiting its metabolism.

Ethosuximide — chemically related to *Phenytoin.* Side-effects resemble those of *Carbamazepine.* Selective against petit mal — drug of choice before advent of sodium *Valproate.*

Diazepam — favoured by iv route in status epilepticus. If a few doses do not abort seizures, iv infusion of large dose of *Phenytoin* may be needed. Large doses of *Diazepam* produce depression of respiration which may demand intubation and ventilation. Not effective by im injection but may be given rectally in babies with febrile convulsions.

Paraldehyde — cyclic trimer of acetaldehyde. Effective by im injection and therefore still used to stop febrile convulsions in babies. Oxidized if stored too long — incompatible with plastic syringes on more than brief contact.

Phenobarbitone — relatively non-selective anticonvulsant. Sedation, general CNS depression, aggressive behaviour in children. Becoming less popular but still widely prescribed — optimum serum concentration probably 20—40 mg/ℓ. If another drug is to be substituted, the exchange must be done gradually over weeks or months.

Primidone — oxidized to *Phenobarbitone in vivo* often producing higher serum concentration than seen in patients prescribed *Phenobarbitone* directly. CNS depressant, anticonvulsant drug in its own right.

No drugs

Many patients with seizures do not need anticonvulsant drugs at all. The seizures may be infrequent, mildly incapacitating (focal motor or sensory), restricted to sleeping hours or precipitated only by unusual or avoidable circumstances (hunger, fever, sleep deprivation).

Intermittent drugs

Seizures may be restricted to the time of the menstrual period. A one-week course of *Acetazolamide* 250—500 mg/day started 7—10 days before the first day of the next period can sometimes prevent these by reducing salt and water retention and raising brain PCO_2.

One drug

Careful adjustment of the dose of one drug is preferable to multiple drug treatment. The more complex the treatment the poorer is patient compliance.

Adequate control of seizures can be achieved in 80–90 per cent of adult patients with grand mal, focal or psychomotor seizures using *Phenytoin* alone. For those few adult patients in whom petit mal absences are troublesome, it is also necessary to use a second drug, for example, *Ethosuximide*, or the drug which is effective against both petit mal and the other types of seizure, sodium *Valproate*.

Serum drug concentration

The response to the anticonvulsant drugs is determined by the serum concentration rather than the dose. The optimum serum *Phenytoin* concentration for a patient is usually 10–25 mg/ℓ.

The regular daily dose required by an adult for such a concentration varies from 200–500 mg. Fine adjustment of dose (25 or 50 mg dosage steps, *Table 5.8*) is sometimes necessary to get this concentration; it is very easy to go straight from a dose which is inadequate to one which is excessive (say from 300 to 400 mg/day). After a dose change it will take about two weeks for the drug concentration to reach its new level.

Very large single doses (for example, 500–1000 mg) are needed to produce a therapeutic concentration quickly in adult patients with a previously low concentration.

Example: A 60 kg man has been taking 300 mg *Phenytoin* daily. He is suffering two or three grand mal seizures per week and his serum *Phenytoin* concentration is only 5 mg/ℓ. He can safely be treated with a single extra dose of 500 mg (5 capsules of 100 mg) and an increase of 50 mg (to 350 mg/day) in his maintenance dose. The response to treatment and the new plateau concentration can be checked 2–4 weeks later.

Two drugs

A small proportion of adult patients do not respond adequately to *Phenytoin* alone. In these a second drug can be added. *Carbamazepine* is favoured particularly in patients with temporal lobe epilepsy, and sodium *Valproate* in patients with grand mal and petit mal attacks.

Table 6.4. *Choice of anticonvulsant drugs in common categories of epilepsy*

	Phenytoin	Carbamazepine	Valproate	Ethosuximide
Grand mal or focal	1	2		
Grand mal with petit mal	2*		1	2*
Petit mal alone			1 or 2	1
Temporal lobe	1 or 2	1 or 2		

1 – first choice, 2 – second choice, * combined.

Sometimes the response to the second drug is useful but commonly we must compromise; it may be better to have a few seizures and be alert than to be fit-free and excessively sedated.

Once or twice daily dosage

With the exception of sodium *Valproate* most anticonvulsant drugs are eliminated very slowly. The serum concentration $t_{1/2}$ varies from about one day (*Carbamazepine*) to four days (*Phenobarbitone*). Thus, there is no need for a midday dose (at work or school). Twice or even once daily dosage is safe, effective and practical.

Family planning

CHOICE OF FAMILY PLANNING METHOD

Reasons for family planning include desire to: (1) increase interval between births; (2) temporarily prevent pregnancy; (3) permanently prevent pregnancy when the required family size is achieved.

Decision on whether to use family planning and which method is influenced by the above and: (1) cultural and religious background, including whether family planning is accepted as a male or female prerogative; (2) efficacy; (3) acceptability; (4) availability; (5) cost.

Modern family planning has had a major influence on individual families but relatively little effect on the populations of most countries.

CONTRACEPTION

'Natural' methods

Lactational amenorrhoea

During lactation first ovulation is delayed and subsequent ovulations less frequent. This is probably related to the high prolactin secretion. Therefore, the interbirth interval is on average increased. This method has a major influence on family size in developing countries.

Withdrawal

Withdrawal of penis from vagina before ejaculation. This method is widely used but of doubtful efficacy.

306

Rhythm method

Knowledge that ovulation occurs about 14 days before next menstrual period and that sperm can survive up to three days in female reproductive tract allows prediction of 'safe' times for intercourse. Prediction of the time of ovulation may be by calculation from the date of the onset of the last menstrual period or by keeping a daily early morning temperature record as body temperature rises following ovulation. A disadvantage of this method is the difficulty in predicting the time of ovulation with any accuracy.

Mechanical methods (*Table 6.5*)

Condom

This method is widely used and with correct use family size, on average, may be reduced to 2—3 children. The 'method' failure rate is low but the 'user' failure rate is higher. There are no adverse effects and no medical involvement.

Diaphragm

This blocks entry of sperm into the cervix. It requires use with spermicidal creams to be moderately effective. There are no adverse effects and, following a preliminary training session, no medical involvement. This method was widely used until oral contraceptives and IUDs became available.

Intrauterine devices (IUDs)

With an IUD in place the blastocyst probably still develops but implantation does not occur. The exact mechanism of action is unknown. It does not prevent ectopic pregnancies. Once fitted it usually remains in the uterus for several years. Occasional problems are expulsion, prolonged uterine bleeding and pelvic inflammatory disease. The efficacy is slightly improved and side-effects reduced if copper wire is wound around the plastic IUD. The mechanism of action of the copper is unknown. This is an effective family planning method.

Chemical methods (*Table 6.5*)

Spermicidal jellies, tablets and foams

These kill sperm by surface tension lowering properties (for example, nonylphenoxypolyethoxyethanol) or binding to sulphydryl groups (for example, phenylmercuric acetate). They are not very effective by themselves.

Hormonal

Combination 'pill': this has a negligible failure rate, any reported failures are likely to be due to missed tablets. They are widely used in developed countries. Recent UK studies suggest caution in their use in women over the age of 35 years or in heavy smokers due to a high incidence of cardiovascular disease compared with non-users.

Progestogen-only: depot injection of medroxyprogesterone acetate or tablets of 19-nor-testosterone derivatives. The mechanism of action is like that of the combination 'pill', primarily to stop ovulation but also affecting the uterus and cervical mucus. The action of the injection form lasts 3–6 months. It causes disturbed menstrual cycles and a delay in the return to fertility. It is very effective and popular in developing countries, especially as it does not affect lactation.

High dose oestrogens: these are effective if taken for about five days pre-implantation. They cause considerable nausea and vomiting.

Surgical methods *(Table 6.5)*

Vasectomy

Vas deferens is divided. It is a minor surgical procedure, usually done as an out-patient procedure under local anaesthesia. Following vasectomy 'sperm antibodies' sometimes appear in the blood (significance unknown). Fertility may be restored in a small proportion of cases.

Oviductal occlusion

Access to oviducts may be gained by abdominal, transvaginal or transcervical routes. The oviducts are either tied or sealed by cautery, clips or bands. Usually,

Table 6.5. *Approximate failure rates of contraceptive methods*

Method	Pregnancy rate per 100 woman years
Oviductal occlusion	About 0.02
Vasectomy	About 0.02
Combination 'pill'	0.03–0.10
Progestogen only 'pill'	1.5–3.0
IUD	1.5–3.0
Condom	4–28
Diaphragm	4–35
Spermidical jellies, etc.	4–38
No contraception	About 80

but not always, it is an inpatient procedure. Very occasional recanalizations and subsequent pregnancies occur. The operation is expensive in medical time and equipment for developing countries.

Hysterectomy

The uterus is usually removed only for medical reasons.

ABORTION

The distinction between a method of contraception (requiring precoital action) and a method of abortion (requiring postcoital action) is not always clear (*see* page 83).

It is estimated there are 125 million livebirths, 40 million spontaneous abortions and 30 million induced abortions annually in the world.

Surgical methods

Vacuum aspiration

Up to about four weeks gestation it is possible to remove the uterine contents with a syringe using a plastic cannula. At this time it will not be certain that the woman is pregnant. Between four and ten weeks more powerful suction is required. After six weeks gestation cervical dilatation is usually required first. These are outpatient procedures.

Dilatation and curettage

Following cervical dilatation, uterine contents can be removed by scraping and suction. This method is used from about six to ten weeks gestation. There is evidence that forced cervical dilatation is followed by a higher spontaneous miscarriage rate.

Hysterotomy

After about 12 weeks gestation the foetus needs to be removed by caesarean section or a chemical method may be used.

Chemical methods

Hypertonic saline solution

Intra-amniotic injection of hypertonic sodium chloride solution causes placental degeneration leading to abortion.

Urea

Causes placental degeneration. Other agents (for example, prostaglandins) may be used in association.

Prostglandins (page 111)

Intra-amniotic prostaglandin $F_{2\alpha}$ or analogues are now preferred to hypertonic saline solution as there is a shorter injection-delivery interval and fewer major complications. Vomiting and diarrhoea are frequent with the prostaglandins.

The chemical methods are used in the second trimester (about 13—26 weeks gestation). Hazards of abortion increase with gestational age.

Drugs and appetite

Drugs play little role in the management of the obese (in whom a suppression of appetite is desired) or of the anorexic.

OBESITY

No patient can lose weight without the persistent exercise of will power. For a considerable time he must consume less energy than he utilizes. It is unusual for patients to maintain a substantial increase in energy expenditure so the problem becomes that of maintaining a substantial reduction in dietary calorie intake.

Drugs have been considered potentially helpful in two ways:

Methylcellulose

Methylcellulose might be swallowed dry, swell in the stomach and provide the physical sensation of a full stomach, thus alleviating one of the unpleasant concomitants of dietary restriction; 10 g daily would be needed but pharma-copoeial preparations swell slowly, only achieving their maximal bulk after leaving the stomach — they are effective bulk purgatives. Further, if compensatory overeating (after weight reduction has been achieved) is to be avoided, the patient's stomach needs to be retrained to feel satisfied at a lesser distension.

Anorectic drugs

These suppress appetite by an action on the hypothalamic appetite centre, and more or less resemble Amphetamine chemically and pharmacologically. Amphetamine itself should never be used for this purpose, its anorectic action is only transient, it has central stimulant and peripheral sympathomimetic actions (including potentiation of catecholamines and antagonism of *Guanethidine*), and in addition causes euphoria tending to encourage drug abuse. It can precipitate psychotic responses.

The non-fluorinated Amphetamine derivatives which have been promoted as anorectics (phentermine, diethylpropion and mazindol) all suffer from the same disadvantages and cannot be recommended.

Only the fluorinated derivative *Fenfluramine* is relatively safe in this respect, it has minimal peripheral and other central sympathomimetic effects, does not interfere with paradoxical sleep but it has its own characteristic CNS toxicity of drowsiness and depression. It should only be briefly used, if at all, at the outset, to help the establishment of new eating habits. Educating the patient about the calorific content of food is vital. Much useful advice can be obtained from popular slimming magazines. Fats and oils have the highest calorific value (9 kcal/g; cal = calorie):
Twice that of sausages, pastry and cheese.
Thrice that of bread and potatoes.
Five times that of beef and chicken.
Eight times that of boiled rice and cottage cheese.
Twelve times that of haddock and cod.
Fruit and vegetables contribute minimally (< 0.2 kcal/g).

Obviously, frying any food will increase its calorie content considerably.

Normality tables of weight

For adults there are two kinds of table: (1) derived from population averages, called 'average' or 'standard' weights for various heights, frames and ages; (2) derived from actuarial studies of the weights associated with minimum mortality, called 'ideal' or 'desirable' weights for various heights and frames. The ideal, unlike the average, weight does not increase with age over 25 years.

Time taken to lose weight

A moderately sedentary person might expend 1800 kcal daily. If two stones over-weight (all of it fat) about 114,000 kcal difference between consumption and expenditure must be accumulated. On a 1000 kcal diet this would take about 140 days.

PRIMARY ANOREXIA NERVOSA

This is a neurotic reaction of adolescent girls characterized by self-starvation, suspension of menstruation and frequently self-induced vomiting and excessive purgation. It is an expression of a morbid fear of 'obesity', but the patient suffers a distorted body image such that they would regard themselves as obese even at their ideal bodyweight. It is said to have underlying it a neurotic fear of adult responsibilities, especially sexual ones. The menstrual arrest is hypothalmic rather than pituitary in origin. Hunger persists and the self-starvation is punctuated by gorging and then self-recrimination. Protein is eaten so anaemias and vitamin deficiencies are rare.

The mother usually asks for help (the patient does not regard herself as ill). Morbidity arises from malnutrition and pH and electrolyte disturbances. Mortality 4–12 per cent from the disease or suicide. It terminates spontaneously after about four years in about 85 per cent of cases but may recur.

Management

In the standard treatment the patient is confined to bed in hospital, persuaded to eat a concentrated high calorie diet (1500 rising to 4000 kcal daily) and not allowed up until a specified weight gain has occurred. *Chlorpromazine* is an adjunct.

Some centres make deliberate attempts to modify behaviour using +ve reinforcements (rewards).

No method can succeed without the patient's co-operation.

Drugs and the blood

ANAEMIA

Anaemia ('lack of blood') means deficiency of haemoglobin. Diagnosis (the only adequate basis for treatment) requires answers to three questions: (1) Is the patient anaemic? (2) What kind of anaemia is it? (3) What is the cause of this kind of anaemia in this patient?

The anaemic patient may show some of the following clinical features. Listless, easily tired. Palpitations, muscle aches and pains, 'blackouts'. Angina pectoris, intermittent claudication, breathlessness on exertion (high output cardiac failure). Pallor of the conjunctivae rather than skin.

Definitive recognition requires measurement of blood haemoglobin content.

There are several different kinds of anaemia to be differentiated.

IRON DEFICIENCY ANAEMIA

Clinical features

Inflamed corners of mouth (angular stomatitis), smooth shiny tongue (sore when eating) and longitudinally ridged, flat (even concave) nails. A suggestive history is of repeated blood loss – menses, drugs irritant to the stomach.

Tests

The blood film shows hypochromic, microcytic cells which vary in size and shape. Serum iron, serum ferritin and bone marrow haemosiderin are all low. Total serum iron binding capacity (transferrin) is high.

Causes

(1) Inadequate intake -- old poor alone, infants fed on cows milk, pregnant women, premature or twin babies.
(2) Inadequate absorption — gastrointestinal surgery, malabsorption syndrome.
(3) Excessive loss — apparent or occult bleeding (*Aspirin* [10—15 per cent of patients with rheumatoid arthritis on 900 mg four times daily lose > 10ml. a day from gastric erosions], Ethanol, *Phenylbutazone, Indomethacin*).

Treatment

The cause, the iron deficiency and the anaemia may need treatment.

Oral iron: about 10 per cent is absorbed from normal diet. This increases in iron deficiency to about 25 per cent. Swallowing more iron increases the amount but reduces the percentage absorbed. A red cell has a life of about 100 days, so the 1 per cent replaced each day needs 25 mg Fe^{2+}. In severe deficiency at least 100 mg Fe^{2+} must be swallowed daily for about five months (for restitution of haemoglobin and stores).

Ferrous sulphate 200 mg = 60 mg Fe^{2+}.

Ferrous gluconate 300 mg = 35 mg Fe^{2+}.

Gastrointestinal side-effects of the therapeutic dose: nausea and epigastric pain are dose-related, 'heartburn', diarrhoea and constipation are less so. If gastrointestinal side-effects are troublesome the following manoeuvres may succeed: take the dose after meal, try other salts (fumarate, succinate), add Ascorbic acid which increases absorption. The only valid indications for parenteral iron are non-compliance or malabsorption. *Iron dextran* or *Iron sorbitol* [sorbitex] im may cause pain and local staining and a significant incidence of hypersensitivity reactions (higher and more severe with the iv route).

MEGALOBLASTIC ANAEMIAS

These are due to defective DNA synthesis.

VITAMIN B$_{12}$ DEFICIENCY ANAEMIA

Clinical features

Sore mouth and tongue. Sterility. Neuropathy and spinal cord degeneration.

Tests

Blood film shows large oval erythrocytes, hypersegmented nuclei in polymorpho-nuclear leucocytes and large platelets.

Bone marrow shows large stem cells of these three peripheral blood cells.

Serum shows unconjugated bilirubin (due to shortened cell life), increased Fe^{2+} and folate but a reduced B_{12}.

Pentagastrin-stimulated gastric acid secretion is absent (achlorhydria in pernicious anaemia).

Cyanocobalamin (^{58}Co) absorption without and with addition of intrinsic factor.

Causes

(1) Low intake – vegans.
(2) Malabsorption: pernicious anaemia; incidence 9 per 10^5 per annum, onset over 40 years. It is due to an autoimmune gastritis or gastrectomy; both these due to lack of intrinsic factor, ileal surgery, fistula, disease or stasis.

Treatment

Hydroxycobalamin (im) 1000 μg six times over three weeks and lifelong maintenance with 1000 μg every three months. Potassium supplements may be needed. Blood transfusion is rarely needed and can precipitate cardiac failure.

FOLIC ACID DEFICIENCY ANAEMIA

Similar clinical features and blood picture to B_{12} deficiency except there is no neurological disturbance. It must be distinguished by history and tests from B_{12} deficiency as an attempt to treat B_{12} deficiency with folate precipitates neuropathy.

Causes

(1) Inadequate intake – commonest (alcoholic, food fad, psychotic, mental defective, old poor alone).
(2) Malabsorption – rare (gluten-sensitive enteropathy).
(3) Increased utilization combined with poor diet. This occurs during pregnancy (incidence 1:200) particularly in the last trimester; routine prophylaxis employs *Iron and folic acid tablets* which contain 100 mg and 350 μg respectively.
(4) Drugs – *Methotrexate* (folinic acid needed to overcome inhibition), *Pyrimethamine, Proguanil*, anticonvulsants (*Phenytoin, Phenobarbitone, Primidone*).

Tests

Decreased red cell folate, jejunal biopsy.

Treatment

Folic acid 5 mg daily by mouth.

APLASTIC ANAEMIA

Causes

(1) Radiation and cytotoxic drugs cause a dose-related aplastic anaemia.
(2) Other drugs and chemicals may induce a hypersensitivity reaction (*Table 6.6*).

Table 6.6. *Hypersensitivity Potential*

	Definite	*Probable*
	Chloramphenicol	Sulphonamides
	Phenylbutazone	*Phenytoin*
	Gold salts	
	Organic arsenicals	*Tolbutamide*
	Potassium perchlorate	*Chlorpropamide*

(3) Idiopathic/myelofibrosis.

Treatment

Withdraw drug if suspected and transfusions of platelets, white or red blood cells as necessary. Bone marrow transplantation.

HAEMOLYTIC ANAEMIA

This is characterized by a shortened red cell life and increased haemoglobin breakdown (may appear in urine). The globin and Fe^{2+} are re-utilized but porphyrin is broken down to bilirubin, conjugated in liver, excreted in bile. Jaundice (acholuric) may occur.

Tests

Marrow shows hyperplasia. Blood shows reticulocytosis (young erythrocytes). Serum shows unconjugated bilirubin.

Causes

(1)　Genetically determined. Glucose-6-phosphate dehydrogenase deficiency —
haemolysis precipitated by oxidants (sulphonamides, *Primaquine*,
Nitrofurantoin).

(2)　Acquired. An autoimmune disease (Coombs' test for IgG antibodies on red
cells +ve) which can be produced by *Methyldopa* (incidence 1:2500).

If many transfusions are needed in treating any anaemia surplus Fe^{2+} can be
chelated with *Desferrioxamine*.

Drugs in joint disease

ARTHRITIS

'Arthritis' is used to describe a variety of inflammatory diseases of the joints and,
not surprisingly, the anti-inflammatory/analgesic/antipyretic group of drugs are
of value principally for symptomatic relief.

Infective arthritis is rare nowadays and antibacterial therapy appropriate for the
causative microorganism is indicated.

Allergic conditions also give rise to arthritis, for example, rheumatic fever, serum
sickness. Rheumatic fever is caused by a sensitization reaction to a β-haemolytic
Streptococcus (usually after a sore throat) and *Aspirin* and bed-rest are the main-
stays of treatment. Serum sickness is so called because it resembles the reaction
which followed injection of antiserum. Nowadays, an allergic reaction to a drug
is the usual cause of the serum sickness syndrome which often requires treatment
with corticosteroids.

The commonest forms of arthritis are osteoarthritis and rheumatoid arthritis.

Osteoarthritis (osteoarthrosis) is a degenerative disease due to wear and tear, and
inflammation plays little part in its pathogenesis. It particularly affects those
over the age of 50 years in their weightbearing joints (spine, hip, knee). Obesity
and injury to a joint aggravate the condition. Movement may be limited. Pain
is variable. Physiotherapy and local heat are often helpful. *Paracetamol* and
Indomethacin are suitable for chronic administration.

Rheumatoid arthritis has a higher incidence in females (ratio 7:1) with a usual
age of onset 20–40 years. The cause of the disease is unknown but it is associated
with the production of abnormal antibodies. In the classical disease the small
joints of the hand are affected. Morning stiffness is a common complaint. The
disease has a remitting course with acute exacerbations followed by quiescent
periods. In severe cases deformity occurs and all joints can be affected.

316

Treatment

General measures

(1) Rest affected joints — use suitable splints.
(2) Active and passive physiotherapy.
(3) Use of heat (radiant heat, paraffin bath).
(4) Encouragement to come to terms with a disease likely to be chronic.

Drug therapy

(1) Anti-inflammatory/analgesic group (*Aspirin, Phenylbutazone, Indomethacin*, ibuprofen, page 117).

This group of agents exerts its therapeutic effects by inhibiting cyclo-oxygenase in a variety of tissues. (Revise the role of prostaglandins in inflammation, page 116). Symptomatic relief can be obtained with any of these drugs, and by adjusting the dose almost the same effect can be obtained from each. Toxicity determines the biggest dose of an individual drug which can be used. Most side-effects are probably related to prostaglandin depletion, for example, gastric erosion, decreased platelet stickiness, salt and water retention, nephrotoxicity, bone marrow depression, asthma. Other side-effects are drug-specific, for example, hypoprothrombinaemia with a high dose of *Aspirin*, potentiation of *Warfarin* by *Phenylbutazone* (pages 217 and 265), hepatic necrosis with an overdose of *Paracetamol*.

Because of the large demand for drugs of this group, continuous research for less toxic drugs is undertaken. More potent derivatives are marketed but are intrinsically better only if they are selective, that is, if they inhibit cyclo-oxygenase in inflammatory tissue at a dose which does not affect gastric mucosal synthesis. (There is the additional problem of high local concentrations of orally administered drug.)

(2) *Penicillamine* (page 119) is the first choice among long-acting drugs. Its effect develops slowly. It acts by immunosuppression. Its toxicity to the kidney and bone marrow (monitor the platelet count and urine protein) is reversible. The maintenance dose should be as low as is compatible with symptomatic control.

(3) Gold salts have been of value in bringing the disease under control, for example, sodium *Aurothiomalate* (page 119). Toxicity is common, especially to the kidney and bone marrow. Dimercaprol chelates gold.

(4) *Chloroquine* (page 119) has been useful as an adjunct to treatment with anti-inflammatory agents. It can cause retinal damage which is usually reversible.

(5) Glucocorticoids in low dosage can provide symptomatic relief in a severe acute attack. In the longer term, with the doses needed to suppress symptoms, a Cushingoid syndrome is inevitable. Osteoporosis is a problem which is accentuated by the underlying disease. Exacerbation of symptoms on withdrawal makes dosage reduction difficult. Glucocorticoids injected into a severely affected joint bypass the systemic route. In general, these drugs are best avoided.

Surgery Correction of deformity and artificial (prosthetic) joints may be required.

GOUT

Gout is a disease featuring recurrent attacks of acute pain and swelling in one joint, typically the big toe, but may involve many joints. It is a disorder of purine metabolism characterized by a raised blood urate (> 0.6 mmol/ℓ) due to the following:

(1) Hereditary predisposition – manifestation unusual under the age of 40 years.
(2) Excessive cell breakdown, for example, lymphoma.
(3) Drugs: (*a*) cytotoxic chemotherapy; (*b*) salicylate (low dose), thiazide diuretics, loop diuretics, Ethanol (by lactate accumulation).
(4) Chronic renal failure.
(5) Starvation (ketoacidosis).

The deposition of urate crystals is responsible for the clinical manifestations. In and around joints it causes arthritis. In the kidney it causes renal damage.

Renal handling of urate is complex. Urate is: (1) filtered at the glomerulus; (2) absorbed in the proximal tubule; (3) secreted in the loop and distal tubule; (4) reabsorbed at these sites.

Net urate excretion depends on the balance of distal secretion and reabsorption. Drugs used to enhance urate excretion (uricosurics) disturb this balance, but only at high doses is excretion increased.

An alternative way to lower blood urate is to inhibit xanthine oxidase, which catalyses the metabolism of purines to urate (via hypoxanthine and xanthine), with *Allopurinol.*

Treatment

Acute gout: symptomatic treatment with an anti-inflammatory drug, initially at high dose which can then be quickly reduced over 3–4 days, for example, *Phenylbutazone, Indomethacin* or *Colchicine* (the last-named is not generally an anti-inflammatory agent but exerts its effect in acute gout by reducing urate crystallization. Its toxicity is related to its antimitotic activity, hence diarrhoea. It can be useful in patients on oral anticoagulants).

Prophylaxis of acute attack

General measures include the following:

(1) Avoid excessive intake of Ethanol.
(2) Eliminate foods known to precipitate an acute attack.
(3) Reduce weight by dietary restriction.

318

Drug therapy

(1) Uricosuric agents (*Probenecid, Sulphinpyrazone*) should not be used if there is renal impairment or a history of urate stones. In the first weeks of treatment: (*a*) fluid intake should be increased to prevent crystallization of urate in the urine; (*b*) anti-inflammatory drugs should be continued as an acute attack may be precipitated.
(2) *Allopurinol* is useful for preventing acute gout and renal impairment in patients with hereditary gout. With hyperuricaemia secondary to the cytotoxic therapy of lymphoma higher doses may be needed. *Allopurinol* may be combined with uricosuric drugs. Administration once daily is adequate.

Drugs and the skin

INFECTIONS

Infestations, page 183; fungal infections, page 189.

Bacterial infections

Staph. aureus

Folliculitis is a small superficial pustule centred on a hair follicle.

Furuncle (boil) is a large, deep, localized collection of pus based on a hair follicle. Stye is a furuncle based on an eyelash follicle.

Acute paronychia (whitlow) is similar to a furuncle but based on a nail fold. A chronic infection here is also common due to bacteria of low pathogenicity, fungi or viruses.

Carbuncle is coalescing deep boils; treat with systemic antibiotic.

Impetigo is a spreading superficial infection of the skin. Because it is superficial topical antibiotics are effective, sodium *Fusidate*, Bacitracin or *Framycetin*. If it is widespread use a systemic antibiotic.

Str. pyogenes

Erysipelas is differentiated from impetigo by an advancing, raised, sharply demarcated edge, thin seropurulent discharge from ruptured vesicles and lymphatic spread. Treat promptly with systemic penicillin (1 per cent suffer allergic acute glomerulonephritis 1—3 weeks later).

Viral infections

Herpes simplex (cold sore) — *Crystal* [gentian] *violet* prevents superinfection, *Idoxuridine* treats the cause (page 203).

Herpes zoster (shingles) — when immunity wanes latent chickenpox virus in the posterior root ganglia spreads down the sensory nerves to invade the dermal segment supplied. Management — analgesics, with *Idoxuridine* for ocular involvement.

Human papilloma virus (warts) — 5—20 per cent regress spontaneously within six months. Treatments which are painful or leave scars are therefore not appropriate. *Salicylic acid collodion paint*, local soaking with Formaldehyde or *Podophyllum resin paint* are chemical alternatives to curettage under local anaesthesia or cryotherapy.

ACNE

Cause

The hair follicles produce too much sebum and too much keratin which is too cohesive. Incidence: 90 per cent in teenagers, declining to 15 per cent at about the age of 25 years; familial tendency. Local sensitivity to androgens.

Clinical features

The pilosebaceous canal is obstructed by a comedone (blackhead). Sebum excessively secreted behind this obstruction blows up the gland. Bacterial colonization and breakdown by lipases lead to a further increase in volume. Rupture initiates an inflammatory response.

Self-management

Sunlight (short of burning) is beneficial in increasing keratin turnover; *Clioquinol* [iodochlorhydroxyquin] (a halogenated hydroxyquinoline) cream is antibacterial.

Treatment

UV irradiation. Keratolytics, for example, benzoyl peroxide, *Resorcinol, Sulphur, Zinc sulphide* [white] *lotion* or tretinoin produce a plug of loosely packed horny cells which unseats the existing comedone. Antibacterial agents, for example, local benzoyl peroxide or oral Oxytetracycline in small doses.

SEBORRHOEIC DERMATITIS

Cause

Excessive sebum secretion (greasy skin) plus low-grade infection.

Clinical features

A recurrent dermatitis with characteristic distribution; scalp shows scaling and hair loss (cradle cap in a baby), in and behind the external ears, eyebrows, nasolabial fold, over the sternum, between the shoulder blades, axillae, pubis and groins.

Management

Cetrimide or *Hexachlorophane* shampoo and *Clioquinol* are antiseptic; *Selenium sulphide* and *Sulphur compound lotion* are irritants causing peeling and kerato-lysis; and if severe *Hydrocortisone* cream.

CONTACT DERMATITIS

Two very different causes operate as follows:

Irritant

Causes — alkali cleaners, abrasives, solvents. Napkin rash is an irritant dermatitis to the ammonia formed by bacterial breakdown of urea. Ensure adequate frequency of napkin changing, cleaning of napkins and use barrier cream.

Sensitization

Causes

Elastic, nickel, rubber, plants.

Antibiotics — penicillins (especially *Ampicillin*), *Streptomycin, Neomycin, Gentamicin, Chloramphenicol, Sulphacetamide*, are all common causes; *Fusidic* acid is an infrequent cause and *Chlortetracycline* a rare one.

Antiseptics — *Iodine* and *Hexachlorophane*; occasionally hydroxyquinolines, rarely *Chlorhexidine*, benzoyl peroxide and *Resorcinol*.

Local anaesthetics — all liable, *Lignocaine* least.

Antihistamines — all liable.

Adhesives — colophony and rubber chemicals but not acrylate monomer.

Vehicles — lanolin (wool fat, wax and alcohol used as emulsifiers in ointments, creams and cosmetics) and parabens (alkylhydroxy-benzoates used as preservatives in creams, lotions and cosmetics).

Incidence

Up to 10 per cent of all patients with dermatitis have allergic contact dermatitis;

1—2 per cent of those with eczema are allergic to lanolin (rare in those with normal skin).

Clinical features

Previous contact with skin is essential for the development of sensitization. Once developed, the whole skin is abnormally reactive, both to skin contact and blood-borne allergen; persists for years and the condition is specific to close chemical analogues of the sensitizer. Occurs more commonly in adults than children and more commonly with damaged skin. Symmetrically distributed rash. History of temporal associations suggests the agent which may then be identifiable by patch testing.

Treatment

Specific — identify the cause and exclude it.

Symptomatic — depends on the stage of skin inflammation.

Acute weeping stage — wet dressings (replace so area never dries) *Calamine lotion, Aluminium acetate lotion.* When weeping stops — *Zinc compound paste* thickly spread over the lesions twice daily.

If dry — *Coal tar paste* (1.5 per cent) or *Zinc and coal tar paste* (6 per cent).

Local anti-inflammatory steroids (systemic if severe); short treatment with intensely active preparation to quickly gain control over the inflammatory process, then a weaker preparation. Secondary infection responds to local *Neomycin* and hydroxyquinolines (which stain clothing).

ATOPIC ECZEMA

Eczema means little more than dermatitis of unknown cause. Incidence is 1—3 per cent, heritable tendency to low itch threshold, deficient sweat and sebum secretion and ready vasodilatation. Scratching produces most of the damage to skin (excoriation, thickening, reddening, exudation, soreness). There is an excessive reactivity of the IgE dependent immune system which is also the basis of seasonal rhinitis and asthma and there are strong associations between all three diseases both in families and individuals. Tend to react to large MW constituents of house-dust, dandruff, kapok, liquorice, tomato, cows milk and egg white.

Clinical features

In infants, begins (at 2—3 months) on face then becomes generalized. Dietary origin relatively common. In childhood (1.5—7 years) flexures are most affected and inhaled allergen is commoner. Tends to decline in steps at puberty and at 18 years.

Treatment

Avoid any demonstrable cause. Bath baby with emulsifying ointment. Maintain control with intermittent weak local glucocorticoids. For infection — antibiotics and hydroxyquinolines. If severe — wet dressings, intermittent intense topical glucocorticoids, *Prednisolone* orally.

PSORIASIS

A genetically transmitted tendency to a ten-times faster than normal epithelial cell proliferation rate.

Incidence

2—3 per cent of population. Onset 25—60 years. Triggered by normal stimuli to cell multiplication, commonly subject to spontaneous remissions and recurrences.

Clinical features

Well defined plaques of red thickened skin covered with loose silvery scales. Commonest sites — scalp, elbows, knees and knuckles.

Management

Sunlight (the 280—320 nm band) is beneficial. Various irritants have been found empirically to hasten remission: *Calamine and coal tar ointment* (0.5 per cent coal tar content), *Coal tar and salicylic acid ointment* (2 per cent coal tar for the scalp) are effective but messy; *Ichthammol cream* is another example but the standard treatment in this irritant group is *Dithranol* [anthralin] *paste* (the dithranol can be prepared at the prescribed concentration in *Zinc compound paste* (zinc and salicylic acid paste, Lassars' paste). Irritant preparations for addition to the bath water have little effect.

Some dermatology clinics offer the combination of long-wave UV irradiation (320—400 nm) with a psoralen (for example, trimethylpsoralen [trioxsalen]; chemicals, naturally occurring in some plant saps, which interact with skin and sunlight to produce phototoxic dermatitis) which, when activated by UV, binds to DNA. Severe cases may also be offered *Methotrexate* in low dosage.

Dilute anti-inflammatory steroid creams (which should be discarded after 2—3 weeks) or a brief treatment with full strength glucocorticoids are also effective but not without danger.

TOPICAL STEROIDS

These are so effective (though only providing symptomatic relief) and so widely used that an appreciation of their limitations is essential. They are non-specifically anti-inflammatory and patients with dermatitis, eczema and psoriasis frequently demand them having heard of their efficiency from other patients.

They are contraindicated in any infected condition (whether fungal or bacterial) for they mask the inflammatory response to, and therefore the signs of, infection. For maximum effect (3−10 per cent of applied dose can enter the skin) the vehicle and diluent are critical; a soft, white, paraffin-based ointment in the simplest satisfactory base, creams, lotions and propylene glycol diluents all inter-fere with activity. The intensity of the effect obtained depends on the potency of the drug used and the dose administered − to avoid undesirable side-effects the least intensity which will control the disease should be used.

Fluocinolone 0.025 per cent and *Betamethasone* 0.1 per cent are equieffective.

Fluocinolone 0.01 per cent is more effective than *Hydrocortisone* 1 per cent.

Local complications

As well as masking the signs of infection, they predispose to infection. They also cause skin atrophy (both dermal and epidermal), telangiectasia (groups of visible dilated small blood vessels), purpura and striae. These effects are maximal with more intensely active preparations, used on the face, in the younger patients and for long treatment times.

Systemic complications

Uncommon toxicity identical to that of systemic glucocorticoids, due to systemic absorption, therefore seen with extensive application, to permeable skin and occlusive dressings.

SUNLIGHT

Sunscreens

The normal skin is burnt by 290−320 nm radiation. *Aminobenzoic acid lotion,* if generously applied, will effectively screen out these wavelengths. Sensitive skins may react to the same wavelength as normal skins, or to the longer wavelengths. Screens for these are *Titanium dioxide paste* which is more effective than *Mexenone.*

Drugs causing sunlight sensitization

Sulphonamides, tetracyclines, *Griseofulvin*, phenothiazines (for example, *Chlorpromazine*), gold salts, Diphenhydramine, protriptyline, *Nalidixic* acid and local tar applications.

'COUGHS AND COLDS'

Bronchial mucosa normally has ciliated columnar cells with few goblet (mucus secreting) cells. Mucus is also secreted by submucous glands (vagal innervation).

Cilia beat rhythmically and move upward a layer of fluid (sol) on which the mucus (gel) floats to be eventually swallowed.

Expectorants increase mucociliary clearance — assessed by measuring the rate of removal of inhaled radioactive microspheres from the lungs.

Menthol may act as irritant but steam inhalation alone is effective.

Guaiphenesin increases mucociliary clearance (usefulness unproven).

Mucolytics (lit: break down mucus) — assessed by measuring sputum viscosity at different shear rates.

Acetylcystein and bromhexine are of uncertain efficacy and the latter may only become effective after 5 day's administration.

Fragmentation of mucus may interfere with ciliary movement.

A cough is abnormal — powerful reflex elicited by irritation of receptors in trachea and bronchi — explosive expiration and increased mucus secretion.

Cough is caused by:
Mechanical stimulation (foreign body, secretions).
Mediators of inflammation (allergy, infection).
Changes in airway calibre.
Distortion of airways.

Inhaled irritants (ether, SO_2, cigarette smoke*, citric acid)

Antitussives (lit: against cough) — assessed by ability to suppress cough induced by a citric acid aerosol.

Only a cough unproductive of sputum should be suppressed. Narcotic analgesics are most effective; for example, *Heroin*. **Codeine** is more potent than the selective antitussive **Dextromethorphan** (page 147).

The common cold (coryza) is a viral infection. Symptomatic relief only is available — a salicylate (antipyretic) plus an indirect sympathomimetic (decongestant); use the cheapest soluble formulation.

Sinusitis (inflammation of the air sinuses within the facial bones and communicating with the nose) is a complication — intranasal *Ephedrine* (or analogue) shrinks mucosa and permits drainage. An antibiotic may be needed.

Allergic rhinitis (hay fever, summer cold) follows exposure to seasonal allergen (for example, pollen). Perennial rhinitis is due to continual exposure to allergens (for example, house dust mite); symptoms throughout the year.

Intranasal **Cromoglycate** or *Beclomethasone* help. Desensitization occasionally cures. Antihistamines cause sedation (beware interaction with Ethanol) and are of uncertain benefit.

---

* Smokers have many more goblet cells and fewer ciliated cells than normal. If they cough up mucus daily they have chronic bronchitis.

Suggested further reading

Albert, A. (1979). *Selective Toxicity*, 6th edition. London: Methuen

Albert, A. (1975). *The Selectivity of Drugs*. London: Chapman and Hall

Bowman, W.C. and Rand, M.J. (1980). *Textbook of Pharmacology*, 2nd edition. Oxford: Blackwell.

British National Formulary, 1982 Number 3. London: British Medical Association and The Pharmaceutical Press

Brotherton, J. (1976). *Sex Hormone Pharmacology*. London: Academic Society of Great Britain

Cooper, J.R., Bloom, F.E. and Roth, R.H. (1978). *The Biochemical Basis of Neuropharmacology*. New York: Oxford University Press

Day, M.D. (1979). *Autonomic Pharmacology. Experimental and Clinical Aspects*. Edinburgh: Churchill-Livingstone

Drug and Therapeutic Bulletin. Hertford: Consumer's Association

Franklin, J.J. and Snow, G.A. (1975). *Biochemistry of Antimicrobial Action*, 2nd edition. London: Chapman and Hall

Garrod, L.P., Lambert, H.P. and O'Grady, F. (1973). *Antibiotic and Chemotherapy*, 4th edition. Edinburgh: Churchill-Livingstone

Goldstein, A., Aronow, L. and Kalman, S.M. (1974). *Principles of Drug Action*, 2nd edition. New York: Wiley

Goodman, L.S. and Gilman, A. (1980). *The Pharmacological Basis of Therapeutics*, 6th edition. New York: Macmillan

Hall, R., Anderson, J., Smart, G.A. and Besser, M. (1975). *Fundamentals of Clinical Endocrinology*. London: Pitman Medical

Hogarth, P.J. (1978). *Biology of Reproduction*. Glasgow: Blackie

Kruk, Z.L. and Pycock, C.J. (1979). *Neurotransmitters and Drugs*. London: Croom Helm

Laurence, D.R. and Bennett, P.N. (1980). *Clinical Pharmacology*. Edinburgh: Churchill-Livingstone

Laurence, D.R. and Black, J.W. (1978). *The Medicine You Take*. Fontana Paperbacks

Lee, J. and Laycock, J. (1978). *Essential Endocrinology*. Oxford: Oxford Medical Publications

Melmon, K.L. and Morrelli, H.F. (1978). *Clinical Pharmacology*, 2nd edition. New York: Macmillan

Prescriber's Journal, Hannibal House, Elephant and Castle, London

Ryall, R.W. (1979). *Mechanisms of Drug Action on the Nervous System*. Cambridge: Cambridge University Press

Smith, S.E. and Rawlins, M.D. (1973). *Variability in Human Drug Response*. London: Butterworths

Tausk, M. (1975). *Pharmacology of Hormones*. Chicago: Year Book Medical Publishers; Stuttgart: Thieme

WHO Expert Committee, (1977) Technical Report Series, 615, *The Selection of Essential Drugs*. Geneva: WHO

Index

Additional references for drug groups marked (*) may be found under individual agents

Abortion, induction of, 309–310
Abortion, habitual, 113
Abscess cavities, drug distribution into, 316
Absences (petit mal) epileptic attacks, 302
Absorption, of drugs,
  acidic drugs, 243
  basic drugs, 247
  bronchial mucosa, 211
  buccal mucosa, 211
  carrier mediated transport, 210
  definition, 209
  delayed release formulations, 212–213
  eye, 215
  injection, 212
  mucous membranes, 210
  nasal mucosa, 211
  rectal mucosa, 211
  sites of absorption, 210–212
  skin, 211–212
  small intestine, 210
  sustained release formulations, 212–213
  tablets and capsules, 210
  water filled pores, 210
Abuse of drugs, 251–255
Accommodation, of the eye, 8–9
Accumulation, of drugs, 228–229
Acetaldehyde, 164
Acetaldehyde dehydrogenase, 165
Acetaminophen, 118
Acetazolamide,
  anticonvulsant, 304
  carbonic anhydrase inhibitor, 105
  drug poisoning, use in, 268
  pKa, 242–243
Acetone, 157

Acetylcholine (*see also* Cholinergic transmission), 15
  arterioles of skeletal muscle, 13
  central neurotransmission, 127
  formula, 20
  ganglionic transmission, 25–27
  hydrolysis, 17, 19, 26, 31, 35, 36
  muscarinic receptors, 31
  effects, summary, 32
  neuromuscular transmission, focally innervated, 19–23
  neuromuscular transmission, multiply innervated, 23–25
  parasympathetic nervous system, in, 4
  peripheral transmitter, summary, 3
  release, 16, 19, 26, 31
  synthesis, 17–19, 26, 31
Acetylcholinesterase, 17, 35
Acetylcysteine, 325
Acetyl kinase, 18
Acetylsalicylic acid (*see also* Aspirin), 118
Achlorhydria, 314
Acidic drugs, 242–245
  absorption, 243, 244
  distribution, 214–215, 230, 244
  examples, 242
  models, of disposition, 230
  pharmacokinetic characteristics, 243
  pKa values, 243
  protein binding, 217
  renal clearance, 220
Acidosis, metabolic, 105–106
Acne, 222, 320
Acromegaly, 75

ACTH-endorphin prohormone, 143
ACTH-releasing factor, 74, 98, 101
Actinomycin D, 204, 206
Action potential,
  acetylcholine release, 19, 20
  conduction, 16
  ganglia, 26, 27
  local anaesthetics, 57
  noradrenergic neurones, 42
Activated carbon, 268
  paraquat poisoning, 221
Active tubular reabsorption, 220
Acupuncture, 145
Acute intermittent porphyria, 162, 258
Addiction, *see* Dependence, physical
Adenylate cyclase, 46, 153
Adipocytes, β-agonists on, 46
Adrenal cortex, 78, 98–101
Adrenal insufficiency, 99, 100
Adrenaline,
  actions, summary, 55
  adrenal medulla, synthesis, 55
  agonist activity, 45
  central neurotransmission, 127
  histamine, functional antagonism of, 72
  hypoglycaemia, 97
  insulin release, 95
  local anaesthetics, combination with, 60
  monoamine oxidase, 53
  pKa, 247
  structure, 47
  therapeutic use, 47, 290
  uptake into neurones, 53
Adrenal medulla, 5, 7
  angiotensin, 102
  phaeochromocytoma, 284
  secretions, 55–56

327

Adrenergic neurone blocking
 agents (*see under* Nor-
 adrenergic neurone
 blocking agents)
α-Adrenoceptors (*see also*
 Agonists, Antagonists
 and tissues location), 45
β-Adrenoceptors (*see also*
 Agonists, Antagonists and
 tissues location), 45–46
*α-Adrenoceptor agonists,
 44–49, 97
*β-Adrenoceptor agonists, 44–49
*α-Adrenoceptor antagonists,
 44–48, 50
 5-hydroxytryptamine,
 antagonism of, 111
 neuroleptics as, 142
 potency ratios, 45
 therapeutic use, 50–51
*β-Adrenoceptor antagonists,
 44–48, 51
 angina, use in, 51, 286
 Digoxin toxicity, 51
 hypertension, use in, 51, 281
 insulin release, 97
 potency ratios, 45
 selectivity (β_1 and β_2
 receptors), 45, 51
 thyrotoxicosis, 51, 92–93
Adrenocorticotrophic hormone
 (ACTH), 74
 corticosteroid release, 98, 100
 diabetes, 97
 steroid synthesis, effect on,
 78
 therapeutic use, 99, 101
Advertising, of drugs, 255
Aerosols, 291
Afferent, neurones, 2
Affinity constant, equilibrium,
 68, 226
 protein binding, 217–218
Age,
 antibacterial drugs, response
 to, 195
 water soluble drugs, disposition of, 231
Agonist,
 description, 68–69
 partial, 69
Agoraphobia, 295
Akinesia, 131
D-Alanine, 172
Alanine racemase, 172
D-Alanyl-D-alanine, 172
D-Alanyl-D-alanine synthetase,
 172
Alcohol dehydrogenase, 164–
 165
Alcoholism (*see* Ethanol
 dependence)
*Alcohols, 164–165
Aldehyde dehydrogenase, 110, 240
Aldosterone, 98, 101
 antagonists, 105–106
 renal function, 103
 synthesis, 77

*Alkylating agents, 175,
 206–207
 antispermatogenic action, 89
 developmental toxicity, 262
 emetic action, 300
 resistance, 207
Allele, 257
Allergens, 288, 321–322, 325
Allergic rhinitis, 325
Allergy, *see also* individual
 disorders, 107, 110, 115,
 148, 257, 287, 316
Allopurinol, 206, 266, 318–319
Alloxan, 97
Alphadolone, 162
Alphaxalone, 162
Althesin®, 157, 162
Aluminium acetate lotion, 322
Aluminium hydroxide, 271
Amantadine,
 antiviral action, 202–203
 Parkinson's disease, 131
Amaranth, model of drug
 disposition, 226
Amethocaine, 56
 pKa and use, 60
Amiloride, 105, 278
Aminoacids, neurotrans-
 mitters, 127
p-Aminobenzoate, 60, 173
Aminobenzoic acid lotion, 324
γ-Aminobutyric acid, 127,
 150, 304
 antagonists, 152
Aminocaproic acid, 123
Aminoglutethimide, 101
Aminohipporate, 215
δ-Aminolaevulinic acid, 259
4-Aminoquinolines,
 mechanism, 179
 resistance, 179
*Aminosugar antibiotics, 199
 distribution, 177, 199, 321
 elimination, 199, 321
 mechanism of action, 177
 neuromuscular blocking
 agents, interaction with,
 23
 resistance, 177, 195
 spectrum, 177
 toxicity, 177, 199
Aminophylline, 153
 absorption, 211
 asthma, 153, 290–291
 diuretic action, 106
 heart failure, 277–278
 pulmonary oedema, 277, 284
Amitryptyline, 55, 135–136,
 299
Albumin, plasma binding, 217–
 218
Ammonium chloride, 106
Amnesia, 164
Amoebiasis, 177, 187–188
Amoxycillin, 197
Amphetamine, 41, 151
 anorexia, 151, 310–311
 central actions, 130, 151
 drug laws, 253

Amphetamine (*cont.*)
 hallucinations, 153
 mechanism of action, 151
 monoamine oxidase, 53,
 151
 narcolepsy, 151
 pharmacokinetics, 249
 pKa, 247
 poisoning, 151
 structure, 48
 therapeutic use, 151, 166
Amphotericin, 178, 190
Ampicillin, 197
 dose, 194
 elimination, 194, 197
 minimal inhibitory concentration, 193
 principal uses, 192
 spectrum, 197
 $t_{1/2}$, 194
 toxicity, 198
Amygdala, 129, 130
Amyl nitrite, absorption, 211
Amylobarbitone, 166
*Anabolic steroids, 87
Anaemias, 312–316
Anaesthesia, 158–160
*Anaesthetics (*see also* local,
 general and inhalation
 anaesthetics), 160–162
Anaesthetic premedication,
 162, 164
*Analeptics, *see* Convulsants,
 152
Analgesia, 145
*Analgesics,
 antipyretic, 154–156
 general anaesthetics, 161
 narcotic, 145–147
Anaphylaxis, 289
 ACTH in, 99
 Adrenaline, 47
 histamine and antihistamines,
 108–109
 5-hydroxytryptamine, 110
Ancylostoma, 185
*Androgens, 80, 86–89, 261–
 262
Androgen antagonists, 88
Androstenedione, 77
Angina, 285–287
Angiotensin II, 98, 101–102,
 128
Angiotensin I, 101
Angiotensinogen, 98, 101
Aniline, pKa, 215
Anopheline mosquito, 188
*Anorectic agents, 96, 151,
 301–311
Anorexia nervosa, 311–312
Anovulation, 113
*Antacids, 265, 270–271
Antagonism,
 competitive, 69–70
 description, 68–69
 functional, 71–72
 indirect, 71
 non-competitive, 70–71
 surmountable, 70

p.g. 241

Antagonism (*cont.*)
unsurmountable, 71
Anterior pituitary, *see*
Pituitary, 74
Anthraquinones, laxatives, 275
Anti-anergic agents, 208
Anti-arrhythmic drugs, 60–64,
275–276
basic nature, 246
Lignocaine, 63–64, 276
local anaesthetics, 60
muscarinic antagonism, 33
Oxprenolol, 63
Phenytoin, 63–64, 276
pKa, 247
Procainamide, 62–63
Propranolol, 63
Quinidine, 62–63
Antibody, 170, 287
*Anticoagulants, 120–123
Anticholinesterase agents (*see*
Cholinesterase inhibitors),
35
*Anticonvulsants, 303–306
benzodiazepines, 164, 304–
305
Carbamazepine, 303, 305–
306
carbonic anhydrase inhibi-
tors, 303, 304
developmental toxicity, 267
Ethosuximide, 304, 305
mechanism of action, 167,
303
membrane stabilization, 303
Phenobarbitone, 304, 306
Phenytoin, 303–306
poisoning, 267–268
Sodium valproate, 305–306
*Antidepressants (*see* Tricyclic
and monoamineoxidase
inhibitors), 135, 136
Antidiuretic hormone ADH, 73
renal function, 103
*Anti-emetics, 109, 205, 300–
301
Antigen-antibody reaction (of
anaphylaxis), 108–109
*Antihistamines, 109–110
basic nature, 246
central actions, 131
Ethanol, interaction with,
264
histamine release, 108
inflammation, 117
pKa, 247
rhinitis, 325
selectivity, 109
side effects, 109
therapeutic use, 109–110
*Antihypertensive drugs, 279–
284
*Anti-inflammatory drugs, 117–
119, 155, 242, 316–319
*Analgesic-antipyretic drugs,
118, 270, 317
Chloroquine, 119
*Corticosteroids, 119, 324
gold compounds, 119, 315

Anti-inflammatory drugs (*cont.*)
gout, 318
Penicillamine, 119
rheumatoid arthritis, 316
*Antimetabolites, 205–206
Antineoplastic drugs, *see also*
Neoplastic disease, 203
Antiparasitic drugs, 169–208
classification, 171
concept, 170
biochemical selectivity, 170
distributional selectivity, 179
Antiparkinson drugs, 33–34,
131–132
Antipsychotic drugs (*see*
Neuroleptic drugs), 139–
142
Antipyresis, 154
*Antipyretic analgesics, 118–
119, 154–156, 292, 325
Antiseptics, 183
Antispermatogenic chemicals,
89
Antitussive agents (*see* Cough
suppressants), 146, 325
Antiviral agents, 202–203,
319–320
Anxiety, 133–134, 158
*Anxiolytics, 158, 163–167,
296–297
anaesthetic premedication,
162
definition, 159–160
insomnia, 158
poisoning, 254, 267
prescribing figures, 255
Aplastic anaemia, 315
Apomorphine, 141, 148
Appetite (*see also* Anorectic
agents), 310–312
Aqueous humour, 9
Arachidonic acid, 112, 113
Arachnid infestation, 169
Area postrema, 131
Aromatic L-aminoacid
decarboxylase, 40, 110,
131
Arrhythmias, cardiac (*see also*
anti-arrhythmic drugs),
61–64
Arsenicals, organic, 315
Arterioles, external genitalia,
13
skeletal muscle, 13, 30
Arthritis, 316–318
Artificial kidney, 221
Ascaris infestation, 178, 179,
185–186
Ascorbic acid, use with iron
preparations, 313
Asparaginase, 206
Aspirin,
anaemia, cause of, 313
anticoagulants, interaction
with, 122, 264
anti-inflammatory action,
118
analgesia, 155, 292
antipyresis, 155

Aspirin (cont.)
cyclo-oxygenase inhibition,
113, 114, 117, 155
gastrointestinal effects,
156, 212, 293, 313
headache, 292
hypersensitivity, 257
migraine, 294
narcotic analgesics, interaction with, 146, 263
pharmacokinetics, 242
pKa, 243
poisoning, 118, 254
prothrombin, 118, 264
respiratory effects, 118, 155
rheumatic fever, 316
rheumatoid arthritis, 316
site of action, 118
social use, 254
solubility, pH dependence,
210
soluble preparations, 156,
293
toxic effects, 118
uricosuric action, 118
Association rate constant, 68
Asthma, 35, 48, 51, 100,
109–110, 148, 153,
287–292
β-adrenoceptor agonists,
288, 290
aetiology, 287–288
allergens, 288
antihistamines, 109, 291
contraindications, 291
corticosteroids, 100, 290
definition, 287
diagnosis, 289–290
epidemiology, 292
extrinsic, 287–289
intrinsic, 288
methylxanthines, 153, 288
muscarinic antagonists, 291
narcotic analgesics, 148, 291
pathogenesis, 288–289
Propranolol, 51, 291
Sodium cromoglycate, 110,
288, 290
status asthmaticus, 291
Astrocytes, 214
Ataractic drugs (*see* Neuroleptic
drugs), 139–142
Ataxia, 159
Atherosclerosis, 114, 285
Athlete's foot, 191
Atopy, 287
ATP
acetylcholine synthesis, 18
noradrenaline storage and
release, 41, 43
methylxanthines, 153
ATPase, magnesium depen-
dent, 41, 275
Atrioventricular node, 10, 14
β-adrenoceptor agonists, 46
heart block, 61
Atrial flutter, 63
Atropine, 19, 25, 31, 33

Atropine (cont.)
anaesthetic premedication,
162
clinical use, 34
competitive antagonism, 70
histamine release, 108
Parkinson's disease, 131
pKa, 247
toxicity, 33, 302
Atropine methonitrate, 33, 249,
291
Autonomic nervous system, 2
effectors, 8–14
parasympathetic division, 2
organization, 4, 14
sympathetic division, 2, 14
organization, 3, 5–8
Autosomal autonomous genetic
idiosyncrasy, 257
Autosomal dominant genetic
idiosyncrasy, 257–258
Autosomal recessive genetic
idiosyncrasy, 257
Azathioprine, 175, 205, 206,
266

Bacitracin,
mechanism of action, 172,
178
toxicity, 182
use, 319
Bacterial infections, 191–201,
216
Bacteriological diagnosis, 192
Bacteriostatic–bactericidal
mixtures, 195
Bacteroides, 178, 192, 193
Barbitone,
dialysis, 221
pKa, 215
*Barbiturates, 157, 165–166
acute intermittent porphyria,
162, 258
anticoagulants, interaction
with, 122
dependence, 166, 254
drug laws, 253
gonadotrophin secretion, 75
narcotic analgesics, interaction with, 146
oral contraceptives, interaction with, 86
poisoning, 152, 166, 254,
268
protein binding and lipid
solubility, 237
structure, 162
therapeutic use, 166
tolerance, 166
tricyclic antidepressants,
interaction with, 135
Basic drugs, 245–250
absorption, 247
distribution, 214–215, 230
models of disposition, 230
renal excretion, 220, 247
Basophils, histamine, 107
Beef extracts, tyramine content, 53

Beclomethasone, 100
anti-inflammatory action,
119
asthma, 290
rhinitis, 325
Belladonna, 131
Bendrofluazide,
disposition of, 242
heart failure, use in, 277
hypertension, use in, 280
mechanism, 104
Bendroflumethazide (*see
Bendrofluazide*), 104
Benserazide, 40, 131
Benzalkonium, 183
Benzene, metabolism of, 224
Benzhexol, 33, 34
Parkinson's disease, 131,
141
*Benzodiazepines (*see also*
Anxiolytics), 163–164,
296–297
central actions, 163–164
depression, aggravation of,
298
drugs, differences between,
164, 296
Ethanol, interaction with,
264
poisoning, 166
structure, 162
Benzoic acid, 191
*Benzothiadiazides (thiazides),
104
Benzoyl peroxide, 320
Benztropine, 131
Benzyl benzoate, 185
Benzylpenicillin, 196, 197
CSF, active transport out
of, 215
dose, 194
elimination, 194, 197, 220
eye, active transport out of,
215
minimal inhibitory concentration, 193
pKa, 243
Probenecid, 197
spectrum, 197
t½, 194
use, principal, 191
Bephenium, 182, 185, 186
Betamethasone, 100, 119, 324
Bethanidine, 42, 54, 60, 282
Bicarbonate ion,
antacid, use as, 270
carbonic anhydrase inhibition,
105
poisoning by salicylates and
barbiturates, 268
renal function, 103
Bicuculline, 152
Bicyclic antidepressants, 135,
136
Biguanides, hypoglycaemics,
96
Bile, drug excretion in, 222
Bilharzia, 185

Biochemical selectivity, anti-
parasitic drugs, 170–179
Biotransformation, of drugs,
see Metabolism, 222–224
Bisacodyl, 275
Bladder (*see* Urinary bladder),
11
Blastocyst, 76, 259–260
Blood coagulation, 120–123
Aspirin, 118
Heparin, 121
mechanism of, 120
oestrogens, 81
oral contraceptives, 86
platelet adhesiveness, 121
thrombus dissolution,
122–123
thrombus formation, 120
Blood, drugs and (*see also*
Anaemia), 312–316
Bone, drug disposition in, 216
Borrelia vincenti, 178
Botulinus toxin, 17
Bradycardia, 10
Bradykinin, 97, 114–115, 117
Bran, laxative, 274
Breast feeding, drug secretion
in, 222
Bromhexine, 325
Bromocriptine, 75, 83, 131
Bronchial glands, 32, 34
Bronchioles, 32
Bronchitis, drugs of choice,
192
Buccal mucosa, drug absorp-
tion, 211
α-Bungarotoxin, 19, 22–25,
31, 71
Bungarus multicinctus, 23
Buprenorphine, 145, 150
Busulphan, 89, 176, 207, 262
Butobarbitone, 166
*Butyrophenones, 140–142,
297

Cadaverine, 220
Caffeine, 152–153
anti-inflammatory action,
119
central stimulation, 152–153
diuretic action, 106, 152
fatigue, 152–153
insomnia, 158
migraine, 294–295
percutaneous absorption, 211
smooth muscle relaxation,
152–153
Calamine and coal tar ointment,
323
Calamine lotion, 322
Calcium antagonists, 287
Calcium flux, 19, 23
Calcium folinate, 206
Calcium ions,
acetyl choline release, 16
action potential, 16, 19
adrenaline release, 55
blood coagulation, 120
chelation, 120, 199, 264

Calcium ions (*cont.*)
  degranulation, 289
  local anaesthetics, 58
  noradrenaline release, 43–44, 54
  precipitation, 120
Calorific values, of foods, 311
Camphor, absorption, 211
Candidiasis, 182, 191
Cannabis,
  drug laws, 253
  hallucinogenic action, 153
  social use, 254
Capacitance vessels, angina, 286
Capsules, disintegration and solution, 210
Carbachol, 19, 21, 24–25, 31–32, 35
  formula, 20
  clinical use, 33
Carbamazepine, 303–304
Carbenicillin, 197
  incompatibility, drug, 265
  principal uses, 192
Carbenoxolone, 271
  diuretics, interaction with, 264
Carbidopa, 40, 131
Carbimazole, 91, 242
  developmental toxicity, 262
  placental transfer, 216
Carbohydrate metabolism, 94, 99
β-Carboline, 164
Carbon, activated, paraquat poisoning, 221
Carbonic anhydrase, 103, 242
*Carbonic anhydrase inhibitors, 105, 303–304
Carbuncle, 319
Carcinoid tumour, 110, 111, 115
Cardiac arrhythmias, 51, 161, 276–277
*Cardiac glycosides, 102, 275–276
  arrhythmias, 61
  mechanism of action, 275–276
  toxicity, 276
Cardiac pacemaker (*see* Sino-atrial node)
Catecholamine, definition (*see also* Sympatho-mimetic), 47
Carrier mediated transport, 67, 210
Cascara, 275
Catatonia, neuroleptic induced, 140, 164
Catechol-O-methyl transferase, 52–53
Caudate nucleus, 129, 130, 141
Cell wall synthesis, parasitic, 170–172
Central nervous system neurotransmitters, 125–130

Central nervous system neurotransmitters (*cont.*)
  acetylcholine, 127, 128, 132, 135–136
  adrenaline, 127
  angiotensin II, 128
  γ-aminobutyric acid, 127, 150, 152, 164
  dopamine, 127, 129–130, 132, 140, 151, 154
  β-endorphin, 128, 143, 145, 153, 154
  enkephalins, 128, 143, 153
  excitatory, 126, 150
  glutamic acid, 127
  glycine, 127, 128, 150
  histamine, 127
  5-hydroxytryptamine, 127, 130, 135, 136, 153, 154
  inhibitory, 126, 150
  noradrenaline, 127, 129–130, 135–136, 151
  proof of transmitter function, 126–127
  somatostatin, 128
  substance P, 128, 155
  taurine, 127
Cephalexin, 194, 198
Cephaloridine, 194, 198
*Cephalosporins, 198
  cephalosporinase, 172
  elimination, 194
  dose, 194
  mechanism of action, 172
  minimal inhibitory concentration, 193
  principal uses, 191
  resistance, 172
  spectrum, 172
  $t_{1/2}$, 194
Cephalosporinase, 172
Cephalothin, 198
Cerebellum, 129
Cerebral cortex, 129, 130
Cerebral palsy, mercury toxicity, 262
Cerebrospinal fluid, active transport, 215
Cervix, oestrogens, 81
Cetrimide, 183, 321
Chalk, 273
Cheese, tyramine content of, 53
Chelation, 119, 199, 268
Chemosensitive trigger zone, 131
  Apomorphine, 141
  Aspirin, 156
  oestrogens, 156
  opiates, 100
Chemotherapeutic index, 170
Chickenpox, 202
Chlamydiae, 170
Chloral hydrate, 157, 165
Chlorambucil, 175, 206, 262

Chloramphenicol, 177, 200
  aplastic anaemia, 259, 315
  allergy, 182
  mechanism of action, 177
  metabolism, 200, 266
  principal uses, 192, 200
  spectrum, 177
  toxicity, 177, 200, 264
  resistance, 195
Chlorate ion, dialysis of, 221
Chlordiazepoxide, 157, 164, 296
Chlorhexidine, 183
α-Chlorhydrin, 89
Chloride ions,
  acetylcholine release, 16
  high ceiling diuretics, 104
  renal function, 103
Chloroform, 66, 157, 159
Chloroquine, 179, 188–189
  amoebiasis, 187
  anti-inflammatory action, 119
  glucose-6-phosphate dehydrogenase deficiency, 259
  mechanism of action, 179, 190
  resistance, 179, 190, 207
  rheumatoid arthritis, 317
Chlorothiazide, 104
Chlorpheniramine, 109
Chlorpromazine, 140–142
  α-adrenoceptor antagonism, 45, 50, 142
  antiemetic action, 141, 297
  antivertigo, 297
  anorexia nervosa, 312
  behavioural effects, 140
  blurring of vision, 142
  extrapyramidal effects, 140–141, 297
  hypotension, 51, 142, 297
  hypothermia, 142
  mechanism of action, 126, 130
  Menière's disease, 297
  metabolism, 224
  muscarinic antagonism, 142
  narcotic analgesics, interaction with, 142, 297
  therapeutic use, 51, 140, 151
Chlorpropamide, 95
  Ethanol metabolism, 165, 266
  hypersensitivity, 315
Chlortetracycline, 199
Chlorthalidone, 104, 280
Cholangiography, 243
Cholecystitis, 197
Cholesterol, synthesis, 77
Cholestgramine, 265
Choline acetyltransferase, 18
Cholinergic transmission, 15–19, 26, 31
Cholinesterase (*see also* Acetyl-cholinesterase), 22, 35–38
*Cholinesterase inhibitors, 36–38

Cholinesterase inhibitors (*cont.*)
  competitive, 36
    basic nature, 246
    pKa, 247
    structural characteristics,
      36
    uses, 38
  non-competitive, 37
    absorption, 38
    insecticides, use as, 180
    poisoning, 268
    use, 38
Choline theophyllinate, 153
Choline, uptake of, 17, 26
  excretion, 220
Cholinoceptors, 17
  muscarinic, 19, 30–35
  nicotinic, 18
    ganglia, 25–30
    skeletal muscle, 18–19,
      21–22, 24–25
Choroid plexus, active trans-
    port, 215
Choriocarcinoma, 174
Chromatin, steroid drugs, 80
Chromogranin, 43
Ciliary ganglion, 4
Ciliary muscle, 4, 8–9, 14, 29,
    32, 34
Cimetidine, 110, 271
Cinchocaine, 35
Cinchocaine (dibucaine)
    number, 35, 258
Cingulate gyrus, 129
Citrate, anticoagulant, 120
Citric acid cycle, 93
Clearance (*see* creatinine
    clearance), 225
  renal plasma clearance,
    219, 225
  total drug clearance, 219
Cleft lip and palate, 262
Clindamycin, 177, 191, 200
Clioquinol, 320, 321
Clomiphene, 75, 83
Clonazepam, 296
Clonidine, 282, 294
Clostridium difficile, 178, 200
Clostridium perfringens, 192,
    193
Clotrimazole, 191
Cloxacillin, 197
  dose, 194
  elimination, 194
  minimal inhibitory concen-
    tration, 193
  principal uses, 191
  t½, 194
Coal tar paste, 322
*Coal tar and salicylic acid
    ointment*, 323
Cocaine,
  central actions, 60, 129–130
  drug laws, 253
  hallucinogenic action, 153
  local anaesthetic action,
    56, 60
  noradrenergic neurone
    blocking agents, 43

Cocaine (*cont.*)
  pKa, 60, 247
  sympathomimetic actions,
    48
  uptake of noradrenaline,
    effect on, 49, 53
Codeine,
  constipative action, 273
  cough suppression, 147, 325
  drug laws, 253
  excitatory–depressant
    ratio, 146
  headache, 292
  histamine release, 147
  potency, 146
  side effects, 318
Colchicine, 318
Colds, 325
Cold sores, 319
Collagenase, 117
Colliculi, superior and
    inferior, 129
Colloid injection, 213
Colistin, 178
Coma, 159
Comedone, 320
Competitive antagonism,
    69–70
Compliance, 194, 254–255
Compound 48/80, 108
Concentration–response
    relationships, 65–66
Condom, contraceptive, 307
Conjugates, metabolites of
    drugs, 220, 224
  tubular secretion, 220
  water solubility, 231
Consciousness, 156
Constipation, treatment of,
    274–275
Constipative agents, 272–273
Contraceptives (*see also* Oral
    contraceptives), 75, 83,
    306–310
Controlled Drugs, 253
Convoluted tubule, function,
    103
Convulsants, 152
Coombs' test, 283, 316
Copper poisoning, 300
Copper sulphate, 300
*Corticosteroids, 98–101
  actions, 99
  ACTH suppression, 100
  anti-inflammatory action,
    99–100
  asthma, 290, 291
  glucocorticoids, 99–100
  gut superinfection, 191
  insulin release, 97
  metabolic effects, 99
  mineralcorticoids, 99–100
  protein binding, 99
  release, 98–99
  side effects, 100–101
  synthesis, 77, 98–99, 101
  t½, 100
  therapeutic uses, 100, 290
  topical use, 324

Corticosterone, 77, 98, 101
Corti, organ of, 199
Corticotrophin (*see* ACTH),
    98–101
Cortisone, 100
Corynebacterium diphtheriae,
    drugs of choice, 191
Coryza, 325
Co-trimoxazole, 174, 194, 196
  dose, 194
  elimination, 194
  principal uses, 192
  t½, 194, 228
Coumarins, 122
Cough, 146, 325
Cranial nerves, 2, 4
Cretinism, 262
Crohn's disease, 196
Cromoglycate (*see also* Sodium
    Cromoglycate), 110, 290,
    325
Cromolyn sodium (*see also*
    Sodium *Cromoglycate*),
Crystal violet, 319
Cushing's syndrome, 100, 317
Cyclic AMP, 153
  thyroid hormone synthesis
    and release, 91
Cyclizine, 300
Cyclo-oxygenase, 112–114
Cycloplegia, 9
Cyclophosphamide, 206
  developmental toxicity, 262
  mechanism of action, 175,
    204
  prodrug, 224
  side effects, 205
Cyclopropane, 66, 159
  cardiac arrhythmias, 161
  neuromuscular blocking
    agents, interaction
    with, 23
  physical properties, 160
  potency, 161
Cycloserine, 172, 184, 195, 210
Cyproheptadine, 109, 111,
    294
Cyproterone, 88, 262
Cystinuria, 119
Cytarabine, 175, 204,
    206
Cytochrome P_{450}, 222, 266
Cytocidal action, 170
Cytoplasmic membrane,
    parasitic, 170, 171, 178
Cytostatic action, 170

Dactinomycin (*see* Actino-
    mycin D), 204, 206
Dapsone, 174
Daunorubicin, 204, 206
Delayed release formulations,
    212–213
Delirium, 132
Dementia, 132
Debrisoquine,
  idiosyncrasy, 257
  local anaesthetic action, 60
  mechanism of action, 42, 54

Debrisoquine (cont.)
  metabolism, 224
  use in hypertension, 282
Dehydroepiandrosterone, 77
Dependence,
  physical, 252–253
    barbiturates, 167, 254
    benzodiazepines, 164
    Chloral hydrate, 165
    definition, 252–253
    Ethanol, 164, 302
    mechanism, 252–253
    opiates, 149
  psychic (mental),
    amphetamines, 151, 152
    benzodiazepines, 164
    cannabis, 252
    Chloral hydrate, 165
    Ethanol, 164
    mechanism, 252–253
    Nicotine, 252
    tobacco, 252
Depolarization,
  end plate, 31
  ganglia, 26
  multiply-innervated muscle,
    23, 24
*Depolarizing neuromuscular
  blockade, 21, 38
Depressants, central, non-
  specific, 156–167
Depression (mental), *see also*
  Antidepressants, 129,
  133–135, 298
Dermatitis,
  contact, 321–322
  seborrhoeic, 320–321
Dermatophytes, 180, 191
Desferrioxamine, 268
Desmopressin, 103
Detergents, histamine release,
  108
Detrusor muscle, 11–12, 14
Developmental toxicity, 259–
  263
Dexamethasone, 119–120
Dextran, 108, 222
Dextromethorphan, 148, 325
Dextromoramide, 146
Dextropropoxyphene, 146,
  262–263
Dextrose injection, 273
Diabetes,
  mellitus, 94–97
  insipidus, thiazides, 104
Dialysance, 221
Dialysis, *see* Plasma and
  peritoneal dialysis, 221
Diamine oxidase, 107
Diamorphine,
  cough suppression, 325
  dependence, 252
  duration of action, 147
  pKa, 247
  potency, 146
Diaphragm, contraceptive,
  307, 308
Diarrhoea, 272–273

Diazepam, 157, 162–164, 296
  amnesia, 164
  anaesthetic premedication,
    162
  anticonvulsant action,
    164, 304
  binding sites, 164
  dependence, 164, 252
  effects, 163–164
  headache, 292
  migraine, 294
  muscle relaxation, 163–164
  rectal absorption, 211
  side effects, 164, 304
  structure, 162
  $t_{1/2}$, 164
Diazoxide
  antihypertensive action,
    104, 281, 284
  hypoglycaemia, 98
  insulin release, 97
  mechanism of action, 104
  protein binding, 218
Dibucaine number, 35, 258
Dichloralphenazone, 165, 265
Dichlorophen, 182
Dicyclomine, 33, 271
Dienoestrol 82
Diethylcarbamazine, 185
Diethyldithiocarbamate, 41
Diethyl-ether (ether), 66
Diethylpropion, 311
Diethylstilbestrol (*see*
  Stilboestrol), 82
Digitoxin, 235–236, 275–276
Digoxin, 275–276
  absorption, 233, 234
  distribution, 234
  dose, 235
  elimination, 234
  high ceiling diuretics, 104
  heart failure, 278
  pharmacokinetic model,
    230, 233–236
  poisoning, 268
  protein binding, 234
  renal clearance, 220, 234
  renal insufficiency, 221
  solubility, 234
  structure, 234
  $t_{1/2}$, 228, 234
  therapeutic index, 228, 234
  thiazide diuretics, 104, 276
  toxicity, 212, 235, 276
Dihydrocodeine, 146
Dihydrofolate, 173
Dihydrofolate reductase,
  170, 173, 174
Dihydrofolate synthetase, 170
3,4-Dihydroxymandelic acid,
  52
Dihydroxyphenylalanine (*see*
  Levodopa), 131
Dihydroxyphenylethylamine
  (*see* Dopamine), 129
Di-iodotyrosine, 89
Dilator pupillae, innervation,
  5, 9
Diloxanide, 188

Dimenhydrinate, 109, 300
Dimethoxymethylamphetamine,
  153
Dimercaprol, 268, 317
Dioctyl sodium sulpho-
  succinate, 275
Diphenoxylate, 148, 273
Diphenylhydantoin (*see*
  Phenytoin), 63–64, 167,
  303–306
Diphtheria, drugs of choice,
  192
Dipipanone, 146
Dipyridamole, 121
Disposition and metabolism,
  of drugs, 209–250
Disposition, drug,
  definition, 209
  causes of drug interactions,
    264–266
  importance of, 209
  models of, 225, 250
Dissociation rate constant, 68
Distribution, drug, 213–219
Distributional selectivity, of
  antiparasitic drugs,
  181–183
Disulfiram,
  aversion treatment in
    alcoholism, 165, 240
  interaction with other
    drugs, 223, 266
  mechanism of action, 41
Dithranol paste, 323
Diuresis, forced, 243, 247
  alkalinization, 268
*Diuretics, 102–106
  acid forming, 106
  aldosterone antagonism,
    105–106
  benzothiadiazides, 104
  carbonic anhydrase inhibi-
    tors, 105
  heart failure, 277–278
  high ceiling (loop), 104, 277
  hypertension, use in, 280
  mercurial, 106
  osmotic, 106
  potassium sparing, 105
  renal insufficiency, 221
  renal function, 102–103
  xanthines, 106
Dopamine, 127
  agonists, 131, 141, 151
  Amphetamine, 151
  bromocryptine, 75
  formula, 127
  Metoclopramide, 75
  Parkinson's disease, 131
  prolactin secretion, 75, 141
  synthesis, 40
  tracts, neuronal, 129–130
  vomiting, 131
Dopamine-β-hydroxylase,
  41, 43
Dose-response relationship,
  65–66, 227–228
Doxapram, 150, 152
Doxorubicin, 206

Doxycycline, 200, 265
Dreaming, 157
Droperidol, 163
Drug interactions, adverse, 264–266
Duodenal ulcer, 110, 269–271
Dysarthria, 159
Dysentery, 273
Dysmenorrhoea, 85, 113, 114
Dyspnoea, 289

Eccrine sweat glands, 13, 14, 29–30, 32, 34
Eclampsia, 30
Eclamptic toxaemia, 284, 302
Ecothiopate, 37, 38
Ectopic focus, cardiac, 61
Ectopic pregnancies, oral contraceptives, 84
Eczema, atopic, 322–323
Edrophonium, 36, 38
Efficacy, drug, definition, 69
Effective concentration ECn, 65
Effective dose EDn, 65
Ejaculation, 11, 78
    ganglion blocking agents, 29
    noradrenergic neurone blocking agents, 282
    prostaglandins, 113
Electrocardiogram (ECG), 285
Electroconvulsive therapy, 21, 134, 298, 302
Electroencephalogram (EEG), anaesthesia, 160
    epilepsy, 302
    non-specific depressants, withdrawal, 166
    petit mal epilepsy, 302
    sleep, 157
Electrolyte balance, *see also* Diuretics, 99, 103
Elimination, drug, 219–224
    active tubular reabsorption, 220
    bile, secretion in, 222
    definition, 209
    enterohepatic secretion, 222
    excretion, 219–222
    glomerular filtration rate, 219, 220
    lungs, excretion in, 222
    metabolism, 222–224
    milk, secretion in, 222
    models and examples, 230, 231–250
    passive tubular reabsorption, 219–220
    rate constant, 226
    renal insufficiency, 221
    renal plasma clearance, 219
    sweat excretion in, 222
    tubular secretion, 220
Embden-Meyerhof pathway, 93
Embryonic stage (of development), 259–260
Emesis, *see* Vomiting, 299
Emetics, in drug poisoning, 267

Emetine, 177, 300
Energy yielding metabolism, parasitic, 171, 178
Endometriosis, 84
Endometrium, 76
α-Endorphin, 143
β-Endorphin (C fragment), 128, 143
    actions, 144
    appetite, 145
    duration of action, 144
    hallucinations, 153
    location, 143
    Naloxone antagonism, 144
    Nitrous oxide analgesia, 153
    physiological role, 144
    prolactin release, 145
    tolerance, 144
γ-Endorphin, 143
End plate potential, 20, 22
Enkephalins, 128, 143–144
    actions, 144
    definition, 143
    duration of action, 144
    hallucinations, 153
    leu-enkephalin, 143
    location, 143
    met-enkephalin, 143
    Naloxone antagonism, 144
    Nitrous oxide analgesia, 153
    physiological role, 144
    structure, 143–144
    tolerance, 144
Entamoeba hystolitica, 178, 187, 188
Enteric coating, of tablets, 210, 212
Enterobius, 179, 186
Enterohepatic circulation, 80, 86, 90, 222
Enuresis, nocturnal, tricyclic antidepressants in, 136
Ephedrine, 41, 325
    monoamine oxidase, 53
    therapeutic use, 50, 290, 294
    uptake, 54, 266
Epididymis, 78
Epidural block, 59
Epilepsy (*see also* Anticonvulsants), 167, 301–306
Epinephrine (*see* Adrenaline), 55
Equilibrium, affinity constant, 68
Erectile tissue, 32, 113
Ergometrine, 300
Ergotamine,
    α-adrenoceptor antagonist, 45, 50
    emetic activity, 300
    therapeutic use, 51, 294
Erythromycin, 177, 198
    dose, 194
    elimination, 194, 198
    minimal inhibitory concentration, 193
    principal uses, 192, 198
    resistance, 195
    $t_{1/2}$, 194

Erysipelas, 319
Erythropoiesis, androgens, 88
Escherichia coli, 192, 193, 273
Eserine (*see Physostigmine*), 36
Ethacrynic acid, 104
Ethambutol, 192, 201
Ethanol, 157, 239–240
    absorption, 210, 239
    anaemia, cause of, 313, 314
    central depression, 159, 239–240
    dependence, 164, 166–167, 252, 254, 265
    developmental toxicity, 263
    distribution, 240
    drug interactions, 264, 266
    elimination, 238, 240
    enzyme induction, 265
    excretion, lungs, 222
    gout, 318
    hepatotoxicity, 164
    mechanism of action, 158–159
    metabolism, 164–165, 240
    pharmacokinetic model, 230, 239–240
    poisoning, 254
    psychosis, 133
    social use, 254
    $t_{1/2}$, 240
    tolerance, 166
    ulcers, gastric and duodenal, 270
Ether (diethyl ether), 66, 157, 159
    induction, speed of, 161
    neuromuscular blocking agents, interaction with, 23, 161
    physical properties, 160
Ethinyloestradiol, 82
Ethosuximide, 304, 305
Ethyleniminium ion, 50, 175, 206
Ethylene glycol, 165, 221
Ethynodiol, 83
Excitation, *cf.* inhibition, 68
Excitatory postjunctional potential, 31
Excretion, of drugs, 219–224
Exocytosis, 16, 43, 55
Exocrine glands, cholinergic receptors, 30
Exophthalmic goitre, *see also* Thyrotoxicosis, 90–93
Expectorants, 325
Eye,
    absorption of drugs, 215
    autonomic innervation, 8–10
Eyelids, sympathetic innervation, 10, 45

Facial nerve nucleus, 4
Factor VII (of clotting), 122
    IX, 122
    X, 122
    XII (Hageman factor) kinin release, 115

Fainting, 13
Fallopian tubes, 81, 84, 113
False transmitter, 18, 42
Family planning, 306–310
Fat metabolism, 94, 99
Febrile convulsions, 302, 304
Fenfluramine, 151, 311
Fentanyl, 147, 163
Ferguson's principle, 66, 158
Ferredoxin, 178, 187
Ferrous gluconate, 313
Ferrous sulphate, 313
  wax coating, 213
Fertilization, 259–260
'Fertility' drugs, 79, 83, 88
Fever, prostaglandins in,
  113, 155
Fibrillation, 63
Fibrinogen, 120
Fibrinolysinogen, 122
Fibrinolysin, 117, 122–123
Filariae, 185–186
First order kinetics, 238
'First pass' effect, 214, 248,
  286
Flaccid paralysis, 22
Flatworms, 185
Flucloxacillin, 194, 197
Flucytosine, 192
Fludrocortisone, 100
Fluid administration, in drug
  poisoning, 267
Flukes, 185–186
Fluocinolone, 100, 324
Fluoride, deposition in bones
  and teeth, 216
Fluorouracil, 175, 192, 204,
  296
Fluoxymesterone, 87
Flupenthixol, 140
Fluphenazine, 141, 142, 213
Focal (partial) epilepsy, 302
Focal motor (jacksonian)
  epilepsy, 302, 305
Focally innervated skeletal
  muscle, 18
Foetal development, 259–260
Folate, 173
Folic acid deficiency anaemia,
  314–315
Folic acid preparations, 314
Folinic acid, 173
Follicle stimulating hormone
  (FSH), 74, 76
  androgens, 87
  gametogenesis, 78
  (and) LH releasing hormone,
    75
  menstrual cycle, 77
  oestrogens, 81
  oocytes, effects on, 76
  progestogens, 84
  steroid synthesis, effect on,
    78
Follicular phase, of menstrual
  cycle, 77
Folliculitis, 319
Food poisoning, 273
Formaldehyde, 165, 320

Formic acid, 165
Forced expired volume s^{-1}
  (FEV$_1$), 289
Fornix bundle, 129
Fourth ventricle, 131
Framycetin, 319
Freon propellant, 291
Frusemide, 104, 277, 284
Fuller's Earth, 268
Functional antagonism, 71–72
Fungal infections, 178, 180,
  191–192
Furuncle, 319

Galactorrhoea, 75, 141
Gallamine, 19, 22, 24
Gametogenesis, 78
Gamma-benzene hexachloride,
  184, 185
Ganglia, 3–7
*Ganglion blocking agents,
  29–30
  actions, summary, 29
  hypertension, use in, 283
Ganglionic transmission,
  25–30, 102
Gas gangrene, drugs of choice,
  192
Gastrectomy, 271
Gastric emptying, 265
Gastric lavage, in drug
  poisoning, 224
Gastric ulcer, 110, 269–271
Gastrointestinal complaints,
  269–275
Gastrointestinal smooth
  muscle, 11
Gastrointestinal tract,
  α-adrenoceptor agonists, 45
  β-adrenoceptor agonists, 46
  ganglion blockade, 29
  muscarinic receptors, 32, 34
*General anaesthetics, 157
  analgesic activity, 161
  biophase for, 158–159
  cardiac arrhythmias, 161
  central effects, 160
  dependence, 166
  developmental toxicity, 263
  distribution, 214, 240–242
  electroencephalogram, 160
  excretion, 222
  hepatotoxicity, 161
  induction, speed of, 160,
    161, 241
  mechanism, 158–159
  metabolism, 166
  muscle relaxation, 161
  neuromuscular blocking
    agents, 23
  oil gas partition coefficients,
    159
  pharmacokinetic model,
    230, 240–242
  physical properties, 160
  potency, 159, 161, 240
  premedication, 162
  recovery, 242
  renal clearance, 219–221

General anaesthetics (*cont.*)
  tolerance, 166
Genetic causes of drug toxicity,
  257–259
Genital apparatus, 32, 45
Gentamicin, 23, 177, 182, 199
  absorption, 232
  dispositional model, 230,
    231–233
  distribution, 214, 232
  dose, 194, 233
  elimination, 194, 232
  incompatibility, drug, 265
  minimal inhibitory concen-
    tration, 193
  principal uses, 192
  renal clearance, 219
  renal insufficiency, 221, 232
  spectrum, 199, 231
  structure, 232
  t$_{\frac{1}{2}}$, 194
  therapeutic index, 228, 231
  toxicity, 177, 232–233
German measles, developmental
  toxicity, 261
Giardia, 190
Glaucoma, 9, 10, 33
  Acetazolamide, 105
  cholinesterase inhibitors, 38
  sympathomimetics, 48
  tricyclic antidepressants, 136
Glibenclamide, 95
Glomerular filtration, 102–103
Glomerular filtration rate, 219,
  220, 225
Glucagon, 93–94, 97
*Glucocorticoids, 99, 265
  eczema, 323
  insulin release, 94
  psoriasis, 323
  rheumatoid arthritis, 317
  selective agonists, 100
  ulcerative colitis, 272
Gluconeogenesis, 46, 93
Glucose, 93–94, 97, 265
Glucose-6-phosphate dehydrogenase, deficiency, 190
  259, 316
Glucuronides, 220, 224
Glutamic acid, 127
Glutamic acid decarboxylase,
  127
Glutamine conjugation, 224
Glutathione conjugation, 224
Glycerin, *see* Glycerol, 106
Glycerol, 106
  suppositories, 275
Glyceryl trinitrate,
  absorption, 211
  angina, 286
  headache, 292
  route, 286
  use, 278, 286
Glycine,
  conjugation with, 223
  neurotransmission, 127,
    128, 150
  tetanus toxin, 128
Strychnine, 128

Glycogen, synthesis, 93
Glycogenesis, 93
Glycogenolysis, 93
Glycol, ethylene, 165
Glycolysis, 93
Gold compounds, 119, 315, 317
Gold sodium thiomalate, 119, 317
Gonadotrophins,
 actions, 78–79
 secretions, effects on, 10, 75–76
Gonorrhoea, drugs of choice, 192
Goitre, exophthalmic, *see also* Thyrotoxicosis, 90–93
Gout, 104–105, 119
Grand mal epilepsy, 301, 304, 305
Graves disease, *see also* Thyrotoxicosis, 90–91
Griseofulvin, 191, 216
 acute intermittent porphyria, 258
 enzyme induction, 223, 265
 mechanism of action, 180
Growth hormone, 74
 bromocriptine, 75
 insulin release, 94, 97
 Phenytoin, effect on release, 75
Growth hormone release inhibiting hormone, 74
Growth onset diabetes, 95
Growth stimulation, androgens, 88
Guaiphenesin, 325
Guanethidine,
 adrenal medulla, 56
 drug interactions, 54
 hypertension, use in, 282
 local anaesthetic activity, 60
 mechanism of action, 41, 42
 pKa, 247
Guinea pig ileum, opiate receptors, 144
Gull's disease, 90
Gynaecomastia, 75

Haemodynamic factor, of drug distribution, 214
Haemolytic anaemia, 315–316
Haemophilus influenzae, drugs of choice, 192–193
Haemorrhoidal veins, 274
Hageman factor (XII), 115
*Hallucinogenic drugs, 153–154
 Cocaine, 54, 153
 cannabis, 153
 definition, 153
 drug laws, 253
 5-hydroxytryptamine antagonists, 153
 lysergic acid diethylamide, 153
 mescaline, 153
 narcotic analgesics, 146

Hallucinogenic drugs (*cont.*)
 neuroleptics, antagonism of, 140
Nitrous oxide, 153
 structure activity relationships, 151
 sympathomimetics, indirectly-acting, 153
 therapeutic use, 153
 toxicity, 154
*β-Haloalkylamines, 50
Halothane, 66, 157
 cardiac arrhythmias, 161
 hepatotoxicity, 161
 induction, speed of, 161
 metabolism of, 166
 neuromuscular blocking agents, interaction with, 23
 physical properties, 160
 potency, 159, 161
 oil gas partition coefficient, 159
Haloperidol, 140–142
Hapten, 257
Hay fever, 100, 109–110, 257, 287, 325
Headache, 292–293
Health education, drug abuse, 255
Heart,
 β-adrenoceptors, 63
 anti-arrhythmic drugs, 60–64, 275–276
 atrial flutter, 63, 64
 atrial paroxysmal tachycardia, 62
 atrio-ventricular node, 10, 32, 61
 bundle of His, 61, 275–276
 cardiac glycosides, 275–276
 ectopic focus, 61
 fibrillation, 63, 64
 ganglion blockade, 29
 innervation of, 10
 Lignocaine, 63–64
 Phenytoin, 63–64
 Procainamide, 62–63
 Purkinje fibres, 62, 64
 Quinidine, 62–63
 sino-atrial node, 10, 32
 ventricular myocardium (muscarinic receptors), 30, 32
 ventricular arrhythmias (β-adrenoceptor agonists), 64
Heart block, 61, 64
Heart failure, 276–278
Helium dilution, 289
Hemicholinium, 17
Henderson-Hasselbalch (acids and bases, dissociation of), 226, 246
Heparin, and antagonists, 107, 121, 231
Heparinase, 121
Heroin (*see also Diamorphine*), 146

Herpes, 202–203
 simplex, 319
 zoster, 320
Herrings, pickled, tyramine content, 53
Hexachlorophane, 321
Hexose monophosphate shunt, 93
Hippocampus, 129
Histamine, 106–110
 actions, 107–110
 anaphylaxis, 108–109
 bronchial muscle, 108
 capillary permeability, 107
 cardiovascular action, 107
 central neurotransmission, 127
 cerebral vasodilation, 107
 gastric secretion, 108–110
 gastrointestinal musculature, 108
 headache, 107, 292
 heart, 107
 inflammation, 116
 location, 106–107
 receptors,
  H_1, 50, 109
  H_2, 109, 272
 release, 23, 33, 108–109
 sensory nerve endings, 108
 storage, 107
 synthesis, 106
 therapeutic use, 109
 uterine smooth muscle, 108
Histaminase, 107
Histidine, 106
Histidine decarboxylase, 106
Hodgkin's disease, 207
Homatropine, 33, 34
Hookworms, 185–186
Human chorionic gonadotrophin, 76, 79
Human menopausal gonadotrophin, 76, 79
Hyaluronidase, 117
Hydralazine, 257, 281, 283
Hydrochloric acid secretion, ulceration, 269
Hydrochlorothiazide, 104
Hydrocortisone, 98, 101
 anti-inflammatory action, 119
 asthma, 290
 topical use, 324
 status asthmaticus, 291
Hydroflumethiazide, 104
Hydrogen ion, in inflammation, 117
Hydroxycobalamin, 314
5-Hydroxyindole acetaldehyde, 110
5-Hydroxyindole acetic acid, 110, 220
17-α-Hydroxyprogesterone, 77
Hydroxyprogesterone hexanoate, 83
5-Hydroxytryptamine, actions, 110–111

5-Hydroxytryptamine (*cont.*)
anaphylaxis, 109
antagonists, 111, 117, 153
bronchial muscle, 111
cardiovascular effects, 111
cerebral circulation, 293
D-receptors, 50, 111
function, 130
inflammation, 116
intestinal smooth muscle, 111
location, 110
metabolism, 110
migraine, 293
monoamine theory of mental disease, 130
M-receptors, 111
neural tracts, 130
neurotransmission, 127
sensory nerve endings, 111
storage, 110
synthesis, 110
uterine smooth muscle, 111
5-Hydroxytryptophan, 110
Hyoscine, 31, 33–35, 300
Hyperaemia, 115
Hypertensin (*see also* Angiotensin), 101
Hypertension (*see also* Antihypertensive drugs), 279–284
β-adrenoceptor antagonists, 51
classification, 279
consequences of, 279
definition, 279
hyperthyroidism, 91
malignant, 279
monoamineoxidase inhibitors, 139
noradrenergic neurone blocking agents, 60
renin-angiotensin system, 102
thiazide diuretics, 104
Hypertensive encephalopathy, 284, 302
Hyperthyroid state (*see also* Thyrotoxicosis), 90–93, 180
Hypnosis, 159
Hypnotics, 163–167
antihistamines, 109
definition, 159–160
poisoning, 267
Hypoalbuminaemia, 218
Hypocapnia, convulsions, 302
Hypoglycaemia, 97–98, 302
Hypokinesia, 131
Hyposensitization, to allergens, 290
Hypothalamus, 129, 130
appetite, 310, 312
body temperature, 154
neurohumours, 74–75
-pituitary axis, 73–75
sex, 262
Hypothyroid state (*see also* Myxoedema), 90–93, 262

Hysterectomy, 309
Hysteria, 133

^{125}I, 92
^{131}I, 92, 131, 208
^{132}I, 92
Ibuprofen, 118, 317
Ichthammol cream, 323
Idiosyncratic reaction (toxicity) to drugs, 255–259
Idoxuridine,
mechanism of action, 175, 183, 203
therapeutic use, 319, 320
Ileostomy, 271
Imidazole-N-methyl transferase, 107
Imidazolyl-acetic acid, 107
Imipramine, 135–136, 298–299
barbiturates, interaction with, 135
behavioural effects, 135–136
cardiovascular effects, 136
central actions, 130, 135–136
depressed patients, effects in, 135
5-hydroxytryptamine uptake, effect on, 135
muscarinic antagonism, 135, 136
noradrenaline uptake, inhibition of, 48–49, 53, 55, 135
noradrenergic neurone blocking agents, 43
normal subjects, effect in, 135
peripheral effects, 136
side effects, 136
sleep, effects on, 135
structure, 135
therapeutic use, 136
Immune stimulants, 208
Immune suppressants, 205
corticosteroids, 99–100
diabetogenic, 97
Immunoglobulin E, 287–289
Impetigo, 319
Implantation, blastocyst, 259–260
Impotence, ganglion blocking agents, 29
Indanediones, 122
Indomethacin, 118–119
anaemia, 313
cyclo-oxygenase inhibition, 113
gout, 318
osteoarthritis, 316
pharmacokinetics, 242
rectal absorption, 211
rheumatoid arthritis, 317
Infertility (*see also* 'Fertility' drugs), 75
Infiltration anaesthesia, 58
Inflammation (*see also* Anti-inflammatory drugs), 100, 115–119

Influenza, 202
Inhibition (cf. Excitation), 68
Injection, routes of, 212, 214
Inocybe patovillardii, 34
Insect infestations, 169, 180, 182
Insecticides, 38
Insomnia, 157–158
Insufflators, 290, 291
Insulin, 93–97, 101, 302
adrenaline, 95
chemical nature, 94
effects, 94
immunogenicity, 97
preparations, summary, 96
release, 94
source, 93
therapeutic index, 228
Insulinase, 96
Insulin injection, 96
Insulin zinc suspension, amorphous or *crystalline*, 96, 213
Interferon, 202, 203, 208
Intravenous anaesthetics, 161–162
advantages, 161–162
distribution, 214
drugs, 162
hazards, 162
Intrauterine device, contraceptive, 307, 308
Intrinsic activity, of drugs, 69
Inulin, 222, 231
Iodide, 89–90, 92
Iodine, absorption, 89
Iodine, aqueous solution, 92
Iodine, radioactive, 92–93
Iodotyrosine dehalogenase, 90
Ipecacuanha emetic draught, 267, 300
Ipratropium, 33, 34, 291
Iproniazid, 298
Iridocyclitis, 34
Iris,
adrenoceptors, 45
innervation, 14, 32
muscarinic receptors, 32, 34
organization, 9–10
Iritis, 34
Iron,
deficiency, 312–313
preparations, 313
ascorbic acid, use with, 313
poisoning, 268, 313
tetracyclines, interaction with, 265
Iron dextran colloidal injection, 213, 313
Iron sorbitol, 313
Ischaemia, 285
Islets of Langerhans, 94–96
Isoniazid, 201
genetic idiosyncrasy, 257
mechanism of action, 201
microsomal enzyme inhibition, 223, 266
principal uses, 192

Isophane insulin, 96
Isoprenaline
  agonist activity, 45, 47
  asthma, 290
  heart block, 64
  neuronal uptake, lack of,
    53
  pKa, 247
  structure, 47
  toxicity, 64, 292
Isoproterenol (*see Isoprenaline*)

Jacksonian (focal motor)
    epilepsy, 302
Joint diseases, 316–319
Juvenile diabetes, 95, 97

k (*see* Association rate constant
    and Dissociation rate
    constants, 68
K_a, *see* Equilibrium affinity
    constant, 68
Kallidin, 114–115, 117
Kallikrein, 97, 114–115
Kanamycin, 177, 192
Kaolin and morphine, 148,
    253, 273
Keratin, fungal infections, 180,
    191
Keratolytics, 320
Kidney function, 102–103
Kininases, 115
Kininogens, 114
Kinins, 109, 114–115, 117
Klebsiella, drugs of choice,
    192, 193
Krebs' cycle, 93, 120

Labour, induction of, 114
Lacrimal glands, 32, 34
  ganglion blockade, 29
  innervation, 4, 13, 14
β-Lactamase, 172, 193, 195
Lactation, suppression of, 83
Lactational amenorrhoea, 306
Lassars' paste, 323
Law of Mass Action, 68
Laxatives, 274–275
Lead poisoning,
  absorption, 211
  deposition in bones and
    teeth, 216
  psychoses, 133
  treatment, 268
Leishmania, 190
Leprosy, 174
Leucocyte emigration
    (inflammation), 116
Leucovorin, *see* Folinic acid, 174
Leukaemia, 203
  asparaginase, 206
  Busulphan, 175, 207
  Chlorambucil, 207
  corticosteroids, 100
  Mercaptopurine, 174–175
  Methotrexate, 174
Levamisole, 208
Levodopa, 126, 131
  absorption, 210

Levodopa (cont.)
  carbidopa, use with, 40
  cerebrospinal fluid, active
    transport, 215
  monoamine oxidase, 53
  side effects, 131
  structure, 40
Levorphanol, 146
Levothyroxine (*see* Thyroxine
    sodium), 91
Lewis's triple response, 107
Leydig cells, 78
Libido, 81, 84, 87
Lignocaine, 42, 56, 247
  absorption, 248
  antiarrhythmic action, 59,
    63–64, 276
  central actions, 64
  distribution, 248
  metabolism, 248
  muscarinic antagonism, 64
  pharmacokinetics, 247–249
  pKa, 60, 220, 247
  renal clearance, 220, 248
  structure, 56
  $t_{1/2}$, 248–249
  therapeutic index, 228
  use, 60
Limbic system, 129
  anxiolytics, 163
  narcotic analgesics, 145
  neuroleptics, 140
  sleep, 157
Lincomycin, 177, 200
  colitis as a side effect, 200
  dose, 194
  elimination, 194
  minimum inhibitory concen-
    tration, 193
  spectrum, 200
  $t_{1/2}$, 194
Liothyronine, 91
Lipid soluble drugs, disposition
    of, 230
  absorption, 236
  blood brain barrier, 214
  cell penetration, 214
  distribution, 236
  eye, 215
  metabolism, 222–224, 236
  models, dispositional, 230,
    236–242
  placenta, 216
  plasma dialysis, 221
  protein binding, 236
  renal clearance, 220
  renal insufficiency, 221
  serous cavities, 216
  small intestine, 210
Lipogenesis, 93
Lipolysis, 46, 93
Liquid paraffin, 275
Liquorice, 271
Lithium carbonate, 299
Liver,
  β-adrenoceptor agonists, 46
  excretion of drugs, 222
  non-specific central depress-
    ants, 161, 164

*Local anaesthetics, 16, 56–60
  action potential, effect on,
    57
  adrenaline, inclusion with,
    47
  antiarrhythmic action, 59,
    63–64, 276
  application, summary, 59
  basic nature, 246
  calcium ions, 58
  central effects, 58
  definition, 56
  dissociation, 249
  epidural block, 59
  hyper- and hypobaric solu-
    tions, 59
  individual agents, 60
  infiltration anaesthesia, 58
  ionization, 56
  ions, effects of, 58
  mechanism of action, 57
  nerve block, 58
  neurones, effects on, 57
  noradrenergic neurone block-
    ing agents, 60
  noradrenergic transmission,
    effects on, 42
  pH, effect of, 249
  pKa, 60, 247
  sensations, differential
    effects, 57
  site of action, 57
  sodium ions, 58
  specific gravity of, 59
  spinal anaesthesia, 58–59
  structure–activity relation-
    ships, 56
  subarachnoid block, 25
  topical (surface) anaesthesia,
    58
*Local hormones, 106–123
Locus ceruleus, 129
Long acting thyroid
    stimulator, 91
Loop (of Henle) diuretics,
    103, 104, 277
Lorazepam, 162, 164, 296
Louse infestations, 180, 182,
    185
Lupus erythematosus, systemic,
    100, 205, 281
Luteal phase, of menstrual
    cycle, 77, 113
Luteinizing hormone (LH)
    74, 76
  androgens, 87
  FSH releasing hormone, 75
  menstruation, 77
  oestradiol, 76
  oestrogens, effects of, 81
  oestrogen and progestogen,
    75
  oocytes, 76
  steroid synthesis, 78
  progestogens, effects on, 84
Lymecycline, 199
Lymphomas, 203
Lymphoreticular organs, 289
Lypressin, 101, 103, 211

Lysine-vasopressin, 101
Lysergic acid diethylamide,
    111, 153
    drug laws, 253
    neuroleptics, antagonism
        by, 140
Lysyl bradykinin, *see* Kallidin,
    114

Macrophages, 116
Magnesium hydroxide, 271,
    275
Magnesium ion,
    acetylcholine release, 16
    laxative action, 275
    noradrenaline release, 44, 54
Magnesium trisilicate, 271
Magnesium sulphate, 275
Malaria, 174, 179, 188–190
Malaoxon, 37, 180
Malathion, 37, 38, 180, 183.
Malignant hyperthermia, 258
Mamillary body, 129
Mammary glands, oestrogens
    effect on, 81
Mania, 129, 299
Manic depressive psychosis,
    133, 299
Mannitol, 106, 222, 231
Mass Action Law, 68
Mast cells, 107, 110, 289
Maturity onset diabetes, 95
Mazes, 134
Mazindol, 311
Mebeverine, 33, 271
Medroxyprogesterone, 83, 308
Mefenamic acid, 118
Megaloblastic anaemia, 313
Meiosis, 78
Melphalan, 175, 207
Membrane potential,
    ganglia, 26
    skeletal muscle, 20–21, 24
Membrane stabilization,
    anticonvulsants, 167, 303
    local anaesthetics, 57
    general anaesthetics, 159
Menière's disease, 297, 301
Meningitis, 177, 192
Menopausal symptoms, 82, 85
Menstrual cycle, 76–77, 113
Mental disorders, 132–133,
    295–296
Menthol, 325
Meperidine (*see Pethidine*), 146
Mepyramine, 109, 247, 300
Mercaptopurine, 204, 266
    developmental toxicity, 262
    mechanism of action, 174–
        175
    use, 206
Mercury, 211, 262, 268
Mescaline, 140, 151, 153
Mesterolone, 87, 88
Mestranol, 82
Metabolism, effects on, 81, 84,
    87, 90
Metabolism, of drugs, 222–224,
    265–266

Metazoal infestations, 169,
    184–186
Metformin, 96
Methacholine, 19, 25, 31
Methadone,
    excitation and depression,
        146
    opiate dependence, use in,
        149
    potency, 146
    structure, 147
Methandienone, 87
Methandrostenolone (*see
    Methandienone*), 87
Methanol, 165
Methaqualone, 166, 253
Methicillin, 197
Methionine, 268
Methisazone, 203
Methohexitone, 162
Methotrexate, 204, 206, 266
    anaemia, 314
    developmental toxicity, 262
    mechanism of action, 174
    resistance, 195
Methoxamine, 45, 47, 53
Methoxyflurane, 159, 161
3-Methoxy-4-hydroxy mandelic
    acid, 52
Methylamphetamine, 151
Methylcellulose, 273, 274, 310
Methyldopa, 41, 44
    absorption, 210
    active tubular reabsorption,
        220
    anaemia, 316
    CSF, active transport, 215
    mechanism of action, 42,
        282
    renal clearance, 220
    therapeutic use, 42, 282
    toxicity, 257
Methyldopa hydrazine, 40
α-Methyl dopamine, 41
Methyl salicylate, 211
α-Methyl tyrosine, 284
*Methylxanthines, 152–153
    actions, 152
    asthma, 290, 291
    diuresis, 106
Methysergide, 111, 294
Metoclopramide,
    antiemetic action, 205,
        301, 295
    drug interactions, 264
    prolactin secretion, 75
Metronidazole, 187, 188, 190,
    200
    aldehyde dehydrogenase,
        165, 266
    mechanism of action, 178
    principal uses, 192
Metyrapone, 101
Mexenone, 324
Mianserin, 136
Michaelis–Menten kinetics, 226
Miconazole, 191
Microsomal enzyme induction,
    166, 222, 265

Micturition, 11
Middle ear infection, drugs of
    choice, 192
Migraine, 111, 293–295
Milk, secretion of drugs in, 222
Mineralocorticoid action,
    99–100
Mineral oil (liquid paraffin),
    275
Miniature end plate potentials,
    17, 20
Miniature synaptic potentials,
    26
Miosis, 9
Misuse of drugs, 251–255
Mite infestations, 182, 183
Mixed function oxidase
    system, 222–224, 265–
    266
Monoamine oxidase, 41, 52–
    53, 110
*Monoamine oxidase inhibitors,
    136–139, 298
    cardiovascular actions,
        137–138
    central actions, 137
    classification, 53
    competitive, 53
    drug interactions, 53, 138,
        266, 298
    non-competitive, 53
    structure activity relation-
        ships, 151
    toxicity, 138
Monoamine theory of mental
    disease, 129
Mono-iodotyrosine, 89–90
Mono-oxygenase system (*see
    Mixed function oxidase
    system*), 222–224
Monosulfiram, 165, 185
Morning sickness of pregnancy,
    301
Morphine, 126, 143–149
    anaesthetic premedication,
        162
    ADH release, 146
    analgesia, 146
    central actions, 146
    constipative action, 148,
        273
    cough suppression, 146
    emetic action, 141
    euphoria, 146
    excretion, 220
    gonadotrophin secretion, 75
    heart failure, 277, 284
    histamine release, 108, 148
    miosis, 146, 148, 149
    monoamine oxidase inhibi-
        tors, 53
    oral absorption, 146
    pKa, 247
    respiratory depression, 146,
        147
    structure–activity relation-
        ships, 144, 147
    tolerance and dependence,
        149, 252–253
    vomiting, 146, 149

Morula, 260
Mosquito, Anophyles, 188
Motion sickness, *see* Travel
    sickness
Motor end plate, 8, 18
α-Motor neurone — Renshaw
    cell, 128
Mucolytics, 325
Mullerian duct, 261
Multiply innervated (slow)
    skeletal muscle, 23–25
Muramyl dipeptide, 208
Murein, 172
Muscarine, 25, 30, 31, 34
*Muscarinic antagonists, 34
    anaesthetic premedication,
        162
    asthma, 291
    basic nature, 246
    Parkinson's disease, 131
    pKa value, 247
    ulcers, 271
Muscarinic receptors, 30–35
    antagonists, 33
    effects on (summary), 32
    antihistamines, 109
    phenothiazines, 142
    potency ratios of agonists
        and antagonists, 31
Muscle relaxants, centrally
    acting, 163–164
Muscle relaxants, peripherally
    acting (*see* Neuromuscular
    blocking agents),
Mushroom (rapid type)
    poisoning, 34
Mustards, nitrogen, 175,
    206–207
Mustine, 175, 206
Myasthenia gravis, 38, 63
Mycobacterium tuberculosis,
    drugs of choice, 192
Mycoplasma, 169, 192
Mydriasis, 9, 34
Myocardial infarction, 285
Myocardial ischaemia, 285
Myxoedema, 90–93

Nails, drug distribution in,
    216
Nalidixic acid, 181, 201
Nalorphine, 145, 150, 247,
    268
Naloxone
    antagonist activity, 145
    endorphins and enkephalins,
        144
    narcotic poisoning, 268
    post-anaesthetic medication,
        162
    use, 149–150
Nandrolone, 87
Napkin rash, 321
Narcolepsy, 151
Narcosis, 143
*Narcotic analgesics, 143–150
    agonist–antagonist ratios,
        145
    analgesic action, 146

Narcotic analgesics (*cont.*)
    anaesthetic premedication,
        162
    barbiturates, interaction
        with, 146
    basic nature, 246
    central actions, 146
    cough suppression, 146,
        147–148, 325
    dependence, 149, 150, 252,
        254
    depressant actions, 146
    drug laws, 253
    duration of action, 147
    endorphins and enkephalins,
        143–144
    euphoria, 146
    excitatory actions, 146
    gastrointestinal effects, 148,
        265, 273
    intracranial pressure, 292
    miosis, 146, 148
    neuroleptanalgesia, 163
    neuroleptics, interaction
        with, 146
    oral absorption, 146
    partial agonists, 145
    peripheral models for
        screening, 144
    pKa, 247
    placental barrier, 216
    poisoning, 147, 148, 254,
        268
    respiratory depression, 146,
        147
    salicylates, interaction with,
        146
    tolerance, 149, 252
    vomiting, 146, 148, 300,
        302
    withdrawal syndrome, 149,
        252
Narcotic antagonists, 149–150
    hallucinogenic action, 153
    precipitation of withdrawal,
        150
    use, 149
Nasal mucosal absorption, 211
Nausea, 299–300
Nebulizers, 291
Neisseria gonorrhoeae, drugs
    of choice, 192, 193
Neisseria meningitidis, drugs
    of choice, 192, 193
Neomycin,
    distribution, 181–182
    intraperitoneal absorption,
        212
    mechanism of action, 177
    percutaneous absorption,
        212
    use, 199
Neonatal respiratory depression,
    150
Neoplastic disease and treat-
    ment, 170, 203–208
    alkylating agents, 175,
        206, 207
    androgens, 88, 207

Neoplastic disease (*cont.*)
    anti-anergic agents, 208
    antibiotics, 206
    antimetabolites, 205
    breast cancer, 82, 83, 88,
        207
    cell cycle, 204
    chemotherapy, 203
    endometrial, 85
    enterochromaffin, 110
    enzymes, 206
    hormones, 207
    immune stimulants, 208
    leukaemias, 100, 174, 175,
        203, 206, 207, 208
    oestrogen antagonists, 83,
        88, 207
    oestrogens, 82, 207
    phaeochromocytoma, 51,
        284
    progestogens, 85
    prostatic tumour, 82, 207
    pyrimidine antimetabolites,
        175
    radiotherapy, 208
    resistance to drugs,
        195, 207
    sites of action, 204
    toxicity of drugs, 205, 264,
        315
    vinca alkaloids, 207
Neostigmine, 36, 38, 162,
    220
Nerve block anaesthesia, 58
Nerve gases, 38
Neuroeffector junctions
    (autonomic); 3–5, 14, 32
    (*see also under* individual
        neurotransmitters and
        tissues), 45–46
Neuroglycopoenia, 98
Neuroleptanalgesia, 163
*Neuroleptic drugs, 139–142,
    297
    α-adrenoceptor antagonism,
        142, 297
    anaesthetic premedication,
        162
    antihistaminic action, 142
    butyrophenones, 140
    choice of drug, 142
    cholestatic jaundice, 297
    extrapyramidal effects, 140,
        297
    galactorrhoea, 141
    hallucinogens, antagonism
        of, 140
    mechanism of action,
        140
    muscarinic antagonism, 142
    narcotic analgesics, inter-
        action with, 146, 297
    neuroleptanalgesia, 163
    phenothiazines, 140
    Reserpine, 139
    side effects, summary, 297
    therapeutic uses, 142, 162
    thioxanthines, 140

Neuromuscular blocking
agents (*see also* competitive and depolarizing
agents), 21–23
anaesthetic premedication,
162
drug interactions, 23
parasites, paralysis of, 178–179
Strychnine poisoning, 152
Neuromuscular transmission,
19–23
Neurones, and local anaesthetics,
57
Neurosis, 133, 295
Neurotic depression, 133
Neutral insulin injection, 96
Niclosamide, 182
Nicotine (*see also* Tobacco),
basic nature, 246
convulsant action, 302
dependence, 252
ganglia, actions at, 25, 27
muscarinic receptors, 31
neuromuscular junction, 21
sympathomimetic actions,
48–49
Nicotinic receptors, definition,
18
ganglia, 25, 27–29
skeletal muscle, 21–25
indirect antagonism,
atropine, 71
sympathomimetic conse-
quences, 48
Nicoumalone, 122, 242
Nictitating membrane, 10, 45
Nifedipine, 287
Nigrostriatal dopaminergic
tracts, 129, 131
Nikethamide, 152, 166, 302
Nimorazole, 178, 187
Niridazole, 188
Nitrazepam, 158, 164, 296
Nitrofurantoin, 181, 201
glucose-6-phosphate dehydrogenase deficiency, 259,
316
spectrum, 181
toxicity, 189, 201
Nitrogen, 159
Nitrogen mustards, 175, 206–
207
Nitrous oxide, 66
analgesic action, 161
endorphins, 153
hallucinogens, 153
induction, speed, of, 161
oil gas partition coefficient,
159
physical properties, 160
potency, 159, 161
'Non-barbiturate' sedatives,
166
Non-competitive antagonism,
70–71
Non-polar drugs (*see also* Lipid
soluble drugs), 320

Non-specific central depressants,
156–167
alcohols, 164–165
anxiolytics, 163–167
barbiturates, 166–167
biophase for, 158–159
Chloral hydrate, 165
dependence, 166–167
drugs, 157
general anaesthetics, 159–
161
hypnotics, 163–167
intravenous anaesthetics,
161–162
mechanism of action, 158–
159
sedatives, 163–167
tolerance, 166–167
Nonylphenoxypolyethoxy-
ethanol, 307
Noradrenaline, 3, 7, 39–56
acetylcholine, functional
antagonism by, 72
α- and β-adrenoceptor
agonist potencies,
45, 46
central actions, 127, 129
Guanethidine, 41, 43
metabolism, 39, 52–53
pKa, 247
release, 39, 43–44, 48–49
Reserpine, 41
storage, 41
structure, 47
synthesis, 39, 40–41
Noradrenergic neurone blocking agents, 42–43
drug interactions, 266
hypertension, use in, 282
local anaesthetic activity, 60
mechanism of action, 43
pKa, 246–247
side effects, 282
therapeutic use, 43, 60, 282
toxicity, 282
uptake, 53
Noradrenergic transmission
(*see also* Noradrenaline),
39–55
central nervous system,
127–130
Guanethidine, 41
local anaesthetics, 42
Methyldopa, 41–42
neurone blocking agents,
42–43
Reserpine, 41, 44
sequence of events, 39
summary of drugs affecting,
54
Tetrodotoxin, 42, 43
Norepinephrine (*see* Noradrenaline), 39
Norethindrone (*see* Norethisterone), 83
Norethisterone, 83
Norgestrel, 83
Normetadrenaline, 52
19-Nortestosterone, 83, 85

Nucleic acid synthesis, of
parasites, 171, 173–176
Nucleus acumbens, 129
Nystatin, 178, 182, 191

Obesity, 151, 310–311
Obsessional neurosis, 133
Occupancy (receptor) theory,
69
Oculomotor nerve nucleus, 4
Oedema, pulmonary, heart
failure, 277
17-β-Oestradiol, 76, 81–83,
85–86
FSH, effects on, 76
LH, effects on, 76
menstrual cycle, 77
oestrogens, actions of,
80, 81
synthesis, 77
Oestriol, 81
*Oestrogens, 80–83, 85–86
Oestrogen antagonists, 83
Oestrogen–progestogen com-
binations, 85–86, 308
Oestrone, 81
Oil gas partition coefficient,
general anaesthetics, 159
Oily solutions, for injection,
213
Oocytes, 76, 261
oogonia, 261
Opiate analgesics, *see* Narcotic
analgesics, 143
Opiate receptors, 144–145
Opiate analgesics (*see* Narcotic
analgesics), 143
Opiate receptors, 144–145
Opioid analgesics (*see* Narcotic
analgesics), 143
Opium, 143
Oral anticoagulants (*see*
Anticoagulants), 122
Oral contraceptives, 308
drug interactions, 265
gonadotrophin release, 75
mechanism of action, 84
oestrogen–progestogen combinations, 85, 308
'once a month' preparation,
114
ovulation, effect on, 75
post-coital, 83
pregnancy rates, 84
progestogens, 84
prostaglandins, 114
*Oral hypoglycaemic agents,
95–96, 242
acute intermittent porphyria,
259
characteristics, 95
mechanisms of action, 96
Orciprenaline, 48, 53, 64, 290
Organic solvents, central
depression, 157
Organogenesis, 260
Organophosphorous cholin-
esterase inhibitors, 36–38,
268

Orphenadrine, 131
Osmotic diuretics, 106
Osteoarthritis, 118, 316
Over-prescribing, 255
Oviductal occlusion, 308–309
Oxazepam, 296
Oxprenolol, 45, 51
  anti-arrhythmic action, 63
  hypertension, use in, 281
  membrane stabilization, 51
  toxicity, 51, 63
Oxtriphylline (*see Choline
  theophyllinate*), 153
Oxygen, 291, 294
Oxyntic glands, innervation,
  13
Oxyphenbutazone, 119, 224
Oxytetracycline, 199, 320
Oxytocin, 73
  absorption, 211
  induction of labour, 114
  therapeutic index, 228

Pacemaker, cardiac (*see* sino-
  atrial node), 10
Pain threshold and tolerance,
  146
Pancreas, 74, 93
Pancuronium, 19, 22, 24
Papaver somniferum, 143
Papilloma virus, 320
Paracetamol, 118
  analgesia, 156, 292
  antipyresis, 156
  cyclo-oxygenase selectivity,
    118
  headache, 292
  metabolism, 265
  osteoarthritis, 316
  phenacetin, metabolism
    from, 224
  poisoning, 268
  site of action, 118
  toxicity, 118, 156
Paradoxical sleep, 157
Paraesthesia, 105
Paraldehyde, 222, 304
Paranoia, 132
Paranoid schizophrenia, 132
Paraquat poisoning, 221, 254,
  268
Parasympathetic nervous
  system, 4, 14, 29–30
Parasympathomimetics, 32
Paravertebral ganglia, 5, 7
Parkinson's disease, 40, 129–
  132, 141
Paronychia, acute, 319
Parotid gland, innervation, 4
Partial agonists, definition, 69
Partition coefficient, 226, 230
Passive tubular drug reabsorp-
  tion, 219
Peak flow meter (Wright's),
  289
Pediculosis, 38, 185
Pediculus humanus, 185
Penicillamine, 268, 317

*Penicillin, 196–198
  allergy, 182, 257
  bile, secretion in, 222
  drugs, 196–197
  mechanism of action, 172
  penicillinase, 172
  pharmacokinetics, 242
  resistance, 172, 196
  sensitivity, 198, 257
  spectrum, 172
  structure–activity relation-
    ships, 196
  therapeutic index, 228
  toxicity, 198, 257
Penicillinase, 172
Penicillin G (*see also Benzyl
  penicillin*), 196–197
Penicillin V, 192, 197, 198
Pentagastrin, 109, 314
Pentazocine, 145, 150, 162
Pentobarbitone, 166
Pentolinium, 19, 25, 30–31, 283
Pentose phosphate shunt, 93,
  189–190
Pepsin, ulcers, 269
Peptide neurotransmitters, 128
Perchlorate, potassium, 92
Peritoneal dialysis, 221
Permeability, drug disposition,
  214
Peroxidases, 89
Perphenazine, 297
Pethidine, 53, 146, 266
Petit mal (absences) epilepsy,
  302, 304, 305
Petrol, 157
Phaeochromocytoma, 51, 53,
  63, 284
Phagocytosis, 116, 170
Pharmacodynamics, 227, 264
Pharmacokinetics, summary,
  250
  accumulation, 228
  classification of drugs,
    summary, 230
    acids, 242–245
    bases, 246–250
    lipid soluble drugs, 236–
      242
    intermediate soluble
      drugs, 233–236
    water soluble drugs,
      231–233
  definition, 209
  dose regimens, 227–230
  drug interactions, causes of,
    264–266
  examples, 229–230
  models, 225–250
  $t_{1/2}$ considerations, 228
  terms and equations, 225–
    226
Phase I and II reactions, mixed
  function oxidases, 224,
  265
Phenacetin, 224
Phenazocine, 146
Phenelzine, 49, 53, 136–139
  cardiovascular actions, 137

Phenelzine (*cont.*)
  central effects, 137
  drug interactions, 138
  food interactions, 138
  idiosyncratic reactions, 257
  mechanism of action, 137
  Reserpine, interaction with,
    137–138
  side effects, 138
  sleep, 137
  tyramine, 138–139
  use, 298
Phenformin, 96
Phenindione, 122
Phenobarbitone, 157, 166,
  167
  anaemia, 314
  anticonvulsant, 304, 306
  enzyme induction, 223, 265
  forced diuresis, 243
  pharmacokinetics, 242
  pKa, 243
  poisoning, 268
  $t_{1/2}$, 306
Phenol, 211, 224
Phenolphthalein, 222, 275
*Phenothiazines, 140–142, 297
  antipsychotic activity, 140
  entero-hepatic recycling, 222
  extrapyramidal effects,
    140–141, 297
  gonadotrophin secretion, 75
  potency, 140
  structure, 140
Phenoxybenzamine, 45, 50
  characteristics of antagon-
    ism, 71
  therapeutic use, 51, 284
Phenoxymethyl penicillin,
  Penicillin V, 197
Phentermine, 311
Phentolamine, 45, 50–51, 70
Phenylalanine, 40
Phenylbutazone,
  anaemia, cause of, 119,
    313, 315
  anticoagulants, 122
  anti-inflammatory actions,
    118–119
  gout, 119, 318
  metabolism, 224, 266
  pharmacokinetics, 242
  pKa, 243
  protein binding, 218, 219,
    265
  rheumatoid arthritis, 119,
    317
  toxicity, 119
  tubular secretion, 220
Phenylethanolamine-N-methyl
  transferase, 55, 127
Phenylephrine, 45, 47, 53
Phenyl mercuric acetate, 307
Phenylpropanolamine, 53
Phenytoin, 63–64, 167,
  303–306
  anaemia, 314
  antiarrhythmic action,
    63–64, 276

Phenytoin (cont.)
anticonvulsant action, 167, 303–305
developmental toxicity, 262
dialysis, 221
dose, 238, 239, 305
enzyme induction, 223
enzyme inhibition, 265–266
glucose, incompatibility, 265
gum hyperplasia, 75, 303
hypersensitivity, 315
hypertensive encephalopathy, 284
insulin release, 97
metabolism, 238
oral contraceptives, 86
pharmacokinetics, 230, 238–239
pKa, 238
protein binding, 238
renal clearance and insufficiency, 220–221
side effects, 64, 303
use, 238
Phocomelia, 261
Pholcodine, 147
[32] Phosphate, 180, 208
Phosphodiesterase, 121, 152–153
Phospholipase A_2, 112
Photophobia, 10
Physostigmine, 36, 38, 247
Phytomenadione (*see* Vitamin K), 122
Phytonadione (*see* Vitamin K), 122
Picrotoxin, 152
Piles, 274
Pilocarpine, 31–33, 247
Pilomotor muscles, 13–14, 29, 45
Piperazine, 178–179, 186
Pituitary gland, 73–76
Pizotifen, 294
pKa
acidic drugs, 242–245
basic drugs, 245–250
definition, 226
Henderson-Hasselbalch, 246
significance in distribution, 214–215, 230
elimination, 220, 230
Placebo analgesia, 145
Placental barrier, 215
Plasma expanders, 102
Plasma dialysis, 221
Plasmin (*see* Fibrinolysin), 122
Plasminogen (*see* Fibrinolysinogen), 122
Plasmodium falciparum and *vivax*, life cycle (*see also* Malaria), 188–189
Platelet adhesiveness, 113, 121
Plethysmography, 289
Plummer's disease, 91
Pneumonia, drugs of choice, 192

Podophyllin compound paint, 320
Poisoning, drug, 267–269
adsorbents, 267–268
barbiturates, 166
emetics, 267
fluid replacement, 267
gastric lavage, 267
incidence, 254, 267
management, principles of, 267–268
narcotic analgesics, 149, 268
Phenobarbitone, 166, 268
salicylates, 168
specific antidotes, summary, 268
statistics, 254
Polar drugs (*see* Water soluble drugs), 231–233
Poliomyelitis, 202
Polycythaemia vera, 180
Polyene antibiotics, 178
Polymyxin, 178, 231
Porphyria, acute intermittent, exacerbation by drugs, 258
Postjunction potential, spontaneous, 26, 31, 44
Post-tetanic potentiation, 167
Potassium chloride,
effervescent tablets, 104
slow tablets, 104
wax matrix tablets, 213
Potassium ion,
acetylcholine release, 16
inflammation, 116
local anaesthetics, 57
loss, thiazides, 104
renal function, 103
supplementation, 104, 277
Potassium perchlorate, 92, 315
Potency, drug, definition, 65
Practolol, 45, 51
Pralidoxime, 38, 268
Prazosin, 50
Prednisolone, 100
asthma, 290–291
anti-inflammatory action, 119
enteric coating, 212
Prednisone, 100, 119
Pregnancy testing, 76, 260
Pregnant mares' serum gonadotrophin, 76, 79
Pregnenolone, 77
Prekallikrein, 115
Presynaptic inhibition, 125–126
centrally-acting antihypertensives, 42, 282
opiates and endorphins, 144
Prevertebral ganglia, 5, 7
Primaquine, 189, 259, 316
Primidone, 304
Proadifen, 223
Probenecid,
CSF, active transport from, 215

Probenecid (cont.)
penicillins, combination with, 197
pKa, 243
tubular secretion, 220
uricosuric action, 243, 319
Procainamide, 62–63
absorption, 212
mechanism of action, 62–63
muscarinic antagonist activity, 33, 63
toxicity, 63
use, 63
Procaine, 56, 60
hydrolysis, 35, 60
pKa, 60, 247
structure, 56
use, 60
Procaine penicillin, 197, 213
Procarbazine, 204, 207
Prochlorperazine, 141–142, 295, 297
Procyclidine, 131
Prodrug,
definition, 170
examples, 174, 175, 180, 190
summary, 224
Progesterone, 76–78, 80, 83–85
*Progestogens, 80, 83–86
abortion, 84
oestrogens, combination with, 85
androgen antagonists, 88
biotransformation, 80
definition, 80
effects, summary, 84
oral contraceptives, 84, 308
preparations, 83
receptors, 80
$t_{1/2}$, 80
use, 84
Proguanil, 174, 190, 314
Prolactin, 74, 76
bromocriptine, 75
Chlorpromazine, 75, 141
dopaminergic mechanisms, 75
Metoclopramide, 75
molecular weight, 76
oestrogens, effect of, 81, 306
opiates, 145
release inhibiting factor, 74
Reserpine, 75
Promazine, 297
Promethazine, 109, 142, 247, 300
Promotion, of drugs, 255
Propantheline, 33, 271
Proparacaine (*see* Proxymetacaine), 56, 60
Propranolol, 51
angina, 286–287
anti-arrhythmic action, 63
anxiolytic action, 294
asthma, 288
hypertension, 281

Propranolol (*cont.*)
  membrane stabilization. 51
  phaeochromocytoma, 284
  potency ratios, 45
  thyrotoxicosis, 92–93
  toxicity, 51, 63
  tyramine, indirect antagonism of, 71
Propylthiouracil, 91
Prostacyclin, 112, 113, 120, 121
Prostaglandin,
  anaphylaxis, 109
  atherosclerosis, 114
  biosynthesis, 112
  classification, 112
  clinical use, 113–114, 310
  inflammation, 117
  metabolism, 112, 113
  pain, 155
  pathological involvement, 113
  reproductive processes, 113
  role. 113
  side effects, 114
  storage, 112
Prostaglandin E_2, 112, 113, 114
Prostaglandin $F_{2\alpha}$, 112, 113, 114
Prostaglandin endoperoxide, 112, 113
Prostaglandin synthetase, 112
Prostanoic acid, 111
Prostate, steroid receptors, 80
Prostate cancer, oestrogens and progestogens, 75
Protamine sulphate, 121
Protamine zinc insulin, 96
Protein binding, of drugs, 216–220
  affinity, calculation of and examples, 217–218
  Chloroquine, 217
  Diazoxide, 218
  glomerular filtration rate, 218
  oral anticoagulants, 122, 217, 219, 265
  oral hypoglycaemic drugs, 265
  Phenylbutazone. 217, 218, 219. 265
  plasma dialysis, 221
  proportion. calculation of, 217
  salicylates, 218
  significance. 216, 218–219, 265
  sites of binding, 217
  sulphonamides, 196, 217–218
  $t_{1/2}$, 218
  tetracyclines, 199
  thiazide diuretics, 104
  Thiopentone. 217
  thyroid hormones, 90
Protein metabolism, 94, 99

Protein synthesis, parasitic, 171, 176–177
Proteolytic enzymes, 108
Proteus, drugs of choice. 192, 193
Prothrombin, 118, 120
Protozoal infections, 169, 184–191
Proxymetacaine, 56, 60
Pseudocholinesterase (*see also* Cholinesterase), 35–36
Pseudomonas aeruginosa, drugs of choice, 192
Psoralen, 323
Psoriasis, 323–324
Psychomotor (temporal lobe) epilepsy, 302, 305
Psychosis, 132, 295
  antipsychotic drugs (*see* Neuroleptics), 139–142
  Amphetamine induced, 151
  biochemical basis, 141
  functional, 133
  hallucinogen induced, 154
  manic depressive, 133
  organic, 132
  paranoia, 133, 151
Pteridine, 173
Ptosis, 10
Puberty, delayed, 87
Pulsus paradoxus, 291
Pupil size, 9–10
Purine synthesis, parasitic, 173–175, 210
Purkinje fibres, 10, 46
Putamen, 129, 130, 141
Putrescine, 220
Pyelography, 243
Pyrazinamide, 192, 201
Pyridostigmine, 36, 38
Pyrilamine (*see Mepyramine*), 109, 247, 300
Pyrimethamine, 174, 190
  anaemia, 314
  resistance, 195
Pyrimidine synthesis, parasitic, 173, 175, 210
Pyrvinium pamoate (*see Viprynium*), 182
Pyrogens, 155

Quadricyclic antidepressants, 135–136
Quaternary ammonium compounds, 249–250
  acetylcholine, 33
  cholinesterase inhibitors. 36
  distribution, 214, 231
  ganglion blocking agents, 30
  muscarinic antagonists, 33
  neuromuscular blocking agents, 22–23
  renal clearance, 219
Quinidine, 33, 62–63
  absorption, 212
  mechanism of action, 62
  muscarinic antagonism, 63

Quinidine (*cont.*)
  pKa, 247
  therapeutic use, 63
  toxicity, 63
Quinine,
  mechanism of action, 179, 190
  pKa, 215, 247
  renal tubular secretion, 220
  resistance, 179, 190
  toxic effects. 118

Rabies. 133
Radioactive iodine, 92–93
Radiotherapy, 208
  anaemia. 315
  emesis. 300
Raphe nuclei. 130
Rapid eye movement (REM) sleep. 157
Rate constants (*see* association and dissociation), 68
Reactive (neurotic) depression, 133
Receptor (*see also* individual transmitters and hormones). definition, 67
  spare, 69
Receptor occupancy theory, 67–72
Rectal mucosal absorption, 211
Rectus abdominis, 23
Redistribution, drug, 214
Referred pain, 292
Renal clearance, of drugs, 219–221
Renal insufficiency, drug elimination, 221
Renal plasma flow, 220
Renal tubular secretion. 220
Renin-angiotensin system, 98, 101–102, 277
Renshaw cell–α-motor neurone circuit, 127–128
Reserpine,
  central actions, 139
  chromaffin cells, 56
  galactorrhoea, 75
  gonadotrophin secretion, 75
  gynaecomastia, 75
  hypothermia, 137
  impotence, 75
  infertility, 75
  mechanism of action, 41, 44, 54, 130, 139
  pKa, 247
  prolactin secretion, 75
  sedation, 137
  side effects, 75, 139
  sympathomimetics, interactions with, 49
Resistance, parasitic, 170, 193, 194–195
Resorcinol, 320
Respiration,
  depressants, 146, 150, 159
  stimulants, 151–153

Respiratory smooth muscle, 11, 46
Retching, 299–300
Reticular activating system, 156, 163
Retinoscopy, diagnostic, 47
Rheumatic carditis, 100
Rheumatic fever, 118, 316
Rheumatoid arthritis, 100, 118–119, 316–318
Rhinitis, allergic and perennial, 325
Rhythm method, contraception, 306
Ribosomes, 70S and 80S, 176
Rickettsiae, 169
Rifampicin,
 enzyme induction, 265
 mechanism of action, 176, 201
 oral contraceptives, interaction with, 86
 uses, 192, 201
Rifampin (*see Rifampicin*), 176, 201
Ringworm, 191
Rotating rod, 134
Roundworm, 178–179, 185–186
Rubella, developmental toxicity, 261

Sacral nerves, 4
Salbutamol,
 absorption, 211
 neuronal uptake, lack of, 53
 structure, 47
 use, 48, 290, 291
Salicylic acid, 191, 196
 absorption, 244
 anti-inflammatory action, 118
 clearance, 245
 distribution, 244
 dose, 244–245
 excretion, 220, 238
 glucose-6-phosphate dehydrogenase deficiency, 259
 metabolism, 244
 pharmacokinetics, 244–245
 pKa, 214, 243
 poisoning, 268
 $t_{1/2}$, 245
Salicylic acid collodion paint, 320
Salivary glands, 4, 13, 14
 muscarinic agonists and antagonists, 32, 34
 ganglion blocking agents, 29
Salmonella typhi, drugs of choice, 192
Sarcoptes scabei, 184
Scabies, 184
Schistosomes, 185
Schizophrenia,
 description, 133
 endorphins, 145
 hallucinogens, 154

Schizophrenia (*cont.*)
 management, 140
 theories of, 145, 151, 154
Schlemm, canal of, 9
Scopolamine (*see* Hyoscine), 31, 33–35, 300
Scotoma, 293
Screening, centrally-acting drugs, 133–134
 anxiolytics, 164
 catatonia, 140
 monoamine oxidase inhibitors, 137
 neuroleptics, 140
 non-specific depressants, 140
 Reserpine offset, 137
 tricyclic antidepressants, 135–136
Sedatives, 159–160, 163–167
 monoamine theory of, 130
 narcotic analgesics, 146
 non-specific depressants, 159
 Strychnine poisoning, 152
Selective toxicity, definition, 170
Selenium sulphide, 321
Seminal vesicles, 12, 14, 29, 45
Senna, 275
Sensitivity, parasitic, 170
Septicaemia, drugs of choice, 192
Septum, 129
Serotonin (*see* 5-Hydroxytryptamine), 110–111
Sertoli cells, 78
Sequential therapy, 174
Serum sickness, 316
*Sex hormones, 76–78, 80
Shingles, 203, 320
Shock, 115
Sino-atrial node, 10, 14, 32, 46
Sinusitis, 325
Skeletal muscle, 18–25, 46
SKF 525-A (*see* Proadifen), 223
Skin, 180, 182–183, 211–213, 216, 319–324
Sleep, 135, 156–158, 296
Sleep-wake cycle, 156
Slow reacting substance of anaphylaxis (SRS-A), 109
Small intestine, drug absorption, 210
Smallpox, 202
Snake venom, histamine release, 108
Sodium acid phosphate, 275
Sodium *Aminosalicylate*, 173–174, 201
Sodium *Aurothiomalate*, 119
Sodium bicarbonate, 270
Sodium chloride, in dehydration, 272
Sodium *Cromoglycate*, 110, 290
Sodium edetate, 120
Sodium *Fusidate*, 182, 319

Sodium ions,
 acetylcholine release, 16
 action potential, 16
 aldosterone antagonists, 105
 angiotensin, 101–102
 Chlorthalidone, 104
 focally innervated skeletal muscle, 18
 local anaesthetics, 57, 58
 multiply innervated skeletal muscle, 23
 renal reabsorption, 103
 thiazides, 104
Sodium nitroprusside, 278, 281, 284, 286
Sodium phosphate, 275
Sodium stibogluconate, 190
Sodium sulphate, 275
Sodium *Valproate*, 304, 305
Somatic nervous system, 2, 3
Somatostatin, 74, 93, 97, 128
Sorbitol, 231
Spare receptors, 69
Spastic paralysis, 25
Sperm, 78–79, 113
Spermatogonia, 78
Spermatids, 78
Spermatogenesis, 78, 87, 88, 261
Spermatocytes, 78
Spermatozoa, 78
Spermicide preparations, contraceptives, 307–308
Sphincter pupillae, 9
Spinal anaesthesia, 58
Spinal nerves, 2
Spinhaler®, 290
Spirometry, diagnosis of asthma, 289
Spironolactone, 101, 105, 271, 277
St. Anthony's fire, 294
Staphylococcus aureus, 192–193, 319
Starling curve, 276
Status asthmaticus, 99, 291
Status epilepticus, 302, 304
Stein–Leventhal syndrome, 75, 83
Stereoselectivity, of drugs, 67
Stilboestrol, 82, 263
Stimulants, central, 150–153
Stokes–Adams syndrome, 64
Stomach, drug absorption, 210
Streptococcus pneumoniae, 192, 193
Streptococcus pyogenes, 192–193, 319
Streptokinase, 123
Streptomycin, 199
 allergy, 182
 distribution, 177, 231
 mechanism of action, 177, 178
 principal uses, 192, 199, 201
 resistance, 177, 195
 spectrum, 177
 toxicity, 177, 199

Streptozocin, 97
Stress, 75, 296
Striatum, 131
Strongyloides, 185
Structurally non-specific
  drugs, 66–67
Strychnine, 126, 128, 152,
  302
Subarachnoid block, 58
Sublingual gland, innervation,
  4, 13
Submaxillary gland, inner-
  vation, 4, 13
Substance P, 128, 155
Substantia nigra, 129
Succinyl choline (*see*
  Suxamethonium), 19, 21,
  24
Sulfadoxine, 189
Sulphacetamide, 183, 196
Sulphadiazine, 196, 243
Sulphamethizole, 173, 196,
  242, 257
Sulphamethoxazole, 174, 196
Sulphapyridine, 196
Sulphasalazine, 196, 272
Sulphate, ethereal, conjugation,
  224
Sulphates (conjugation)
  tubular secretion, 220
Sulphinpyrazone, 319
Sulphobromophthalein, 222
Sulphonamides, 173–174,
  196
  acute intermittent porphy-
    ria, 259
  allergy, 182
  anaemia, 315, 316
  derivatives, pharmacologi-
    cally useful, 242
  elimination, 196
  glucose-6-phosphate dehydro-
    genase deficiency, 259,
    316
  hypoglycaemia, 95
  mechanism of action, 173
  metabolism, 196
  percutaneous absorption,
    212
  pharmacokinetics, 242
  Procaine, interaction with,
    60
  protein binding, 196, 218
  renal toxicity, 196
  resistance, 196
  spectrum, 173–174
  structure, 173
  toxicity, 189
  Trimethoprim, combination
    with, 174
Sulphones, 174, 189
Sulphonylureas, hypoglycaemic
  agents, 95
Sulphur, use in acne, 320
Sulphur compound lotion, 321
Sulthiame, 223
Sunlight, 320, 323–324
Surface anaesthesia, 58

Surface/mass ratio (infants
  and adults), 211
Surmountable antagonism, 70
Suspensions, for injection, 213
Sustained release formulations,
  212–213
Suxamethonium, 19, 21, 24
  anaesthetic premedication,
    162
  atypical cholinesterase, 35,
    257–258
  clinical uses, 21
  drug interactions, 23
  hydrolysis, 22, 35
  malignant hyperthermia,
    258
  structure, 21
Sweat, secretion of drugs in,
  222
Sympathetic nervous system,
  5–8, 14
  cholinergic transmission,
    postganglionic, 30
  cholinergic transmission,
    preganglionic, 28–29
  noradrenergic transmission,
    7, 39–55
Sympathomimetic, definition,
  (*see also* Adrenoceptor
  agonists), 46
*directly acting, 44–48
  basic nature and pKa,
    246–247
  cardiac arrhythmias, 61
  indirect comparison
    with, 49
  monoamine oxidase
    inhibitors, 53
*indirectly acting (centrally
  acting), 41
  cardiac arrhythmias, 53
  cold, symptomatic
    treatment of, 325
  directly acting, compari-
    son with, 49
  drug laws, 253
  hallucinogenic actions,
    153
  monoamine oxidase
    inhibition, 53, 266
  noradrenergic neurone
    blocking agents, 43
  psychosis, antagonism by
    neuroleptics, 140,
    151
  structure activity relation-
    ships, 48, 151
  therapeutic use, 151
Synapse, definition (*see also
  under* individual transmitters). 3
Syphilis, drugs of choice, 192
Syrup of *Ipecacuanha*, 267

$t_{1/2}$, calculation and signifi-
  cance, 226–228
Tablets, disintegration of, 210
Tachycardia, 10
Taenia saginata, 186

Tamoxifen, 83, 88
Tannic acid, percutaneous
  absorption, 212
Tapeworm, 182, 185–186
Tardive dyskinesia, 297
Taurine, 127
Teeth, drug deposition in, 216
Temazepam, 296
Temperature, body, 154
Temporal lobe (psychomotor)
  epilepsy, 302, 305
Testosterone, 77–78, 84,
  86–88
Testosterone esters, 86
Testosterone propionate, 86
Tetanus toxin, 128
Terbutaline, 290
Tetracaine (*see Amethocaine*),
  56, 60
Tetracosactrin, 99, 101
Tetracyclines, 199–200
  Candida superinfection,
    191, 200
  chelation, 199, 216, 263,
    264, 265
  dose, 194
  elimination, 194, 199
  mechanism of action, 179
  minimal inhibitory concen-
    tration, 193
  placental transfer, 216
  principal use, 192
  protein binding, 199
  resistance, 179, 195
  spectrum, 179, 199
  $t_{1/2}$, 194, 228
  toxicity, 182, 200
Δ^9 Tetrahydrocannabinol, 153
Tetrahydrofolate, 173, 174
Tetrodotoxin, 16, 17, 42, 60
Thalamus, 129
Thalidomide, 261
Theobromine, 106, 152
Theophylline, 106, 152, 290
Theophylline ethylenediamine
  (*see Aminophylline*), 106
Therapeutic index, 228
Thermoceptors, 154
Thermodynamic activity, of
  drugs, 66
Thermostat, 154
Thiabendazole, 185
*Thiazides (benzothiadiazides),
  104, 277
  antihypertensive action,
    104, 280
  Carbenoxolone interaction
    with, 264
  carbonic anhydrase, 104
  diabetes, 104
  Digoxin, use with, 104
  gout, precipitation of, 259
  insulin release, 97
  mechanisms of action, 104
  potassium loss, 104, 264
  protein binding, 104
  side effects, 104, 280
  tubular secretion, 220
  uric acid excretion, 104

Thiopentone, 66, 157, 166
  anaesthetic action, 162
  dialysis, 221
  distribution, 214
  dose, 236
  duration of action, 237
  metabolism, 237
  pharmacokinetic model,
    230, 236–237
  protein binding, 237
  redistribution, 237
  renal clearance, 220
Thioridazine, 141
Thioxanthines, 140
Threadworm, 178–179, 182,
  185–188
Throat infections, drugs of
  choice, 192
Thrombin, 120
Thrombosis,
  dissolution, 122
  formation, 86, 114, 120
Thromboxane A$_2$ and B$_2$,
  112, 113, 120
Thromboxane synthetase, 112
Thrush, 191
Thymidylate synthetase, 175
Thyroglobulin, 89–90
Thyroid gland, 89–93, 180
Thyroid hormones (*see also*
    Thyroxine and tri-
    iodothyronine, 89–93
Thyroid stimulating hormone
  (TSH), 74, 90–91
Thyroid stimulating hormone
  releasing hormone, 74,
  90–91
Thyrotoxicosis, 51, 63, 90–93
Thyroxine, 89–93, 210, 220
Tinea pedis, 191
Tinnitus, cinchonism, 63
Titanium dioxide paste, 324
Tobacco,
  angina, 285
  asthma, 288
  bronchitis, 325
  developmental toxicity, 263
  poisoning, 254
  social use, 254, 265
  ulcers, gastric and duodenal,
    270
Tolbutamide,
  hypersensitivity, 315
  mechanism of action, 95–96
  protein binding, 265–266
Tolerance,
  acute, 239
  mechanisms, 253
  microsomal enzyme induc-
    tion, 223
  non-specific central depress-
    ants, 166
  opiates, 149
  sympathomimetics, 151
Tolnaftate, 191
Topical anaesthesia, 58
Total drug clearance, 219
Toxaemia of pregnancy, 113,
  284

Toxicity, 255–259, 264–266
Toxoplasma, 190
Tranexamic acid, 123
Tranquillization, 159
Tranquillizers,
  major (*see* Neuroleptics),
    139–142, 297
  minor (*see* Anxiolytics),
    158, 163–167, 296–297
Transcortin, 99
Translocation (protein synthe-
  sis), 176–177
Transpeptidation, 172
Tranylcypromine, 53–54,
  136–139, 151, 298
Travel sickness, 35, 109, 141,
  299–301
Treponema pallidum, drugs
  of choice, 192
Tretinoin, 320
Triamterene, 105, 278
Tribromethanol, 211
Tricarboxylic acid cycle, 93
Trichloroethanol, 165
Trichomonas vaginalis, 178,
  186
Triclofos, 165
*Tricyclic antidepressants,
  135–136, 298–299
  basic nature, 246
  mechanism of action, 130
  muscarinic antagonism, 33,
    265
  noradrenergic neurone
    blocking agents, 43
  overdose, 299
  peripheral effects, 136
  screening, 135–136
  structure, 135
  uptake inhibition, 55, 266
Triethylcholine, 16, 17, 18
Trifluoperazine, 141, 297
Trigone, of bladder, 11–12,
  14, 45
Trihexyphenidyl HCl (*see
  Benzhexol*), 33, 34
Tri-iodothyronine, 89–93
  Thyroxine, production from,
    90
Trimeprazine, 142
Trimethoprim, 174
Tripsoralen, 323
Trophoblast, 76
Tropicamide, 33, 34
Trypan blue, 214
Trypsin, histamine release, 108
Tryptaminergic neurotrans-
  mission (*see* 5-Hydroxy-
  tryptamine)
Tryptophan, 110
Tryptophan-5-hydroxylase,
  110
Tuberculosis, 174–175, 192,
  201
Tubocurarine, 19, 22, 31
  anaesthetic premedication,
    23, 162
  aminosugar antibiotics,
    interaction with, 23

Tubocurarine (*cont.*)
  anticholinesterase agents,
    interaction with, 23, 38
  focally innervated skeletal
    muscle, 23
  ganglia, 25
  histamine release, 23, 108
  multiply innervated skeletal
    muscle, 24
Twitch (skeletal muscle), 18
Typhoid, drugs of choice, 177,
  192
Tyramine, 41, 48–50, 138–139
  foods containing, 53, 294
  monoamineoxidase inhibi-
    tors, 138–139, 294
  migraine, 294
  structure, 48
  uptake, 53
Tyrosine, 40, 89
Tyrosine hydroxylase, 40, 284

Ulcerative colitis, 196, 271–272
Ulcers, gastric and duodenal,
  110, 269–271
Ultraviolet radiation, 320, 323
Unsurmountable antagonism,
  71
Uraemia, 300, 302
Urate, in gout, 318
Urea, 106, 210, 310
Uric acid excretion, 104–105
Urinary antiseptics, 181
Urinary bladder, 11
  α-adrenoceptors, 45
  ganglion blocking agents, 29
  muscarinic receptors, 32, 34
Urinary tract infections, 192,
  193, 200
Urticaria, 109
Urokinase, 123
Uterine smooth muscle, 46, 113
Uterus, 80–81, 84

Vaccines, 202
Vagal nerve nucleus, 4
Vagina, 81, 84
Valproate, sodium, 304–305,
  306
Vascular smooth muscle, 12
Vas deferens,
  α-adrenoceptor agonists, 45
  innervation, 12, 14
  ganglion blockade, 29
  opiate receptors, 144
Vasoactive intestinal poly-
  peptide, 128
Vasodilators, 280
Vasectomy, 308
Ventilation, artificial, in
  poisoning, 267
Ventricular arrhythmias, 64
Ventricular myocardium, 10
Vestibular disease, 297
Vidarabine, 203
Viloxazine, 136
Vinca alkaloids, *Vinblastin*
  and *Vincristine*, 204, 207
Viprinium embonate, 182, 186

Viral infections, 169, 202–203, 319–320, 325
Vitamin B_{12} anaemia, 313–314
Vitamin K and antagonists, 118, 122
Vomiting, *see also* Anti-emetics, 299–300
  Apomorphine, 141, 148
  depressants, 299
  dopamine, 131, 148
  chemosensitive trigger zone, 131
  Emetine, 300
  gastrointestinal irritation, 300
  narcotic analgesics, 146, 148, 300
  parasympathetic mechanisms, 299
  respiratory muscles, 299
  vomiting centre, 131, 299

Warfarin
  developmental toxicity, 263
  drug interactions, 122, 264, 266
  metabolism, 122
  pharmacokinetics, 242

Warfarin (*cont.*)
  protein binding, 122, 219, 265
  vitamin K antagonism, 122
Warts, 320
Wasp venom, histamine release, 108
Water filled pores, drug absorption, 210
Water soluble drugs,
  blood brain barrier, 214
  cell penetration, 214
  examples, 231–233
  eye, 215
  models, dispositional, 230, 231–233
  peritoneal dialysis, 221
  placenta, 216
  plasma dialysis, 221
  renal clearance, 219–220
  renal insufficiency, 221, 232
  serous cavities, 216
  small intestine, 210
Wax matrix tablets, 213
Whitlow, 319
Withdrawal method, contraception, 306

Withdrawal syndrome,
  non-specific depressants, 167, 252
  opiates, 149, 252
Wolffian ducts, 261
Worm infestations, classification, 169, 185
Wound infections, drugs of choice, 192

Xanthine oxidase, 318
*Xanthines (*see* Methyl-xanthines), 106, 152–153
Xenobiotic, definition, 222
Xenon, 66, 159

Yeasts,
  extracts, tyramine content, 53
  infections, Candida, 191

Zero order kinetics, 238
Zinc and coal tar paste, 322
Zinc compound paste, 322, 323
Zinc insulin, 94
Zinc sulphide, in acne, 320
Zygote, 260